Health and social organization

There is a growing recognition, that the most powerful determinants of health in modern populations are to be found in social, economic and cultural circumstances. These include: economic growth, income distribution, consumption, work organization, unemployment and job insecurity, social and family structure, education and deprivation and these are all aspects of 'social organization'. In *Health and Social Organization* these issues are examined by leading British and North American researchers. They bring together an array of evidence from the social sciences, epidemiology and biology.

Medical services and health damaging behaviour have been the main concerns of public health policy and interventions in recent decades. *Health and Social Organization* starts by briefly examining the strengths and weaknesses of these approaches to improving the population's health. Most of the contributions, however, focus on a particular aspect of social organization and its relationship to health.

Health and Social Organization will be essential reading for politicians and policy-makers, professionals working in the NHS and health authorities, practitioners in epidemiology and public health and nurses, as well as for students in medical sociology, social policy and social psychology.

David Blane is Senior Lecturer, Charing Cross and Westminster Medical School; **Eric Brunner** is Senior Research Fellow, Department of Epidemiology and Public Health, University College London; **Richard Wilkinson** is Senior Research Fellow at the Trafford Center for Medical Research, University of Sussex and Associate Director, International Centre for Health and Society, University College London.

Health and social organization

Towards a health policy for the twenty-first century

Edited by David Blane, Eric Brunner and Richard Wilkinson

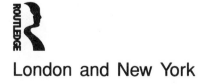

London and New York

First published 1996
by Routledge
11 New Fetter Lane, London EC4P 4EE

Simultaneously published in the USA and Canada
by Routledge
29 West 35th Street, New York, NY 10001

Typeset in Times by
Florencetype Limited, Stoodleigh, Devon

Printed and bound in Great Britain by
Redwood Books, Trowbridge, Wiltshire

British Library Cataloguing in Publication Data
A catalogue record for this book is available from the British Library

Library of Congress Cataloging in Publication Data
A catalogue record for this book has been requested

ISBN 0–415–13069–7 (hbk)
    0–415–13070–0 (pbk)

Contents

Figures

Tables

Contributors

Dr Mel Bartley
Social Statistics Research Unit, City University, London

Dr David Blane
Academic Department of Psychiatry, Charing Cross and Westminster
Medical School, London

Professor Mildred Blaxter
School of Economic and Social Studies, University of East Anglia,
Norwich

Dr Eric Brunner
Department of Epidemiology and Public Health, University College
London

Dr Derek Cook
Department of Public Health Sciences, St George's Hospital Medical
School, London

Professor George Davey Smith
Department of Epidemiology and Public Health, University of Bristol

Maria Evandrou
Department of Epidemiology and Public Health, University College
London

Amanda Feeney
Department of Epidemiology and Public Health, University College
London

Professor Peter Fonagy
Sub-department of Clinical Health Psychology, University College
London
The Anna Freud Centre, London

Dr Clyde Hertzman
Department of Health Care and Epidemiology, University of British Columbia, Vancouver

Professor Michael Marmot
Department of Epidemiology and Public Health, University College London
Director, International Centre for Health and Society

Scott Montgomery
Social Statistics Research Unit, City University, London

Dr Jerry Morris
Health promotion Sciences Unit, London School of Hygiene and Tropical Medicine

Dr J. Fraser Mustard
Canadian Institute for Advanced Research, Toronto

Dr Chris Power
Department of Epidemiology and Biostatistics, Institute of Child Health, London

Professor S. Leonard Syme
School of Public Health, University of California, Berkeley

Dr Alvin R. Tarlov
Department of Health Policy and Management, Harvard University

Professor Michael Wadsworth
MRC National Survey of Health and Development, Department of Epidemiology and Public Health, University College London

Ian White
Medical Statistics Unit, London School of Hygiene and Tropical Medicine

Richard Wilkinson
Trafford Centre for Medical Research, University of Sussex, Brighton
Associate Director, International Centre for Health and Society

Preface

THE INTERNATIONAL CENTRE FOR HEALTH AND SOCIETY

The publication of this volume marks the launch of the International Centre for Health and Society. The Centre aims to provide policy-makers and the public at large with a scientific understanding of the social, economic and cultural determinants of a nation's health status. To this end, it combines the varied talents of biological and social scientists, epidemiologists, sociologists, psychologists, economists, as well as medical and health professionals.

Based at University College London, the Centre brings together an accomplished group of researchers who have played a leading role in the growing understanding of the relationship between social organization and health. In addition to its own research staff it includes a collaborative network of scientists from the United Kingdom, North America and Europe, many of whom have kindly contributed chapters.

Only recently has it become clear how closely patterns of health mirror the social characteristics of a society, including the social and economic divisions within it. Indeed, health is an indicator of a society's well-being. The Centre's research has pointed to the salience of the social and physical environment in which people work: to income, education, the organization of work, to family functioning and people's psychosocial well-being as important determinants of health. Population health is predicated on widely shared economic prosperity, on the development of a supportive community life and on investment in people.

Beyond the boundaries of conventional health services, these issues are the central challenges which health policy in the twenty-first century will have to meet. A start can be made now, and there are a number of policy proposals which may be expected to benefit both the health of individuals and the prosperity of society.

By tracing the social and health costs of divisive or sub-optimal patterns of social and economic development, the Centre's work will help to identify the social foundations for health, prosperity and well-being. A great deal of work remains to be done. In order to discover the most effective ways of improving the population's health, research must continue to map out the cumulative impact of social circumstances on biological processes throughout life.

The chapters which follow show not only the range and detail of the new Centre's interests, but also its conceptual strengths and the richness of the empirical data sources available to it. We believe that the programme of research set out in this book has the power to transform public health policy and to make a dramatic contribution to the welfare of populations throughout the world.

The establishment of the International Centre for Health and Society owes a special debt to Fraser Mustard, President of the Canadian Institute of Advanced Research, who nursed it into being over several years. Without the generous gift of his time, imagination, encouragement and advice, it would not exist. We have also benefited from the steadfast support of Sir Derek Roberts, Provost of University College London, who has not only given his time, but has made the Centre's development a priority. Al Tarlov has also been enormously helpful at key points and has repeatedly crossed the Atlantic from his base in Harvard for our benefit. As a non-profitmaking and non-political organization, the Centre has received financial support from the Baring Foundation, The Paul Hamlyn Foundation and the Lord Ashdown Charitable Settlement. Individual research projects have been funded from a wide variety of sources including the Medical Research Council and the Economic and Social Research Council. We are grateful to all these bodies for making this endeavour possible.

Chapter 1

The evolution of public health policy
An anglocentric view of the last fifty years

David Blane, Eric Brunner and Richard Wilkinson

The British and North American contributors to this volume share an approach to health and health policy which goes beyond medical care and individual behaviour. Each in their somewhat different ways regards the social structure as a major determinant of population health. This perspective has guided their research, which in many cases stretches back over several decades. Some of the contributors present a synthesis or overview of their research endeavours, while others report specific pieces of work. The thinking of all, however, has been shaped by post-war developments in public health research, so it is appropriate, by way of an introduction, to describe briefly the main features of this intellectual history. As the editors of the volume we are conscious that our introduction is anglocentric and may omit important details. Nevertheless we believe it provides a useful map of how we have come to understand that the social structure will be central to effective health policy in the twenty-first century.

PUBLIC HEALTH THROUGH MEDICAL TREATMENT?

At the end of the Second World War confidence in medical science had rarely been higher. It seemed obvious to contemporaries, if not to the public health profession, that the decline in infectious disease mortality owed much to the progress of medical science. Although the first sulphonamides had been developed before the war, it was the wartime mass production of penicillin which promised effective treatment for a host of infectious diseases that had been the scourge of previous generations. Similarly, although immunization against diphtheria had been available since the 1930s, wartime development of immunization raised the possibility of protecting whole populations against some diseases. Not only were these new forms of treatment and prevention effective but – and this was presumably important to policy-makers in countries, like Britain, where post-war circumstances were straitened – they were considered affordable.

It is understandable, given this background, that the provision of universally available medical care was seen as a vital part of policy for improving health standards throughout society. In many countries this development coincided with a political enthusiasm for social justice which had its roots in wartime experience and the desire not to return to pre-war conditions. In Britain the National Health Service was established to provide free medical care for all, financed by central government revenues. Its founders expected that the population would become healthier as a result. They anticipated an early surge in demand, due to the backlog of untreated disease. Once it had been treated, however, they predicted a steady decline in the demand for medical care. Most commentators also assumed that social inequalities in health would be steadily eroded by this combination of medical science and egalitarian health care reform.

Prior to the establishment of the National Health Service health and welfare services directed towards much of the urban working class had been administratively intertwined. In 1948 almost 80 per cent of the country's hospital beds were provided by municipal hospitals run by local government (Webster 1988). These hospitals had developed out of the provision made by the Poor Law Boards of Guardians to provide accommodation for the sick poor. This was the basis of what had been a wider integration. School medical inspections were combined with supplementary feeding, which had been introduced before the First World War. 'By 1938 the School Medical Service was engaged in diverse activities, ranging from special schools, school meals and milk, physical education, to inspection and treatment of minor ailments.' (Webster 1988: 6). Similarly, antenatal and child welfare clinics were able to provide subsidized milk and health foods as well as medical care. The separation of the sick from welfare recipients could also appear arbitrary; '... of the 149,000 residents in Poor Law Institutions in England and Wales in 1939, nearly 60,000 (40 per cent) were classified as sick' (Webster 1988: 5).

In Britain as early as 1937 the independent research unit, Political and Economic Planning, had recommended that 'Medical and allied services should be financially and administratively divorced from social insurance and the Poor Law, and unified into one national system providing services to the whole population on the basis of common citizenship.' The decision to separate medical care, under the new National Health Service, from welfare and preventive services stemmed primarily from the desire to create a service for everyone which was not seen as an outgrowth of services to the poor. Despite usually being reformed in tandem and despite their additive impact on health, welfare and health systems became increasingly separated, administratively, professionally and intellectually.

Although the British National Health Service was innovative in the comprehensive free cover it provided to the whole population, as Beveridge pointed out, a number of other countries, including Denmark,

France, Germany, Hungary, Romania, Norway, New Zealand and the Soviet Union had also taken important steps towards ensuring that the benefits of medical care were more widely applied.

HEALTH INEQUALITIES AND THE WELFARE STATE

Attempts to widen access to medical care were usually accompanied by other social reforms which might be expected to affect health. In Britain full employment policies and post-war developments in welfare provision, including house building programmes, income support and social insurance, were introduced around the same time as the National Health Service. In Canada a similar series of programmes were put in place between 1947 and 1971: universal, comprehensive, tax-funded medical care; a generous unemployment insurance scheme; the Canada Pension Plan; and the Canada Assistance Plan, which gave the country a welfare system more European than American in scope.

The expansion of the welfare state might have been expected to narrow social class differences in health, and when the 1951 decennial figures were released that is what they seemed to show had happened. So much so that the normal inverse mortality gradient had been replaced by a W-shaped distribution (Table 1.1, first row). Subsequently, however, these figures were 'adjusted' by the Registrar General. Paradoxically, his correction seems to have been prompted primarily by an assumption that the figures must be wrong because they did not show the usual inverse gradient between social position and mortality. With some justification he transferred 'company directors' (who may have included everyone from small self-employed tradesmen to large employers) from social class I to social class II. More fundamentally, and with no apparent justification, he weighted the 1951 occupations by their populations in the previous census in 1931. To show he was aware of the dubious method by which he had managed to produce the desired class gradient in mortality he said, 'My colleague who did these sums for me, in letting me have these figures ... added a comment which seems to me very apt: "Ain't science wonderful!" ' (Logan 1959: 20).

The adjusted figures (Table 1.1, second row), which show class differences in mortality widening rather than narrowing in 1951, became the ones normally quoted. A few years before Logan, in 1955, Illsley had published a paper which seemed to show that most of the social class differences in infant mortality were due to selective social mobility. Analyses from the Aberdeen Maternity and Neonatal Data Bank, set up in 1951, demonstrated that taller and presumably healthier mothers tended to marry upwards, while shorter ones married down. The implication was that social class mortality differentials were not primarily a reflection of the health effects of the different circumstances in which people currently

Table 1.1 Standardized mortality ratios for social classes, men aged 20–64
years, England and Wales, 1951

	Social classes				
	I	II	III	IV	V
From the Decennial Supplement	98	88	101	94	118
As adjusted by Logan (1959)	86	92	101	104	118

lived. Thus Logan's adjusted 1951 figures on social class mortality differentials gave the impression that the mortality differences were unresponsive to the provision of free medical care and the development of the welfare state, while selective social mobility seemed to provide some explanation of why they were not.

PREVENTION THROUGH THE MODIFICATION OF INDIVIDUAL BEHAVIOUR

What then appeared as the failure of social class mortality differences to respond to the expanding welfare provisions contributed to the belief that social policy was no longer such an important part of preventive health policy. Bartley traces the separation between epidemiology and social policy research to the 1950s. Using quotes from Titmuss, Morris and Heady, whose research had been at the forefront of the integrated approach, she argues that the 'present health education philosophy can be traced in direct line of descent to the belief that pre-war poverty and inequality had been banished by the welfare state and new types of explanations were needed to account for the failure of class inequalities in health to diminish' (Bartley 1985: 290).

These tendencies were also strengthened by the growing prosperity of the immediate post-war decades. The third quarter of the twentieth century was a golden age for American and European capitalism. The almost continuous growth of real incomes, low unemployment and greater equity seemed to have banished the kind of poverty that might have harmed health. To many, the provision of food supplements, free school meals and milk seemed increasingly irrelevant and was gradually discontinued.

In this new world health became the almost exclusive province of medical science. Social policy was redirected to serve exclusively social objectives, and behavioural risks were investigated as a means of prevention. The rise in the number of deaths from lung cancer, which, in 1951, surpassed the number of deaths from tuberculosis, also called for a behavioural approach to prevention. In the same year Doll and Hill started their monumental study of the health effects of smoking among British doctors. By 1954 the link between smoking and lung cancer was clear.

Interestingly, this was the rediscovery of an association first observed by medical scientists in 1930s Germany but submerged in the exigencies of war (Davey Smith *et al.* 1995).

Research proceeded over the next decade or two to lay the foundations of the behavioural approach to the prevention of degenerative diseases. The physical activity/inactivity hypothesis emerged from a large-scale study of men in a wide variety of occupations when it was found that postmen were protected from heart attacks in comparison with clerks and telephonists. Bus conductors running up and down stairs on double-decker buses were similarly protected in comparison with their drivers. The first Whitehall study of 17,000 civil servants, started in the late 1960s, was also used initially to explore behavioural risk factors. In 1970 Ancel Keys reported the first international correlations between heart disease mortality and fat consumption. These were among the first results to come from the Seven Countries study, a massive and continuing project to investigate the health effects of diet and other behavioural factors in America, Japan, Greece, Italy, former Yugoslavia, Holland and East Finland. Pilot trials began in 1957, and the full study a year later. Its aim was to 'relate differences in incidence among cohorts to the average or general characteristics of the men in the cohorts, including their living habits' (Keys 1980).

A few epidemiological studies continued to monitor the importance of structural and psychosocial as well as behavioural factors. The Alameda County study in northern California which followed residents between 1965 and 1974 was one of them. Based at Berkeley, this study showed that social support and material circumstances were associated with mortality risk (Berkman and Syme 1979). Another study at Berkeley showed that coronary risk rose with the level of acculturation among Japanese-Americans (Marmot and Syme 1976). In Britain the 1946 and 1958 birth cohort studies continued to study the impact of a wide range of social and economic variables and the Whitehall study was used increasingly to illuminate socioeconomic differences in health (Marmot *et al.* 1978).

THE BEHAVIOURAL IMPASSE

During the late 1970s several studies were established to quantify the health gains which result from changing the behaviours which earlier research had identified as hazardous. One of the most important was the 361,662-strong Multiple Risk Factor Intervention Trial (MRFIT) in the United States. The level of mortality improvement which would result from successful behavioural change was predicted and, on the basis of the best available knowledge and using unprecedented resources, a programme of behaviour change was launched. The results were disappointing. Sustained behavioural change proved difficult to achieve even among highly motivated high-risk individuals. Even where behaviour was successfully changed, the ensuing improvement in mortality proved smaller than predicted. In addition, the researchers came to realize that each individual adopting the desired behaviours would probably be quickly replaced by a new recruit to the health-damaging behaviours (see Chapter 2).

Results from the first Whitehall study in Britain were consistent with those from MRFIT. Both mortality risk and the prevalence of health-damaging behaviours increased from the top to the bottom grades of the civil service hierarchy. However, grade differences in smoking, blood pressure, obesity and exercise were found to account for only a minority of the grade differences in mortality (Marmot *et al.* 1978). Serum cholesterol was found to predict future heart disease among individuals in the study, but mean cholesterol levels were found to be higher in the higher employment grades. Fat intake, which is merely one of the determinants of blood cholesterol, therefore did not appear to be part of the explanation of occupational differences in heart disease in these men. As well as being unexpectedly hard to change, behaviour seemed to have less effect on health than predicted. This may have been partly a consequence of inadequate measurement. Reliance on a single collection of self-reported smoking habits, for example, cannot hope to capture a precise estimate of a lifetime's exposure. But the results of intervention studies were almost uniformly unimpressive.

In a discussion of the difficulties of using behaviour change as an approach to population health, Rose calculated that the advantages to the individual of various forms of behavioural change were very small (Rose 1981). He concluded that if Framingham men were to modify their diet enough to reduce their cholesterol levels by 10 per cent up to the age of 55, forty-nine out of fifty would eat differently every day for forty years without having avoided a heart attack by doing so. Similarly, to save the life of one male British doctor '399 would have worn a seat belt everyday for forty years without benefit to their survival.' Elsewhere (Rose 1985) he states that even if people are in the lowest risk category for all the behavioural risk factors their most likely cause of death is still heart disease.

If the gains to individuals from prevention through behaviour change are so small even among the most important causes of death, they are likely to be even smaller in relation to the prevention of less common causes. Nor will more research into behavioural factors necessarily solve the problem: more money and effort has gone into research into the causes of heart disease than into any other illness.

Rather than being new, the attempt to improve health by changing individual behaviour can be seen as a development of earlier attempts to combat infectious disease through food hygiene and personal cleanliness. Indeed, in terms of sexually transmitted disease the continuity is clear. As a recipe for health the dos and don'ts of personal behaviour have a strong resonance with traditional morality: against drinking and smoking, in favour of sexual fidelity, and against sloth and gluttony.

The behavioural approach to prevention had other important ideological implications. By focusing attention on individual choices, this persp-ective left unchallenged the assumption that the post-war reforms had eliminated the structural causes of disease. 'Victim-blaming' implied that individuals freely chose these health-damaging behaviours, they could be held responsible for the consequent disease, and the health implica-tions of forms of social and economic organization were hidden from view. The debate on the relationship between behavioural and structural fact-ors in health has much in common with the agency/structure debate in sociology.

THE RETURN OF STRUCTURE

During the last decade or two there has been a growing interest in the preventive possibilities of the relationship between people's health and features of the social and economic environment which are largely beyond the control of individuals. The shortcomings of over-reliance on behav-iour change as an approach to prevention is only one of the factors behind this development.

The pressure to find some more effective approach to the prevention of chronic and degenerative disease was maintained by the tendency for the burden of illness to rise as the population ages. Because so much of this burden is now degenerative rather than infectious disease, the costs of treatment are higher. This has led to problems of funding medical care in different countries regardless of the public–private split. The most important factor pointing to the preventive potential of social and economic policy has been a growing recognition of the scale and causes of social inequalities in health.

Another important factor which fuelled the growing interest in the influence of the social and economic structure on health was the rediscov-ery of poverty in the midst of post-war affluence. Michael Harrington in the United States and Peter Townsend and Brian Abel-Smith in Britain published seminal studies of relative poverty in the 1960s (Harrington 1962; Abel-Smith and Townsend 1965). While economic growth and the welfare state had substantially reduced the scale of absolute poverty, the effects of relative poverty could not be ignored. The gradual rise in unemployment and increase in the proportion of the population living in relative poverty attracted increasing concern over the next decades. There is little doubt, however, that it fed into the rediscovery of social class differences in health in the late 1970s. They were documented anew in the 1971 Decennial Supplement, which was published in 1978 and raised many of the crucial research issues. The Black Report on *Health Inequalities*, published in 1980 (see DHSS 1980), summarized knowledge in this area and focused researchers' attention on the possible causes of these socioeconomic variations in health. It put the issue on the public policy agenda and acted as a stimulus to research and policy development throughout the developed world. Substantial research effort has gone into these issues, not only in Britain but also in The Netherlands, Scandinavia, Canada, the United States and a growing list of other developed countries. The issues are also being addressed in a number of less developed countries, particularly in Brazil, where the scale of material and health inequalities is especially alarming. Very important in terms of the growing interest in the health effects of the socioeconomic structure was the evidence that health inequalities were not diminishing with the decline in absolute poverty brought about by economic growth. Widening occupational differences in mortality were documented in Britain by the Black Report and have since been reported in the United States by educational level and in France by occupational class.

This and other research has demonstrated that health inequalities are not fixed or invariant; they vary substantially over time and between countries. Reports that even in an advanced country like Britain there are now two-, three- or even fourfold differences in mortality between social groups are evidence of a problem which demands attention. Such health differences are increasingly seen as an indication of the 'excess mortality' which arises as the health cost of social and economic organization. Where it might once have been thought that health inequalities were a reflection of remnants of absolute poverty, which would disappear under the impact of rising prosperity, the fact that the differences have widened has shown that they are not going to disappear of their own accord in the course of economic development. Health remains highly sensitive to socioeconomic circumstances even in the most affluent societies.

Although the study of occupational health recognized the importance of the environment from its outset, it sought to identify specifically occupational health hazards as distinct from the increased risk associated with general differences in the socioeconomic environment. The British occupational mortality tables, for many years the main source of information on class and health, were developed primarily to study occupational health hazards. Most of the variation in health, however, turned out to be between social classes rather than between occupations within the same social class (Fox and Adelstein 1978). This suggested that, despite the undoubted importance of specifically occupational hazards, the more important influences on health were factors more generally associated with socioeconomic status.

PROGRESS IN METHODS

A clearer understanding of the structural sources of health inequalities owes a great deal to improvements in their measurement and in tackling a number of other methodological problems. Britain's long run of social class mortality data encouraged researchers to look at trends in health differences over time. Initially there were serious doubts about whether it was possible to compare mortality differences from one period to the next. The class distribution of the population changed, the class classification of occupations was revised every ten years, and there were doubts about how accurately the occupations given on death certificates could be related to the population in each occupation as recorded in each census (the source of the so-called numerator/denominator bias in death rates). However, rather than relying on comparisons between top and bottom classes, measures such as the *slope index of inequality* (Pamuk 1985) allowed the mortality gradient to be measured across the whole of society, taking into account changes in the distribution of the population between classes. Pamuk showed that periodic changes in the allocation of occupations to classes made little difference to the overall picture of trends in mortality differentials. At the same time the OPCS longitudinal study showed that the problem of numerator/denominator bias (encountered when relating deaths in occupations as stated on death certificates to denominator populations in occupations given at census) did not substantially alter the picture of the size of mortality differentials. It took a sample of people from census returns so that each death could be related to the information which the deceased had provided at census instead of relying on the occupation as stated by the next of kin on the death certificate. In this way information on the socioeconomic characteristics of the deceased came from the same source as the information on the population denominators.

Further attention was also paid to the possibility, first raised in the 1930s, that health inequalities might be largely a result of selective social mobility (Wilkinson 1986). Two studies which had followed cohorts of children from their births in 1946 and 1958 showed that although poor health does have an adverse effect on people's life chances and social mobility, it does not make a very large contribution to the observed class differences in mortality (Power and Peckham 1990). A similar conclusion emerged from a study of social mobility consequent on illness later in life (Fox 1985). Bartley has pointed out that if the health of mobile groups is somewhere between that of the class they come from and that of the one they go to, mobility could even narrow differentials.

The pathways by which social structure has an impact on health are important in the policy debate. Such questions of mechanism are being addressed in the Whitehall II study (Marmot *et al.* 1991) of 10,308 male

and female civil servants. Conventional risk factors were a poor explanation of coronary risk differences in the first Whitehall study, and Whitehall
II was set up in 1985 to study structural, psychosocial and biological factors
simultaneously within one large cohort. Investigation of the psychosocial
properties of the Whitehall hierarchy, for example the distribution of
control and decision-making responsibility, potentially adds to the explanation of inequalities in coronary risk. An adverse work environment and
low occupational status (Brunner *et al.* 1993) are linked with metabolic
disturbances, which are not explained by obesity, smoking, alcohol consumption or exercise patterns.

As a result of these different pieces of research the view that socioeconomic differences in health were a reflection of differences in the
circumstances in which people lived and worked became generally
accepted. In the United States over the same period, there was growing
recognition that racial differences in health were largely reducible to
differences in socioeconomic circumstances. It is interesting that the ideological doubts about the validity of socioeconomic differences in health
on each side of the Atlantic were almost the opposite of each other. The
suggestion in Britain that the differences were due to social mobility was
a suggestion that they were an artefact of the social fluidity of the population. In the United States the concern with racial origins was a concern
with biological fixity and genetics. In their opposite ways both served to
suggest that health was a property of individuals independent of their
social and economic circumstances.

THE LIMITATIONS OF MEDICAL CARE

After the post-war confidence in the power of medical care, several studies
have forced a re-evaluation of the comparative strength of medical and
environmental factors as determinants of population health. The view that
medical science did not play an important part in the decline in death
rates since the nineteenth century has been particularly influential.
McKeown and Lowe's *Introduction to Social Medicine* (published in 1966),
showed that most of the decline in mortality from infectious diseases came
before medical care had any effective form of treatment or immunization.
Now that medicine has effective methods for combating many of the infections, the disease burden in the developed countries has shifted towards
the degenerative diseases, where medical science remains less competent.
Relationships between medical care and measures of population health
are hard to find. Even among the small proportion of modern causes of
death where medical competence is greatest, mortality rates appear to be
influenced more by environmental than by medical factors (Mackenbach
et al. 1990). Given that effective methods of treatment provide some reference point, if not a ceiling, for costs, the lack of effective methods for

treating so many modern conditions has provided an important stimulus to the escalation of medical costs.

This is a dramatic change from the belief in the middle of this century that medicine had affordable and effective ways of combating disease. But although it is important to recognize the overwhelming influence of the socioeconomic environment on population health, the power of medical care to improve the quality of life should not be disregarded. Surgery for things such as hernias, cataracts, prostate, varicose veins and hip joints may not be glamorous or do very much to improve life expectancy, but they are important to the quality of life of old people.

THE POLICY CHALLENGE

In a sense we have come full-circle. The post-war settlement in Britain, of which the Beveridge reforms were an integral part, was assumed to have dealt with the structural determinants of health and its unequal social distribution. In the Beveridge Report of 1942 the proposal for 'a national health service for the prevention and cure of disease and disability by medical treatment' (p. 158) was part of a broader plan for social progress. Beveridge's plan had five components: 'the attack on want . . . , on disease, ignorance, squalor and idleness' (p. 6). The National Health Service was designed to deal with disease, but disease was only one of 'the five sources of misery' which were to be eliminated by the reforms. Interestingly, the best measures of health inequalities now available suggest, when applied retrospectively, that health inequalities reached their narrowest around 1950 (Pamuk 1985). There can be little doubt that the massive post-war house-building programme, full employment and what was probably the lowest-ever proportion of the population in relative poverty made an important contribution to the reduction in health differentials. Indeed, there is evidence that mortality differentials have widened in periods when relative poverty has increased, and narrowed when relative poverty has diminished (Wilkinson 1989).

It is instructive to compare the United States and Canada in the light of their different histories of welfare and health care reform. Analyses in the late 1980s show that proportionally fewer Canadians than Americans had an income below half the average income level in each country. Moreover the incomes of the poorest 76 per cent of Canadians were higher than those of their American counterparts, whilst those of the richest 24 per cent were lower (Wolfson 1995). During the post-war period, life expectancy changes occurred in parallel with the emerging Canadian welfare state. In 1950 life expectancy in the United States was higher than in Canada (United Nations 1982). Over the following decades this relationship reversed, such that, by 1987, life expectancy for Canadian males and females was 1.7 and 1.6 years higher than for their American counterparts (WHO 1989). It would be difficult to attribute these changes to universal medical care alone. Among the post-war welfare reforms it was the latest to emerge and the national system was not in place until 1971, while the relative gains in life expectancy began much earlier than this.

The need for an integrated approach to health is a theme which runs throughout this book. Earlier we highlighted the growing separation between the administration of health and other welfare services. Before health services were removed from local authority control the provision of school health checks was integrated with other medical services on the one hand and with the provision of supplementary food on the other. No doubt this form of integration would still have advantages, particularly in the organization of community care for psychiatric patients and the elderly, where decisions about housing, social and medical care have to be closely co-ordinated.

However, preventive research has been set a new task. We face a quite different burden of diseases, arising in a different social and economic context in which deprivation takes on new patterns. The task of preventive research is to identify the links between the socioeconomic environment and human biology in this new context. The chapters of this book give a clear indication of this new integration. A society which nurtures people's skills and abilities throughout the population, which provides economic opportunities for all, and fosters a cohesive and integrated social environment, would do more for health than curative medical services are able to.

Since the 1950s in Britain, as in most of the developed world, living standards have risen, mortality rates have fallen, but Beveridge's attack on the causes of social disadvantage has not been sustained. Levels of unemployment and the numbers in relative poverty have increased, particularly since the 1970s, and house building programmes have been markedly reduced. More recently, with the development of a 'flexible' labour force, job insecurity and consequently financial insecurity have increased. The 1980s brought accelerating social divisions throughout much of the developed world. They were most marked in the English-speaking countries, particularly New Zealand, Britain and the United States. The income gap between the high-paid and low-paid widened rapidly and the rate of divergence in Britain has been surpassed only by that in New Zealand (Joseph Rowntree Foundation 1995). Between 1977 and 1992 top wages in Britain grew by 50 per cent and median wages by 35 per cent, but low wages ended the period lower in real terms than in 1975. For households in the United Kingdom without a full-time earner the picture is similarly drastic. In 1979 such households had an income distribution which clustered around the same point as households with a full-time employee. By 1990/1 net incomes in the latter households had risen, but among the increased number of households with no full-time employee average incomes had fallen, so that the two distributions overlapped only at the margin. At the same time, health inequalities widened and death rates actually rose among young adults in the most economically deprived areas of Britain (Phillimore *et al.* 1994; McLoone and Boddy, 1994). Also related to increasing social polarization is the re-emergence, almost exclusively among the poorest sections of society, of tuberculosis in several countries, including the United States and Britain (Bhatti *et al.* 1995).

Despite these alarming developments, there are grounds for optimism. Some of the policies which are already accepted within the political mainstream can be expected to have beneficial, if unintended, consequences for health. Raising the educational level of the population is primarily a response to the economic challenge facing developed economies, but it will probably also increase collective and individual well-being, and tap into the human capital which is now being wasted. Similarly, the new emphasis on social cohesion (Benzeval *et al.* 1995) is a response to escalating rates of behaviours which are individually and socially destructive, but it is also likely to benefit health. In addition one can hope that the growing contrast between the time pressure and work stress among the employed population and the increasing number of jobless may find a resolution which will benefit the health of both groups.

The chapters in this volume suggest other areas which health policy could usefully address. Taken together the chapters document links in a chain which runs from biology to personal circumstances, from family, education and work to the wider social and economic structure and the need for social investment and the conditions for future prosperity. By showing how the various facets of social organization impact on individual and population health, they raise a challenge to policy-makers. The scale and variety of the challenge covers areas as diverse as income distribution and work, education and the environment.

Income distribution. Absolute income levels affect the poor health associated with poverty, while relative income differences are related to the gradient in mortality and morbidity which stretches across all levels of the social hierarchy. Observational data show that improvements in infant mortality and life expectancy have been more rapid in countries with smaller income differentials (Wennemo 1993; Wilkinson 1994). The conclusion that a nation's health benefits from the levelling of incomes challenges conventional assumptions, although this has not always been the case. The evidence suggests that it may take exceptional circumstance to gain any substantial increase in equity. The World Bank argues that the effects of American occupation after the war, crises of legitimacy, and threats from communist rivals or neighbours were among the reasons for the increases in equity in Asian countries such as Japan, Korea, Taiwan, Malaysia, Hong Kong and Singapore (World Bank 1993). In Britain income equity was substantially improved during the two World Wars (Milward 1984). Titmuss said that during the Second World War the social hierarchy was reduced to gain 'the co-operation of the masses' in the war effort (Titmuss 1958). Despite the fact that medical resources were over-stretched and production capacity was diverted to the war industries, civilian life expectancy continued to improve during the two World Wars more rapidly than during the rest of the twentieth century (Winter 1988).

The traditional response to proposals for greater equity in the absence of national crisis has been to suggest that it is inimical to economic growth and that the best way to increase prosperity is to forget the differentials and pursue the most rapid growth possible: to enlarge the national cake rather than worry about how it is cut up. However, there is increasing evidence from both time series and cross-sectional studies that greater equity is associated with faster economic growth (Persson et al. 1994). All eight of the high-performing Asian economies reduced their income differences between 1960 and 1980 (Birdsall et al. 1994). Other studies have found that investment tends to be higher and productivity growth faster in countries where income differences are smaller (Alesina and Perotti 1993; Glyn and Miliband 1994).

Work. The realization of human potential through economic activity continues to be a preoccupation of those concerned with social and eco-nomic change. There are pressing problems with the quantity and quality of work, both of which have strong influences on many health-related factors, including income, social networks and self-esteem. Redistribution of work to reduce unemployment and to increase equity is a key consid-eration. The nature of work, as the Whitehall studies show (see Chapters 13 and 15), is strongly related to health prospects. In industrialized coun-tries occupation remains a key source of income, social identity and status. The defining role of work in adult life may need to change if the years of working life are to be compressed into a briefer period of adulthood. A new attitude to time, private and social, and new social roles may be required if these changes in the world of work are to be translated into a more even distribution of well-being.

Education. Education is a key factor not only in promoting greater equity but also in greater personal fulfilment and health for all individ-uals. Above their role in imparting skills and knowledge to individual students, educational institutions serve to transmit and develop cultural identity and concepts of social responsibility. Higher education has a special place in the national life, since it fosters innovation, which in turn sustains economic effectiveness. The recent expansion in UK university admissions is striking, having almost doubled between 1985 and 1992. A further positive development was the increase during this period in women's participation in higher education, which for the first time approached that of men. Social class participation rates also indicate a trend towards the equalization of educational opportunity, but here there is continuing evidence of a structural bias in favour of the children of professional fathers (AUT 1995). In 1992 of those offered places in the 'old' UK universities, as opposed to the recently converted polytechnics, two-thirds were from social classes I and II, which together comprise little more than a quarter of the population.

Environment. The connections between the physical environment and health are now receiving increasing research and policy attention. Urban regeneration and environmental improvements, including measures to deal with the problems of inner-city transport and atmospheric pollution, offer the prospect of socially useful employment and a health-promoting strategy in direct line of descent from the nineteenth-century public health tradition.

The development and implementation of detailed policies to tackle the linked problems of health inequalities and the population's health require the efforts of policy-makers and political will. The chapters which follow describe and analyse the nature of the problems and the broad implications of research findings. They indicate a pressing need to act on the public health front in its widest sense.

REFERENCES

Abel-Smith, B. and Townsend P. (1965) *The Poor and the Poorest,* London: Bell.

Alesina, A. and Perotti, R. (1993) *Income Distribution, Political Instability, and Investment,* NBER Working Paper 4486, Cambridge, Mass.: NBER.

Association of University Teachers (1995) AUT response to Department for Education review of higher education, London: AUT.

Bartley, M. (1985) Coronary heart disease and the public health, 1850–1983, *Sociology of Health and Illness,* 7: 289–313.

Benzeval, M., Judge, K. and Whitehead, M. (1995) *Tackling Inequalities in Health: an Agenda for Action,* London: King's Fund.

Berkman, L.F. and Syme, S.L. (1979) Social networks, host resistance and mortality: a nine-year follow-up of Alameda County residents, *American Journal of Epidemiology* 109: 186–204.

Bhatti, N., Law, M.R., Morris, J.K., Halliday, R. and Moore-Gillon, J. (1995) Increasing incidence of tuberculosis in England and Wales: a study of the likely causes, *British Medical Journal* 310: 967–970.

Birdsall, N., Ross, D. and Sabot, R. (1994) Inequality and Growth Reconsidered, paper prepared for American Economic Association, Boston, Mass.

Brunner, E.J., Marmot, M.G., White, I.R., O'Brien, J.R., Etherington, M.D., Slavin, B.M., Kearney, E.M. and Davey Smith, G. (1993) Gender and employment grade differences in blood cholesterol, apolipoproteins and haemostatic factors in the Whitehall II study, *Atherosclerosis* 102: 195–207.

Davey Smith, G., Strobele, S. and Egger, M. (1995) Smoking and death: public health measures were taken more than 40 years ago, *British Medical Journal* 310: 396.

Department of Health and Social Services (1980) *Inequalities in Health,* report of a research working group chaired by Sir Douglas Black, London: DHSS.

Fox, A.J. and Adelstein, A.M. (1978) Occupational mortality: work or way of life? *Journal of Epidemiology and Community Health* 32: 73–8.

Fox, A.J., Goldblatt, P.O. and Jones, D.R. (1985) Social class mortality differentials: artefact, selection or life circumstances? *Journal of Epidemiology and Community Health* 39: 1–8.

Glyn, A. and Miliband, D. (1994) Introduction, in D. Miliband and A. Glyn (eds) *Paying for Inequality: the Economic Cost of Social Injustice*, London: Rivers Oram Press.

Harrington, M. (1962) *The other America: Poverty in the United States*, New York: Macmillan.

Illsley, R. (1955) Social class selection and class differences in relation to stillbirths and infant deaths, *British Medical Journal* 2: 1520–1524.

Joseph Rowntree Foundation (1995) *Inquiry into Income and Wealth chaired by Sir Peter Barclay*, York: Joseph Rowntree Foundation.

Keys, A. (1980) *Seven Countries: a Multivariate Analysis of Death and Coronary Heart Disease*, London: Harvard University Press.

Logan, W.P.D. (1959) Occupational mortality, *Proceedings of the Royal Society of Medicine* 52: 463.

Mackenbach, J.P., Bouvier-Colle, M.H. and Jougla, E. (1990) 'Avoidable' mortality and health services: a review of aggregate data studies, *Journal of Epidemiology and Community Health* 44: 106–111.

McKeown, T. and Lowe, C.R. (1966) *An Introduction to Social Medicine*, Oxford: Blackwell.

McLoone, P. and Boddy, F.A. (1994) Deprivation and mortality in Scotland, 1981 and 1991, *British Medical Journal* 309: 1465–1470.

Marmot, M.G. and Syme, S.L. (1976) Acculturation and coronary heart disease in Japanese-Americans, *American Journal of Epidemiology* 104: 225–247.

Marmot, M.G., Rose, G., Shipley, M. and Hamilton, P.J.S. (1978) Employment grade and coronary heart disease in British civil servants, *Journal of Epidemiology and Community Health* 32: 244–249.

Marmot, M.G., Davey Smith, G., Stansfeld, S., Patel, C., North, F., Head, J., White, I., Brunner, E.J. and Feeney, A. (1991) Health inequalities among British civil servants: the Whitehall II study, *Lancet* 337: 1387–1393.

Milward, A.S. (1984) *The Economic Effects of the Two World Wars*, London: Macmillan.

Pamuk, E. (1985) Social class inequality in mortality from 1921 to 1972 in England and Wales, *Population Studies* 39: 17–31.

Persson, T. and Tabellini, G. (1994) Is inequality harmful for growth? Theory and evidence, *American Economic Review* 84(3): 600–621.

Phillimore, P., Beattie, A. and Townsend, P. (1994) Widening inequality of health in northern England, 1981–91, *British Medical Journal.* 308: 1125–1128.

Power, C. and Peckham, C. (1990) Childhood morbidity and adulthood ill health, *Journal of Epidemiology and Community Health* 44: 69–74.

Rose, G. (1981) Strategy of prevention: lessons from cardiovascular disease, *British Medical Journal* 282: 1847–1851.

Rose, G. (1985) Sick individuals and sick populations, *International Journal of Epidemiology* 14: 32–38.

Titmuss, R.M. (1958) War and social policy, in R.M. Titmuss (ed.) *Essays on the Welfare State*, London: Unwin.

United Nations (1982) *Levels and Trends of Mortality since 1950*, London: HMSO.

Webster, C. (1988) *The Health Services since the War* 1, London: HMSO.

Wennemo, I. (1993) Infant mortality, public policy and inequality – a comparison of 18 industrialised countries, 1950–85, *Sociology of Health and Illness* 15: 429–446.

Wilkinson, R.G. (1986) Socio-economic differences in mortality: interpreting the data on their size and trends, in R.G. Wilkinson (ed.) *Class and Health: Research and Longitudinal Data*, London: Tavistock.

Wilkinson, R.G. (1989) Class mortality differentials, income distribution and trends in poverty, 1921–1981, *Journal of Social Policy* 18(3): 307–335.

Wilkinson, R.G. (1994) Health, redistribution and growth, in A. Glyn and D. Miliband (eds) *Paying for Inequality: the Economic Cost of Social Injustice*, London: Rivers Oram Press.

Winter, J.M. (1988) Public health and the extension of life expectancy, 1901–60, in M. Keynes (ed.) *The Political Economy of Health and Welfare*, Cambridge: Cambridge University Press.

Wolfson, M. (1995) Statistics Canada, personal communication.

World Bank (1993) *The East Asian Miracle*, Oxford: Oxford University Press.

World Health Organization (1989) *World Health Statistics Annual*, London: HMSO.

Part I

The policy problem

Chapter 2

To prevent disease
The need for a new approach

S. Leonard Syme

One of the major tasks of epidemiology is to identify risk factors for disease. Our failure in this mission can be illustrated by examining the case of coronary heart disease. Since the end of the Second World War, coronary heart disease has been studied perhaps more aggressively than any other disease. During this period of tremendous international effort, a large number of seemingly important risk factors have been identified. The three that everyone agrees on are cigarette smoking, high blood pressure and high serum cholesterol. Dozens of other risk factors also have been proposed but not everyone agrees about them. Included here are such risk factors as obesity, physical inactivity, diabetes, blood lipid and clotting factors, stress, and various hormone factors. When *all* of these risk factors are considered together, they account for about 40 per cent of the coronary heart disease that occurs (Marmot and Winkelstein 1975).

How is it possible that, after fifty years of massive effort, all of the risk factors we know about, combined, account for less than half of the disease that occurs? Is it possible that we have somehow missed one or two crucial risk factors? While this is of course possible, it should be noted that the relative risk of the new factors would have to be enormous to account for the other 60 per cent of the coronary heart disease that occurs. It seems not very likely that we have missed one or two risk factors of such enormous power and importance. And, it must be said, our record of success in the area of coronary heart disease is one of the very best; the results for other diseases are far less impressive. This is not to suggest that the risk factors we *have* identified are unimportant. They *are* important and they have been useful in the prevention of coronary heart disease but, clearly, there are other very important issues involved that we do not yet understand.

The second problem we face in epidemiology is that, even when we *do* identify disease risk factors, it has proven very difficult for people to make changes in their risk behaviour (Leventhal and Cleary 1980; Dekker 1975; Syme 1982). Even in the Multiple Risk Factor Intervention Trial

(MRFIT), highly motivated men in the top 10 per cent risk category for coronary heart disease were able to make only minimal changes in their eating and smoking behaviours in spite of intensive intervention over a six-year period (Multiple Risk Factor Intervention Trial Research Group 1982).

The third problem we have in epidemiology is that even when people do successfully change their high-risk behaviours, new people continue to enter the at-risk population to take their place. For example, every time we helped a man in the MRFIT project to finally stop smoking, it is probable that, on the same day, one to two children in a school yard somewhere were for the first time taking their first tentative puffs on a cigarette. So, even when we do help high-risk people to lower their risk, we do nothing to change the distribution of disease in the population because, in one-to-one programmes like MRFIT, we have done nothing to influence those forces in the society that caused the problem in the first place.

There are several ways to think about these problems. One way is to continue along the same path but to develop more innovative and more rigorous research designs. Another approach is to improve measurement and assessment methods. Another is to think more creatively about the statistical methods we use to analyze data: we tend to rely on linear, multivariate statistical methods when we might be better served by such alternative approaches as 'grade of membership' or other non-linear methods. Another alternative is to include in our conceptual models not just individuals but the social and cultural environment in which individuals live and work. It is to this last idea that the remainder of this chapter is devoted.

We epidemiologists tend to study individuals in order to find causes of disease even though it is clear that this will not be helpful in understanding the distribution of disease in the population. This point was forcefully made at the turn of the century by the French sociologist, Emile Durkheim (Durkheim 1951). Durkheim studied suicide – a behaviour that clearly is the result of problems experienced by individuals. Indeed, suicide might be considered as one of the most personal and intimate behaviours possible. In spite of this, Durkheim noted that suicide rates exhibited a patterned regularity over time and place. Thus, he said, suicide rates are consistently higher in certain countries and in certain groups, over time, even though individuals come and go from those groups. If the causes of suicide are rooted in the individual, how can it be that there exists a patterned regularity in groups? Durkheim reasoned that there must be something about the group that somehow promotes a higher or lower rate in the group. This factor would not, of course, account for *which* individuals in the group committed suicide but it would account for the fact that the *rate* in the group was consistently high or low.

The value of this approach is that it can lead to a more effective programme for the promotion of health and the prevention of disease.

This is not to deny the importance of working with individuals one at a time: that clearly is worthwhile and important. But it is at least as important to recognize that this approach is very limited because it does nothing about those forces in society that cause our problems in the first place and that will continue to provide a fresh supply of at-risk people, forever. If epidemiology is to be useful in developing approaches to health promotion and disease prevention, it will need to study the community and the population. As matters now stand, almost all epidemiologists study large numbers of individuals in communities. This is not epidemiology. It is clinical medicine in large groups.

There are at least two reasons for our focus on individuals instead of communities. One reason is that the clinical tradition is so pervasive it overwhelms all other approaches. In the United States it certainly has overwhelmed the National Institutes of Health (NIH). One can apply for money from the NIH to study arthritis and metabolic disease, heart disease, cancer, and eye disease, but one cannot request funds to study health at the National Institutes of Health, since only diseases of clinical relevance are funded. There is of course nothing wrong with categorical support but it is unfortunate that almost all the funds for research go to clinical categories and not to public health categories. Of course, it does not help that we in public health do not have a well reasoned and useful set of categories to offer.

The second reason is more subtle and perhaps even more important. It may be that a community approach to infectious disease is easier to develop because most of us are exposed to infectious agents whether or not we want to be. A contaminated water or food supply puts all of us at risk, as does toxic air or infected mosquitoes. It is clear that public health agencies should look after these things on behalf of us all and this clearly is a public health issue. In contrast, the way we eat, drink, smoke, drive, sit, run and work can be seen as being our own affair and not anyone else's business. These behaviours, it could be said, are private matters and are not the province of public health concern. In this view, we are responsible, each of us as individuals, for the heart disease, cancer, and AIDS that we get. It is my opinion that this line of reasoning is one of the prime reasons for our current neglect of a social environmental approach to health promotion and for our adoption of a clinical, one-to-one perspective, including our adoption of a clinical disease classification scheme.

Infectious disease epidemiologists grouped together different clinical entities based on their similarities in modes of transmission. Thus different clinical conditions were grouped together according to whether they were waterborne, airborne, vectorborne or foodborne. These environmental classifications may not be of direct value in the treatment of sick people, but they certainly are of value in identifying those aspects of the environment to which interventions could be directed. What classification categories do we have today that are equivalent to those of waterborne, foodborne, airborne, and vectorborne? We cannot come up with a very long list. What we need are categories that organize our knowledge in appropriate and relevant ways. We have in epidemiology not devoted much attention to this issue. One approach might be to think about a system based on risk factors, since that is at the heart of the problem. Cigarette smoking diseases are one possibility, for example, but as Sylvia Tesh (1988) has noted, we then continue to focus attention on smoking as an individual problem when what we probably really intend is to focus on tobacco as the issue.

Our determined focus on the individual has made it difficult to understand several important issues. One such issue is to explain the large, dramatic decline in death rates from coronary heart disease in a number of countries where the rate used to be very high. In the United States, coronary heart disease mortality rates have plummeted over 40 per cent since 1968. Many people have tried to explain this decline in terms of lower smoking rates, better control of hypertension, lower-fat diets, increased levels of physical fitness, better medical care of patients with coronary heart disease, and so on, but none of these explanations has been satisfactory (Ragland, Selvin and Merrill 1988; Havlik and Feinlieb 1979). In fact all of the explanations considered together account for less than half of the decline. But far more puzzling is that *all* causes of death have declined about the same amount (with the exception of smoking-related cancers). We can perhaps try to explain the decline of mortality from one or another specific disease, but it is difficult to explain the decline of *all* diseases. Our vocabulary and training do not permit an easy explanation of this problem.

How can we go about developing a more appropriate and useful epidemiology – an epidemiology focused more on communities than on individuals? One approach, following Durkheim, is to take advantage of patterned regularities in morbidity and mortality rates. The most impressive patterned regularity of all is social class. Everyone knows, and has known for hundreds of years, that people lower down in social class have higher rates of virtually every disease and condition (Haan, Kaplan and Syme 1989). In spite of this universal recognition, we know almost nothing about the reasons for this phenomenon. The list of possible explanations is long and well known. It includes poverty, bad housing, unemployment, poor nutrition, inadequate medical care and low education. We do not know the relative importance of these various factors because we do not study social class. Social class is of such overwhelming power that we epidemiologists, in our research, typically 'hold it constant' so that we can study other things. If we did not do this, social class would swamp all other factors and we would not be able to see the role of any other issues.

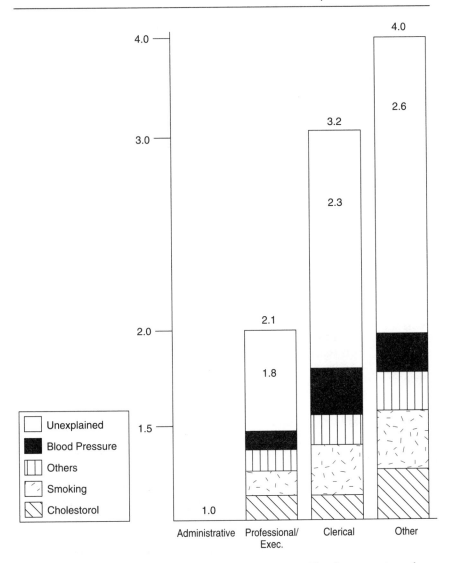

Figure 2.1 Heart disease among British civil servants. The figure on top of each column is the unadjusted relative risk; that within the column is the adjusted relative risk. (Marmot *et al.* 1978)

In consequence, we know virtually nothing about the various subcomponents associated with social class.

But there is another, even more important, reason for our failure to study social class: we do not feel that there is anything that can be done about it. Social class, we say, is a product of vast historical, economic and cultural forces and, short of revolution, it is not something one targets for

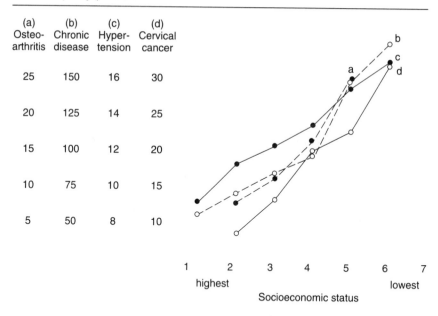

(a) Osteo-arthritis	(b) Chronic disease	(c) Hyper-tension	(d) Cervical cancer
25	150	16	30
20	125	14	25
15	100	12	20
10	75	10	15
5	50	8	10

Figure 2.2 Gradients of common chronic diseases as reported from developed countries. (a) Percentage diagnosed osteoarthritis (Cunningham and Kelsey 1984). (b) Relative prevalence of chronic disease (Townsend 1974). (c) Prevalence of hypertension (Kraus *et al.* 1980). (d) Rate of cervical cancer per 100,000 (De Vasa and Diamond 1980)

intervention. So we give up and instead urge people to lower the fat content of their diet. The problem with this view is that it is based, not on facts, but on speculation. If research were to show that people in the lower social classes had higher rates of disease because they were poor, one might agree that intervention would be difficult. But we have no evidence that lack of money is in fact the major culprit, and without solid facts it seems premature to conclude that social class is too difficult to consider or deal with.

The work of Marmot and his colleagues provides an example of how this problem might better be approached. Professor Marmot and his group (1978) have shown in their study of British civil servants that those at the very bottom of the civil service hierarchy have heart disease rates four times higher than those at the top (Figure 2.1). After adjusting for such heart disease risk factors as blood pressure, serum cholesterol, smoking, physical activity, and so on, the difference between the groups is still three-fold. But in this study they show that those one step down from the top of the hierarchy, civil servants who are professionals and executives (such as doctors and lawyers), have heart disease rates that are twice as high as those at the very top: upper-class directors of agencies, almost all of

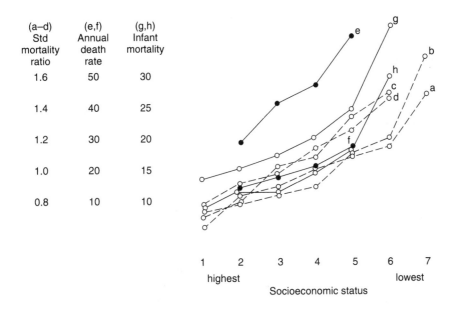

Figure 2.3 Mortality rates from chronic disease as reported from developed countries. (a) Standardized ratio of observed to expected deaths among men (Kitagawa and Hauser 1973). (b) Standardized ratio of observed to expected deaths among women (Kitagawa and Hauser 1973). (c) Standardized ratio of observed to expected deaths among men (Adelstein 1980). (d) Standardized ratio of observed to expected deaths among women (Adelstein 1980).
(e) Annual death rate among men, per thousand (Feldman, Makuer *et al.* 1989).
(f) Annual death rate among women, per thousand (Feldman, Makuer *et al.* 1989). (g) Infant mortality per thousand live births, male (Susser *et al.* 1985).
(h) Infant mortality per thousand live births, female (Susser *et al.* 1985)

whom have been educated at Oxford and Cambridge, and whose career usually ends with a knighthood.

It is not surprising that those at the bottom have higher rates of disease than those at the top, but it is surprising that doctors and lawyers, one step down from the top, also have higher rates. Doctors and lawyers are not poor, they do not have bad houses or bad medical care, and they do not have poor education or poor nutrition. It is not just that those at the bottom have the highest rates of heart disease: there is a gradient of disease from the top of the British civil servant hierarchy to the bottom.

It might be thought that this finding is somehow unique to the British civil service. It is not. We recently completed a review of this issue and we found a similar gradient almost everywhere in the developed world and for virtually every disease that has been studied (Figures 2.2–3). The problem posed by this finding is the following: we can imagine why those at the bottom have higher rates of disease but how can we explain a gradient? How can we explain the finding that those one or two steps from the top have higher rates of disease even though they do not suffer from the problems experienced by those at the bottom? People one or two steps from the top do not experience poverty, or poor nutrition, or problems of access to medical care, or bad housing, or poor education.

The only hypothesis I have been able to come up with is that as one moves down the social class hierarchy one has less control of one's destiny (Syme 1989). By this I mean less opportunity to influence the events that affect one's life. This is not an original idea. Many scholars have studied the concept of mastery, self-efficacy, locus of control, learned helplessness, controllability, predictability, desire for control, sense of control, powerlessness, hardiness, and competence. However, it is important not to over-interpret the fact that so many investigators have suggested the importance of control for health and well-being. In fact, few of these scholars are using the same term in exactly the same way; each use tends to have a special focus and each has been found to be of value in explaining different disease outcomes. For this reason, it is an exaggeration to claim that they are variations on one theme. On the other hand, it is intriguing that so many different investigators, from different backgrounds and with different research objectives, should come up with ideas that are so similar to one another.

More recently a group of epidemiologists led by Robert Karasek from the United States and Tores Theorell from Sweden have shown that rates of coronary heart disease are higher among workers who experience not only high job demands but low discretion and little latitude in dealing with the demands (Karasek and Theorell 1990). The work of these researchers is especially impressive because previous studies of job stress had for decades failed to establish a link between job pressures and health even though the issue had been examined intensively. When the concepts of control and discretion were included in the research, important findings at last emerged and in fact are now being replicated by many others around the world.

I do not know whether the idea of control is correct or not, but I do know that some idea like it is necessary to deal with the difficult problems we face in trying to prevent disease. We need an idea that will help us understand why disease rates are higher in certain groups than in others – over time – even though people come and go from those groups.

Since we do not at present have a better idea than that of control, we are using it in helping us understand the health of bus drivers in San Francisco, California. Several previous studies have noted that bus drivers have a higher prevalence of hypertension, as well as diseases of the gastrointestinal tract, respiratory system and the musculoskeletal system as compared with workers in other occupations (Winkleby, Ragland, Fisher and Syme 1988). These results have been obtained from studies of different transit systems, under different conditions, in several countries. Based on these findings, it has been suggested that certain aspects of the occupation of bus driving may create an increased risk of disease for workers in that occupation.

From a clinical view point it is of value to identify drivers with disease in order to treat them. It would also be of value to teach drivers about better posture, more healthful eating habits and alternative ways of dealing with job stress. However, from an environmental perspective, it would perhaps be more useful to identify those aspects of the job itself that might be changed.

In our study of drivers their exposure to noise, vibration and carbon monoxide fumes is being monitored but particular attention is being paid to the social environment of the driver. For example, in preliminary studies of drivers, the 'tyranny of the schedule' has been forcefully brought to our attention. Drivers must keep to a specific schedule, but in almost every instance, the schedule is arranged without realistic reference to actual road conditions, and in fact cannot be met. If this and other characteristics of the job that are associated with disease can be identified, it may be possible to introduce interventions, not merely among bus drivers, but directly on those environmental factors associated with the job. For example, it might be that by changing the way in which schedules are arranged the bus company would be able to earn more money than it loses through absenteeism, sickness, accidents, and in particular, turnover of employees.

In the case of bus drivers, a clinical focus on hypertension, gastrointestinal diseases, respiratory conditions, or musculoskeletal disorders clearly is useful. However, from an environmental and preventive perspective, it might be useful to group together these different diseases and conditions associated with common work exposure so they can be studied as related phenomena. If this is not done, the circumstances they share will not likely be appreciated.

We also are using the concept of control in another way. We have developed a Wellness Guide that informs people about their options regarding life problems and that then guides them to resources that might be of help. The guide covers thirty-two life problems that involve birth and babies, adolescence, adulthood and old age as well as such problems as food, housing, work and money. We recently have distributed 100,000 copies of this guide to low-income mothers in a Women, Infants and Children Nutritional Supplement Programme. An evaluation of the usefulness of the guide in empowering these mothers to control their lives is now being completed. This evaluation compares the creativity and resourcefulness of 1,189 mothers who either received or did not receive the guide. Preliminary results indicate that the guide is a powerful mechanism for improving the ability of people to influence the life events that impinge upon them.

Whether or not these ideas are useful, they represent an effort to solve a major problem in epidemiology – one not now being addressed very well: can we identify a set of risk factors that will help explain the major, patterned differences in diseases rates seen between groups over the world? The well recognized risk factors help to explain why one individual gets sick instead of another but these factors do not as nicely explain differences between groups. If we are to develop an effective preventive approach to disease, more attention will need to be given to those forces in society that initiate the disease process.

REFERENCES

Dekker, E. (1975) Youth culture and influences on the smoking behavior of young people, in *Smoking and Health*, Proceedings of the Third World Conference, Washington, D.C.: United States Department of HEW, Public Health Service.

Durkheim, E. (1951) *Suicide: a Study of Sociology*, ed. and trans. G. Simpson, Glencoe, Ill.: Free Press.

Haan, M.N., Kaplan, G.A. and Syme, S.L. (1989) Socioeconomic status and health: old observations and new thoughts, in J.P. Bunker, D.F. Gomby and B.H. Keherre (eds) *Pathways to Health: the Role of Social Factors*, Palo Alto, Cal.: H.J. Kaiser Family Foundation.

Havlik, R.J. and Feinleib, M. (ed.) (1979) *Proceedings of the Conference on the Decline in Coronary Heart Disease Mortality*, Washington, D.C.: National Institute of Health.

Karasek R. and Theorell, T. (1990) *Healthy Work: Stress, Productivity, and the Reconstruction of Working Life*, New York: Basic Books.

Leventhal, H. and Cleary, P.D. (1980) The smoking problem: a review of the research and theory in behavioral risk modification, *Psychology Bulletin* 88: 370–405.

Levy, R.I. (1981) The decline in cardiovascular disease mortality, *Annual Review of Public Health* 2: 49–70.

Marmot, M. and Winklestein, W., Jr (1975) Epidemiologic observations on intervention trials for prevention of coronary heart disease, *American Journal of Epidemiology* 101: 177–181.

Marmot, M.G., Rose, G., Shipley, M. and Hamilton, P.J.S. (1978) Employment grade and coronary heart disease in British civil servants, *Journal of Epidemiology and Community Health* 3: 244–249.

Multiple Risk Factor Intervention Trial Research Group (1982) The Multiple Risk Factor Intervention Trial – risk factor changes and mortality results, *Journal of the American Medical Association* 248: 1465–1476.

Ragland, K.E., Selvin, S. and Merrill, D.W. (1988) The onset of decline in ischemic heart disease mortality in the United States, *American Journal of Epidemiology* 127: 516–531.

Syme, S.L. (1989) Control and health: a personal perspective, in A. Steptoe and A. Appels (eds) *Stress, Personal Control and Health*, New York: Wiley.

Syme, S.L. and Alcalay, R. (1982) Control of cigarette smoking from a social perspective, *Annual Review of Public Health* 3: 179–199.

Tesh, S.N. (1988) *Hidden Arguments: Political Ideology and Disease Prevention Policy*, New Brunswick, N.J.: Rutgers University Press.

Winkleby, M.A., Ragland, D.R., Fisher, J.M. and Syme, S.L. (1988) Excess risk of sickness and disease in bus drivers: a review and synthesis of epidemiologic studies, *International Journal of Epidemiology* 17: 124–134.

Chapter 3

The significance of socioeconomic factors in health for medical care and the National Health Service

Mildred Blaxter

The question of the significance of socioeconomic factors is a difficult one for health services, full of paradoxes and dilemmas. The problems arise because the more it is shown that variation in morbidity and mortality is associated with social factors – with poverty, with working circumstances, housing, the environment, social stress – the more it seems that health services, of themselves, can have little relevance. It is obvious that the toll of deprivation can produce burdens for health and social care, but less clear that medicine can do anything to *prevent* inequalities. This line of argument has been strong ever since the movement associated with the name of McKeown (1976a, b) suggesting that the decline in mortality in western Europe in the eighteenth century was due to rising standards of living and nutrition, or perhaps to trends in the relationship between pathogen and host, and not to any advances in medical science.

Moreover, the more sophisticated our research into the etiology of ill health becomes, the more we realize we are not now talking about specific ills with specific and single causes, but rather with general susceptibilities, and with lifelong interactions of the individual and the environment. And the more complex this knowledge grows, the more that medicine – best equipped to deal with specific disease, not general ill health – feels impotent.

An alternative view, pointing to socioeconomic differences in the way that people voluntarily lead their lives, stressing self-responsibility and education, is equally difficult. At present medicine can be seen to be struggling with this. If much ill health is the sufferer's own fault, if individuals are culpable contributors to their own misfortune, how do we distinguish the deserving from the undeserving? Should all be given equal service?

Thus, from both sides of the environment/behavioural debate, medicine has problems: unable to alter socioeconomic disadvantage, and equally unable, on the whole and despite an increasing involvement in health promotion, to change life styles. Thus it is little wonder that medicine may resign itself to treating whatever comes before it, defining socioeconomic differences as outside its sphere of influence.

However, even this has its problems. What comes before it in modern Western societies is largely chronic diseases, or the degenerative conditions of an ageing population, for which the effectiveness of medicine is limited. Another consequence is that it fosters a widespread sense of unmet need. We may not all succumb to the diseases of poverty, but most do suffer degenerative disease eventually, and of course the poor earlier than the rest. Thus potential costs escalate and the funding of services which seem open-ended is seen almost everywhere as a problem.

However, to keep on emphasizing that the need for health care outstrips a society's ability or willingness to pay for it seems unhelpful. The need for health care will *always* outstrip the ability to provide it, since needs are in a sense infinite. Everyone would like to live for ever. Needs – and expectations – change historically: society defines what need is and cuts its coat according to its cloth. The width of that cloth – the proportion of resources devoted to health – is a political question, and not one being addressed here. There is an argument which suggests that there is a trade-off between health care spending and economic growth, and that less spending on health care would mean more of other things which contribute to health and well-being (Lavis and Stoddart 1994). This begs many questions, but in any case, it seems illogical to claim that because demand for health resources outstrips supply, therefore the social distribution of those resources is not relevant. A further argument may be that it is intrinsically possible to have too much health care: medicine can have iatrogenic consequences (Illich 1976), or, on the analogy of defence spending, just as an excess creates the dangers it hopes to guard against, so 'too much' health care affects 'social' auto-immune systems (Evans 1994).

The conclusion of this, that health services can do little to affect inequality in *health*, is perhaps a counsel of despair. Of course medicine cannot prevent inequality, but at the very least it can alleviate its consequences. To fail to acknowledge this is perhaps also an abrogation of responsibility. What might be an alternative view, in the specific context of a reorganized NHS?

Many have commented that one of the disappointing features of the NHS and community care reforms has been the lack of any real discussion of the relevance of social determinants of health (Whitehead 1994). This is not necessarily true at local levels, where the duty placed on public health to assess the health of the population and their needs has resulted in a flurry of surveys and initiatives (Whitehead 1989). Sometimes this has only fuelled the feelings of impotence, however – what is a public health department to do if a community insists on defining its most important health problems as vandalism, or loneliness, or poverty? The lists of the *outcomes* of such local exercises are usually confined to relatively minor features of service provision, far removed from the lists of problems that people themselves identify. The assessment of health needs is a difficult issue, and there is concern that very different interpretations are developing of its purpose (Scott Samuel 1992).

EQUITY

The aims of a reorganized health service are summarized as efficiency, effectiveness and equity, and each will be considered in turn. Equity – equal provision for equal need – was a principle on which the NHS was founded, and there need be no argument about the genuine intention of everyone concerned to approach it as nearly as possible. It has, however, to be noted that equity in health care and equality in health are not at all the same thing. It is probably true that the NHS *was* also seen as promoting greater equality in health between social groups and, especially, geographical areas. But fifty years ago inequality was indeed clearly caused to some extent by inequitable health care. Few would argue that this is any longer true to a significant extent.

Equity was and is largely defined as equity of access. As Klein (1989) has argued, no service can offer equal *treatment* for equal need: it can only offer equal access to doctors, who will inevitably apply different criteria of need and different kinds of treatment. Equality in access does not necessarily mean equality either in treatment or in its outcomes. The arguments that went back and forth in the 1970s and 1980s attempting to relate utilization of services to relative need, discussing, particularly, consultation rates in primary care (e.g. Forster, 1976; Collins and Klein 1980; Le Grand 1982; Blaxter 1984), are now dated and were in any case inconclusive.

However, renewed discussion of concepts of equity began to take place in the context of the reorganized NHS (Pringle 1989; Bevan *et al.* 1989; Jacobson *et al.* 1990; Dahlgren and Whitehead 1992). The commitment of the service in its earlier decades to tackling geographical inequalities in care was, it was thought, lacking in more recent policies. There were suggestions of some channelling of resources away from less affluent regions, and within regions away from deprived inner-city districts (Moore 1992; Judge and Mays 1994). Some studies (e.g. Findlay *et al.* 1991) have shown residents of poorer areas having less access to particular services.

Originally it was thought that dangers to equity arose particularly from the development of fundholding in general practice. The uptake of fund-holding, attracting associated resources, was strongest at first in more prosperous areas (Glennerster *et al.* 1992). The possibility of what was called cream-skimming was feared: perhaps there would be an incentive to be selective about cases or social groups likely to add disproportionately to costs. New forms of contract in primary care offered the opportunity for new services, but if the funding of these depended on the achievement of uptake targets they were easier to reach in more prosperous areas than among poor populations. Thus troubled families and the chronic sick might suffer a new inverse care law (Coulter 1992; Gillam 1992). This fear, as Le Grand (1993) has noted, derived partly from the experience of US Health Maintenance organizations, and there is in fact little evidence that it has materialized in practice.

In the last few years there have been a large number of empirical studies, especially of general practice, in, for instance, South England (Glennerster et al. 1993), West Midlands (Duckworth et al. 1992), Oxford (Coulter and Bradlow 1993), South East Thames (Corney 1994), Northern Region (Newton 1993), and the initial programme in Grampian and Tayside (Howie et al. 1993). Though this research has been piecemeal and often no more than descriptive, in general a summary of its results relates to the disadvantage of the patients of non-fundholders, particularly in terms of admission for hospital treatment (Beecham 1994), rather than to any discrimination by fundholders.

Other equity problems have been identified, such as the way in which the actions of fundholding general practioners may destabilize services for other, perhaps more needy, patients (Whitehead 1993). The most widespread concern, however, relates to the long-term care of the elderly and chronic sick. The decrease in NHS long-stay beds, and the transfer of responsibility and funding for non-acute care to local authorities, have led to many problems. It is suggested that mechanisms for the funding of community care do not respond to actual needs, and that there is wide and inequitable local variation (ACHCEW 1990; Challis and Henwood 1994; Judge and Mays 1994).

All these aspects of reorganized primary care and community care services are continuously changing, and may represent transitional problems. However, a first point of any agenda for health service research and practice with relevance to inequalities in health ought to be careful and continuous monitoring, with questions of equity seen as central.

Even if access to primary care is equitable, however, this does not necessarily ensure equity in referral to specialist care. It is known that there is in fact wide variation in GP referral behaviour, independent of patient conditions, and some evidence of social differentiation (e.g. Blaxter 1984; Noone et al. 1989; Ham and Mitchell 1990; Hoskins and Maxwell 1990). Some research on this is certainly taking place or being encouraged, especially in the different programmes coming forward from the Advisory Groups for the NHS R&D programme.

For instance, in the report on the interface between primary and secondary care, it is noted that there is little evidence of a systematic relationship between population health needs and patterns of referral, and there is a concentration of untreated morbidity amenable to specialist intervention in particular groups of the population. Evidence has been offered by, e.g. Roland and Coulter (1992), Wilkin (1992), and Payne and

Roy (1994). Recognized concentrations of needs in inner cities, among ethnic minorities, or in areas of high unemployment do generate higher utilization rates in primary care, but not, on the whole, more referrals to specialists. This R&D programme's recommended identification of areas of mismatch, and the testing of methods of increasing referrals, are a direct *health service* attack on inequalities.

EFFECTIVENESS

Many of the other chosen areas of this and the other Advisory Groups relate to the second aim of the revised service: effectiveness. A favourable aspect of the NHS reforms, it was thought, was the emphasis on quality standards, greater attention to health outcomes, and more monitoring of the effectiveness of interventions. The important point here is the necessity of including social variables in the medical audit and the evaluation of outcomes (Majeed *et al.* 1994). Sporadic studies for many years have shown clearly that survival after particular diagnoses, or after surgery, differs by social variables. Among the most interesting, for instance, has been the work based on the OPCS longitudinal study (Leon and Wilkinson 1989). Survival from cancer and heart disease appears to be consistently better among those at the upper end of the social scale: among cancers, the survival disadvantage may be more consistent than the incidence disadvantage. For instance, 'standardized fatality ratios' 1971–6 for those with malignant neoplasm, in the period up to 183 days since registration, were found to be 87 for non-manual men and 103 for manual (and 119 for those not ascribed to a class because of inadequately described occupation). It has also been shown that social class differences in survival are small for cancers with poor prognosis, but much larger for cancers where the prognosis is good, if owner occupiers and council tenants are compared. Median survival time from diagnosis of lung cancer was 0.27 years for owner occupiers and 0.25 years for council tenants, for instance, but for cancer of the larynx it was 5.87 years for owner occupiers and 4.39 years for council tenants (Kogevinas *et al.* 1991). In such studies it is difficult to know, of course, whether these differences represent a slower rate of progress of the disease, or a differential probability of apparent recovery, and whether they are due to the timing of presentation, to clinical factors, treatment, after care, or perhaps differences in host response.

However, more recently Cannon *et al.* 1994 studied the relationship between socioeconomic deprivation and pathological prognostic factors in women with breast cancer, and found that differences in survival, across all age groups, were not accounted for by the women presenting with more advanced or more malignant tumors. The authors point out that if the reasons for socioeconomic differences in survival could be identified and eliminated a greater number of lives could be saved than the number expected from the national breast cancer screening programme. Theoretically, 336 lives per year could be saved in the west of Scotland by breast screening programmes. If the survival gradient by deprivation category could be eliminated, 475 would be expected to survive for five years.

One of the problems of the evaluation of outcomes, of course, is the crudity of tools of measurement apart from mortality. It is possible that social differentiation in morbidity duration and disability requires more attention than differences in mortality: we need to consider functional status and quality of life as outcomes. These concepts are not easy to define and quantify, but great strides have been made in recent years, recognizing the multidimensional nature of health, and avoiding the simplicities of counting years of life or counting symptoms – and it should be noted that, again, some of these issues are indeed being addressed in one of the NHS R&D programmes, and there is work going on in many departments and institutes of public health.

Outcomes are social as well as clinical, and the social affect the clinical. So, though clinicians are still resistant to what are seen as soft measures, they must be persuaded of the relevance of the subjective experience of medical interventions. There is certainly a need for more attention to be paid to the interplay between statistical and qualitative methods in defining health needs and health outcomes, and for the results of qualitative studies to be made more convincing to health purchasers.

EFFICIENCY

The third area of policy, efficiency, is relevant because health services have a responsibility to direct priorities where there is most potential for improvement, most health gain for the nation. Indeed, this is another of the hopes of the reorganized NHS. The responsibility of purchasers for assessing health needs suggests the possibility of positive discrimination. One approach, not just at the local level, might be to choose priorities among particular problems or diseases that exhibit social variation. It has to be recognized that in a sense these are the conditions where there is hope of being able to do something, hope of health gain: the conditions with the least social variation are the most intractable, since they do not offer the same potential for change.

Inequality is still to a degree a geographical phenomenon. There are many strong gradients from the north and Scotland to the south in health-related indices. For some diseases and measures, internal migrants acquire the health status of their new region, and for some they do not. Some of the variation appears to be associated primarily with income levels and some is more clearly environmental. Urgently, more study is needed of the factors contributing to these specific – and frequently changing –

patterns, to tease out the extent to which protective or detrimental effects are truly area effects or simply a reflection of the individual characteristics of those who live there. The efficient distribution of health service resources depends on an understanding of these relationships.

As research adds to our knowledge of social variation and its possible causes, the wider policy implications must be considered. For instance, a new phase of research has looked back to the importance of factors operating in early life and indeed before birth (Barker 1990; Ben Shlomo and Davey Smith 1991). The maturing birth cohort studies are very relevant (Power *et al.* 1991; Wadsworth 1991). If this paradigm shift from a life-style model to an early life one is accepted, then the policy implications are clear. A challenge is presented to the contemporary focus on health education or attempts at adult life-style change. Obviously the emphasis must be on the health of infants, or on that of mothers, or even directed earlier at adolescent girls.

In any efficient health policy attention must be paid to the *distribution* of risk factors, not just their frequency. Improvement in services which is applied across a population will not necessarily reduce social inequalities in health and may in fact widen them (Reading *et al.* 1994). This has been demonstrated, for instance, in the prevention of childhood accidents, the prevention of coronary heart disease and other smoking-related conditions, the reduction of teenage pregnancies, and screening for cervical cancer. A screening programme may be held to be successful, but if those who are not reached are precisely those most likely to be at risk it is not an efficient programme. Inequality in the uptake of preventive services can be changed, but only if the explicit aim of a programme is to reduce inequality, not simply general improvement (Marsh and Channing 1988). The understanding of the cultural, behavioural and structural causes that lie behind class-related differences is an essential prerequisite for efficient preventive medicine.

Finally, it might be asked how health services could be persuaded to adopt any agenda such as this for research and practice. Two reasons could be offered, one in the self-interest of the medical professions and one issue of principle. The first is that the more social–health interactions are understood the easier it is to judge what health services actually can do and are doing. Quite rightly, objections are being raised to crude league tables of mortality and other outcomes as a means of judging services. But it is not really sensible to complain about the meaninglessness of a hospital's mortality rates until and unless outcome studies include social factors to make them less problematic.

At a perhaps more important level, attempts must be made to try to depoliticize the topic of inequalities in health. Health services must not stand aside because social inequalities are seen as a political arena. Rather, all the knowledge, and power, and influence, and professional standing of medicine in all its branches ought to be used to keep the issue, and the research it requires, centrally on the public agenda. Medicine and health services have, at the very least, a strong duty of advocacy.

REFERENCES

Association of Community Health Councils for England and Wales (1990) *NHS Continuing Care for Elderly People*, London: ACHCEW.

Barker, D.J.P. (1990) The fetal and infant origins of adult disease, *British Medical Journal* 301: 1111.

Beecham, L. (1994) Fundholders' patients are treated quicker, *British Medical Journal* 308: 11.

Ben Shlomo, Y. and Davey Smith, G. (1991) Deprivation in infancy or adult life: which is more important for mortality risk?, *Lancet* 337: 530–534.

Bevan, G., Holland, W. and Mays, N. (1989) Working for which patients and at what cost?, *Lancet* 1: 947–949.

Blaxter, M. (1984) Equity and consultation rates in general practice, *British Medical Journal* 288: 1963–1967.

Cannon, A.G., Semwogerere, A., Lamont, D.W., Hole, O.J., Mallon, E.A., George, W.D. and Gillis, C.R. (1994) Relation between socioeconomic deprivation and pathological prognostic factors in women with breast cancer, *British Medical Journal* 307: 1054–1057.

Challis, L. and Henwood, M. (1994) Equity in community care, *British Medical Journal* 308: 1496–1499.

Charlton, J., Hartley, R., Silver, R. and Holland, W. (1983) Geographical variation in mortality from conditions amenable to medical interventions, *Lancet* 2: 691–696.

Collins, E. and Klein, R. (1980) Equity and the NHS: self-reported morbidity, access, and primary care, *British Medical Journal* 281: 1111–1115.

Corney, R. (1994) General practice fundholding in S.E. Thames RHA, *British Journal of General Practice* 44: 34–37.

Coulter, A. (1992) Fundholding general practices: early successes, but will they last?, *British Medical Journal* 304: 397–398.

Coulter, A. and Bradlow, J. (1993) Effects of NHS reforms on general practitioners' referral patterns, *British Medical Journal* 306: 433–437.

Coulter, A. and McPherson, K. (1985) Socioeconomic variations in the use of common surgical operations, *British Medical Journal* 291: 183–187.

Dahlgren, G. and Whitehead, M. (1992) *Policies and Strategies to promote Equity in Health*, Copenhagen: WHO.

Dixon, J. (1994) Can there be fair funding for fundholding practices?, *British Medical Journal* 308: 772–775.

Duckworth, J., Day, P. and Klein, R. (1992) The First Wave: a Study of Fundholding in General Practice in the West Midlands, University of Bath: Centre for the Analysis of Social Policy.

Evans, R.G. (1994) Health care as a threat to health: defense, opulence and the social environment, *Daedalus* 123: 21–42.

Findlay, I.N., Dargie, H.J. and Dyke, T. (1991) Coronary angiography in Glasgow: relation to coronary heart disease and social class, *British Heart Journal* 66: 70.

Forster, D.P. (1976) Social class differences in sickness and GP consultation, *Health Trends* 8: 29–32.

Gillam, S. (1992) Provision of health promotion clinics in relation to population need: another example of the inverse care law, *British Journal of General Practice* 42: 54–56.

Glennerster, H., Matsaganis, M. and Owens, P. (1992) *A Foothold for Fundholding*, London: King's Fund Institute.

Glennerster, H., Matsaganis, M., Owens, P. and Hancock, S. (1993) GP fundholding: wild card or winning hand?, in R. Robinson and J. Le Grand (eds) *Evaluating the NHS Reforms*, London: King's Fund Institute.

Ham, C. and Mitchell, J. (1990) A force to reckon with, *Health Services Journal* 100: 164–165.

Ham, C., Hunter, D.J. and Robinson, R. (1995) Evidence-based health policy, *British Medical Journal* 310: 71–72.

Hoskins, A. and Maxwell, R. (1990) Contracts and quality of care, *British Medical Journal* 300: 919–922.

Howie, J., Heaney, D. and Maxwell, R. (1993) Evaluation of the Scottish shadow fundholding project: first results, *Health Bulletin* 51: 94–105.

Illich, I. (1976) *Medical Nemesis: the Expropriation of Health,* New York: Random House.

Jacobson, B., Smith, A. and Whitehead, M. (1990) *The Nation's Health,* London: King's Fund Institute.

Judge, K. and Mays, N. (1994) Allocating resources for health and social care in England, *British Medical Journal* 308: 1363–1366.

Klein, R. (1989) *The Politics of the NHS*, London: Longman.

Kogevinas, M., Marmot, M.G., Fox, A.J. and Goldblatt, P.O. (1991) Socioeconomic differences in cancer survival, *Journal of Epidemiology and Community Health* 45: 216–219.

Lavis, J.N. and Stoddart, G.L. (1994) Can we have too much health care?, *Dadedalus* 123: 43–60.

Le Grand, J. (1982) *The Strategy of Equality*, London: Allen & Unwin.

Le Grand, J. (1993) Evaluating the NHS reforms, in R. Robinson and J. Le Grand (eds) *Evaluating the NHS Reforms*, London: King's Fund Institute.

Leon, D. and Wilkinson, R.G. (1989) Inequalities in prognosis: socioeconomic differences in cancer and heart disease survival, in J. Fox (ed.) *Health Inequalities in European Countries*, Aldershot: Gower.

McKeown, T. (1976a) *The Role of Medicine: Dream Mirage or Nemesis?*, London: Nuffield Provincial Hospital Trust.

McKeown, T. (1976b) *The Modern Rise of Population*, New York: Academic Press.

Majeed, F.A., Chaturvedi, N., Reading, R. and Ben-Shlomo, Y. (1994) Monitoring and promoting equity in primary and secondary care, *British Medical Journal* 308: 1426–1429.

Marsh, G.N. and Channing, D.M. (1988) Narrowing the gap between a deprived and an endowed community, *British Medical Journal* 296: 173–176.

Mooney, G. (1983) Equity in health care: confronting the confusion, *Effective Health Care* 1: 179–184.

Moore, W. (1992) Cash allocation formula is unfair to socially deprived districts, *Health Service Journal* 102: 5.

Newton, J. (1993) Fundholding in the Northern Region: the first year, *British Medical Journal* 306: 375–378.

Noone, A., Goldacre, M., Coulter, A. and Seagoroatt, V. (1989) Do referral rates vary widely between practices and does supply of services affect demand?, *Journal of the Royal College of General Practitioners* 39: 404–407.

Payne, N. and Roy, J. (1994) Is hospital use a proxy for morbidity?, *Journal of Epidemiology and Community Health* 48: 74–78.

Power, C., Manor, O. and Fox, J. (1991) *Health and Class: the Early Years*, London: Chapman & Hall.

Pringle, M. (1989) The quality divide in primary care: set to widen under the new contract, *British Medical Journal* 299: 470–471.

Reading, R., Colver, A., Openshaw, S. and Jarvis, S. (1994) 'Do interventions that improve immunisation uptake also reduce social inequalities in uptake?, *British Medical Journal* 308: 1142–1144.

Roland, M. (1992) Measuring appropriateness of hospital referrals, in M. Roland and A. Coulter (eds) *Hospital Referrals*, Oxford: Oxford University Press.

Roland, M. and Coulter, A. (eds) (1992) *Hospital Referrals*, Oxford: Oxford University Press.

Scott Samuel, A. (1992) Health gain versus equity, *Health Visitor* 65: 176.

Wadsworth, M.E.J. (1991) *The Imprint of Time*, Oxford: Clarendon Press.

Whitehead, M. (1989) *Measuring Health and Lifestyles*, London: Health Education Authority.

Whitehead, M. (1993) Is it fair? Evaluating the equity implications of the NHS reforms, in R. Robinson and J. Le Grand (eds) *Evaluating the NHS Reforms*, London: King's Fund Institute.

Whitehead, M. (1994) Who cares about equity in the NHS?, *British Medical Journal* 308: 1284–1287.

Wilkin, D. (1992) Patterns of referral: explaining variation, in M. Roland and A. Coulter (eds) *Hospital Referrals,* Oxford: Oxford University Press.

Chapter 4

The social pattern of health and disease

Michael Marmot

A SOCIAL VIEW OF HEALTH AND DISEASE

Conceptions of the causes of ill health show marked historical changes. With the recognition of the social problems attendant on industrialization, investigators in England and France studied the influence on health of poverty, occupation, housing and other factors. In Germany a group of physicians, Virchow prominent among them, subscribed to the view that social and economic conditions have an important effect on health and disease and must be subjected to scientific investigation (Virchow 1958). These investigations should form the basis of health policy (Morris 1974).

With the rise of scientific medicine and enormous breakthroughs in basic biological science, these insights tend to have been lost. When I was a medical student in the 1960s, the idea that appendicitis or stomach cancer might have environmental causes never appeared to have occurred to our teachers. By then, at least, lung cancer was related to smoking, but if our teachers had any knowledge of the social distribution of smoking and lung cancer they did not feel it important enough to pass on to the young. One was aware of diseases of affluence, but not of the fact that they were more common among the least affluent members of industrialized society.

The increase in understanding of the molecular basis of biology can, without hyperbole, be described as a scientific revolution. Allied to this, is the belief of many clinicians that the most important determinant of life expectancy has been chosen for their patients, namely by who their parents were. Departures from this genetic model of disease causation usually only go so far as to emphasize the importance of 'bad behaviour' such as smoking, drinking and unsafe sex.

In fact, health and disease are socially patterned. Rates of occurrence of disease states vary according to social and economic conditions, culture, and other environmental factors. This is true today, as it was during the major social and economic changes that came with industrialization. Not only do they vary, but the evidence suggests that variations in rates of

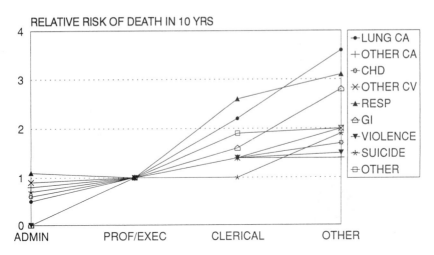

Figure 4.1 Mortality by employment grade among British civil servants. *CA* cancer, *CHD* coronary heart disease, *CV* cardiovascular, *Resp* respiratory, *GI* general infection. (Marmot *et al.* 1984a)

occurrence of disease are actually determined by social and economic factors. It is the purpose of this chapter to demonstrate this variation and to present a framework for understanding its causes. Detailed exploration of the causes will be taken up in other chapters.

SOCIAL, ECONOMIC AND CULTURAL DIFFERENCES IN DISEASE WITHIN COUNTRIES

Our own exploration of this area began with the Whitehall study of British civil servants. Figure 4.1 shows mortality from a range of causes in the first Whitehall study (Marmot *et al.* 1984a). When we began this work, it seemed unlikely that social class differences would be as large in civil servants as they were in the country as a whole. These were all non-industrial civil servants in office-based jobs. At that time their jobs were stable, with high security of employment, and presumably free from chemical and physical industrial hazards. We were surprised, therefore, to discover that the nearly threefold difference in mortality between bottom and top grades of the civil service was larger than the difference between the top and bottom social classes in national mortality data (OPCS 1978; Fox and Goldblatt 1982). This presumably reflects the precise hierarchical classification of occupations within the civil service.

To investigate the causes of these social differentials, we launched a second study of civil servants, the Whitehall II study (Marmot *et al.* 1991;

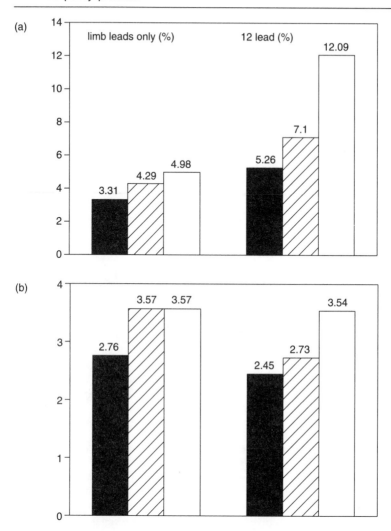

Figure 4.2 Prevalence of cardiorespiratory morbidity and smoking among men aged 40–54 in the Whitehall I (1967–9) and II (1985–8) studies, age-adjusted percentages. (a) Possible and probable ischaemia. (b) Angina.
Black columns show administrative grade; shaded columns, professional and executive; white, clerical/office support staff. (Marmot *et al.* 1991)

Pilgrim *et al.* 1992; Stansfeld and Marmot 1992a, b; Brunner *et al.* 1993; Marmot *et al.* 1993; North *et al.* 1993; Roberts *et al.* 1993; Stansfeld *et al.* 1993, 1995a). Figure 4.2 shows that there were gradients in morbidity and health behaviour (smoking) in Whitehall I and Whitehall II, in addition to the mortality gradients (Marmot *et al.* 1991). There is no suggestion

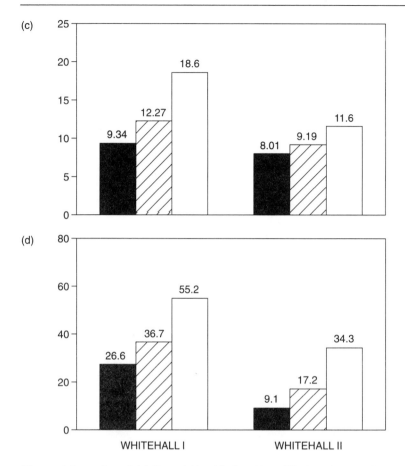

Figure 4.2 continued (c) Bronchitis. (d) Smoking. Black columns show administrative grade; shaded columns, professional and executive; white, clerical/office support staff. (Marmot *et al.* 1991)

that these gradients in morbidity were somehow due to the British civil service being atypical. Figure 4.3 shows, for both men and women, social gradients in self-reported health and depression in Whitehall II and in two large American studies, the Wisconsin longitudinal study and the National Survey of Families and Households (Marmot *et al.* 1995b). Neither of the two American studies is based on an occupational cohort. The first has followed up a cohort of high-school seniors from 1957 in the American state of Wisconsin. The second is a national household survey.

There are two points worth emphasizing from these data. First, there is a gradient in morbidity and mortality. Each group has worse health than the one above it in the hierarchy. The task for explanation here is not why is there a link between poverty and ill health but why is there a

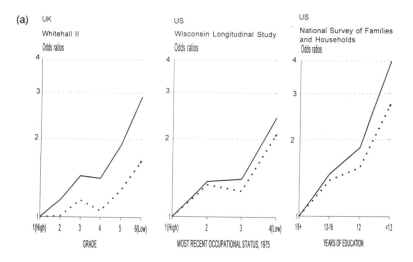

Figure 4.3a Odds ratios of average or worse self-reported health in men according to measures of socioeconomic status in three studies, adjusted for age, parents' social class, intact family (Wisconsin longitudinal study and US National Survey), IQ at school (Wisconsin longitudinal study), work, social circumstances and alcohol (Whitehall II). (Marmot *et al.* 1995a)

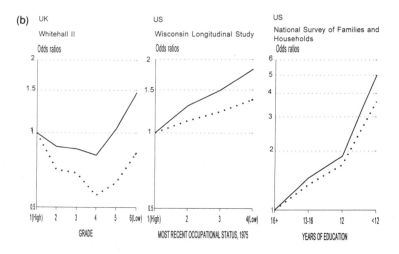

Figure 4.3b Odds ratios of average or worse self-reported health in women according to measures of socioeconomic status in three studies, adjusted for age, parents' social class, intact family (Wisconsin longitudinal study and US National Survey), IQ at school (Wisconsin longitudinal study), work, social circumstances and alcohol (Whitehall II). (Marmot *et al.* 1995a)

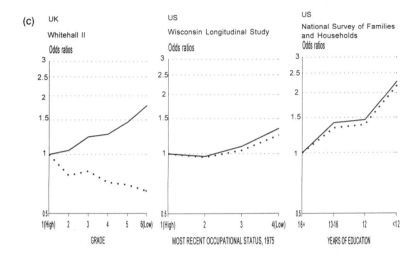

Figure 4.3c Odds ratios of self-reported depression in men according to measures of socioeconomic status in three studies, adjusted for age, parents' social class, intact family (Wisconsin longitudinal study and US National Survey), IQ at school (Wisconsin longitudinal study), work, social circumstances and alcohol (Whitehall II). (Marmot *et al.* 1995a)

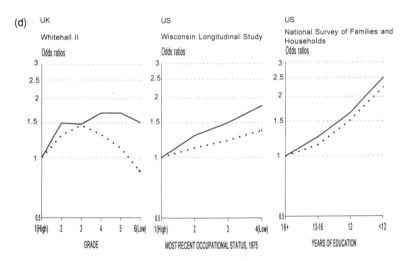

Figure 4.3d Odds ratios of self-reported depression in women according to measures of socioeconomic status in three studies, adjusted for age, parents' social class, intact family (Wisconsin longitudinal study and US National Survey), IQ at school (Wisconsin longitudinal study), work, social circumstances and alcohol (Whitehall II). (Marmot *et al.* 1995a)

social gradient that runs across the whole of society. In the higher grades of the civil service there is no poverty, yet those who are near the top have worse health than those at the top, and the gradient continues all the way down. Similarly, in the Wisconsin longitudinal study, the participants in the cohort were white high-school graduates, thus excluding the quarter of the population that did not graduate from high school at that time.

This is not to imply that there is no longer a problem of poverty in wealthy countries. On the contrary, young black men in Harlem, in New York City, for example, have six times the US average mortality (McCord, 1990). Interestingly, although the relative risk of violent death was large, the greatest contributor to the absolute excess in mortality was cardiovascular disease. Income levels in Harlem are less than a third of the US average. The definition of poverty in wealthy countries has been much debated. One part of the debate has centred on whether poverty should be measured in absolute or in relative terms. The Rowntree Report on income and wealth in Britain produced both measures (Joseph Rowntree Foundation 1995). As a relative measure, it reported the percentage of the population that had incomes below half the average, after allowing for housing costs. This fell to a low point of 7 per cent of the population in 1977 and rose to 24 per cent in 1990. In absolute terms, the bottom tenth of the distribution had a 17 per cent fall in real income between 1979 and 1991, the second bottom 10 per cent had no change. This contrasted with a 36 per cent rise in average incomes. However, only the top three-tenths of the distribution had incomes rising as fast as the average (Joseph Rowntree Foundation 1995).

We have, therefore, two types of problem to understand and address. First, the relation between inequality and ill health (Wilkinson 1986); second, the relation between poverty and ill health (World Bank 1993).

The second point arising from these Whitehall analyses is the generality of the findings across causes of morbidity and mortality. Specific diseases have specific causes. Cutting across these, there may be a predisposition to ill health that is related to position in the social hierarchy. In Figure 4.1 the gradient in mortality according to civil service employment grade is shown for most of the major causes of death (Marmot *et al.* 1984a). There are similar gradients for various measures of morbidity and for the general measure of self-reported health. A particular demonstration of the general importance of environment in the patterning of disease comes from the study of migrants (Marmot *et al.* 1984b). In general, disease rates among migrants reflect influences from the country of origin and the country of destination. There are some genetic abnormalities such as thalassaemia or sickle cell disease. Apart from these, we observe a pattern of disease in migrants that resembles that of the old country in the early years after migration, and comes to resemble that of the new country with the progress of time. Men of Japanese ancestry living in the United States have rates of coronary heart disease intermediate between the low rates in Japan and the high rates in the United States (Syme *et al.* 1975). Japanese men in Hawaii have lower rates than those in California (Marmot *et al.* 1975).

There has been much debate as to the extent to which ethnic differences in disease can be attributed to socioeconomic factors. In the United States, for example, it appears that the bulk of the black/white differences in health can indeed be accounted for by social and economic factors (Pappas *et al.* 1993). Comparing ethnic groups is not the same as comparing migrants and non-migrants. The position of blacks in the United States may indeed be largely determined by socioeconomic circumstances. This appears not to be the case for migrants to England and Wales. Figure 4.4 examines mortality from ischaemic heart disease by country of birth and social class in England and Wales. The high mortality in immigrants from the Indian sub-continent and the low mortality in immigrants from the Caribbean persist within social classes and hence cannot easily be attributed to socioeconomic circumstances. Indeed, there is a suggestion that the social class pattern of mortality in the South Asian and Caribbean immigrants differs from the inverse relation between social class and mortality seen in the country as a whole (Marmot *et al.* 1995c).

These migrant data illustrate an important point about the influence of social circumstances. Because social factors are more distant in the causal chain than biological processes, their effects may be contingent on other circumstances. There is evidence, for example, that the social class distribution of heart disease changes with level of economic development (Marmot 1992:3). With the emergence of ischaemic heart disease as a major cause of death, it appears at first to be more common in higher socioeconomic groups. Subsequently, the social class distribution changes to the one more commonly seen now in industrialized countries, with higher rates in lower socioeconomic groups.

This changing social class pattern presumably means either that important causal factors have changed their social class distribution or that the relative importance of different factors has changed. For example, the social class distribution of smoking appears to have reversed. It now shows a clear social gradient, with high rates in low socioeconomic groups (see Figure 4.2 for example). Other things may not have changed their social class distribution. The disadvantage of low social position in terms of psychosocial factors related to inequality may not have changed. These psychosocial factors may not have led to an increased risk of ischaemic heart disease in the absence of important causes, such as high intake of saturated fat, smoking, sedentary life style and obesity. This emphasizes the importance of studying the links between social, economic, cultural and other determinants of ill health.

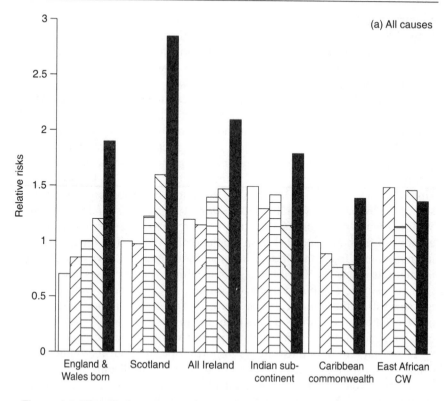

Figure 4.4 Mortality by country of birth and social class, 1979–85. (a) All causes. (Marmot *et al.* 1995b)

MEASURES OF SOCIAL INFLUENCES ON HEALTH

In the United States, social position is usually referred to as socioeconomic status and is commonly measured as some combination of occupation, income and education. In Britain much of the evidence for the relation between social position and ill health has come from analyses using the Registrar General's social classes (OPCS 1978). This classification is based on grouping occupations into social classes. It has continued to be widely used for the pragmatic reason that it is a potent predictor of a wide range of health outcomes. It regularly attracts criticism because the basis of the grouping is unclear (Goldblatt 1990). Goldthorpe has contrasted three different systems of measuring social stratification. The first is based on the prestige of occupations. The second is based on social status and is a measure of whether members of a social group are treated as equals. The third is social class. Goldthorpe's preference is for a measure of social class that locates individuals in households within the economic sphere (Erikson and Goldthorpe 1992).

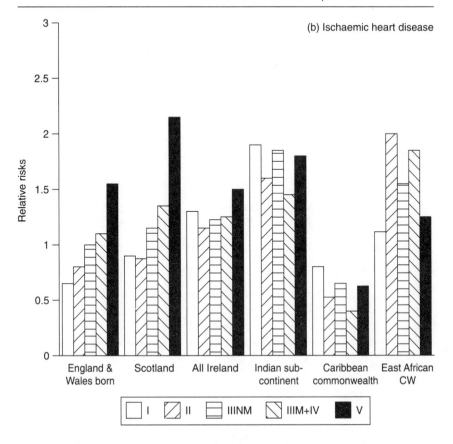

Figure 4.4 continued Mortality by country of birth and social class, 1979–85.
(b) Ischaemic heart disease. (Marmot *et al.* 1995b)

There are at least two reasons for wishing to be precise about social classification. The first relates to the pragmatic issue of better prediction, the second to understanding. The argument is that a measure that has a clear conceptual base and higher validity is more likely to convey meaning when attempting to interpret a correlation. This is desirable but maybe illusory. Education has appeal as a measure because it appears to convey what it is about social position that may be causally related to increased risk. If education were then shown to be a stronger predictor than, say, occupational prestige, this could lead to the presumption that it is education, not factors related to occupation, that is more important in the causal chain leading to ill health. This may be an over-interpretation. If it were the case that education was measured more precisely than occupational prestige, that alone could account for its stronger predictive power.

Table 4.1 Rate ratios[a] for short and long spells of sickness absence, by employment grade and level of education

Measure	Men		Women	
	Short spells[b]	Long spells[c]	Short spells[b]	Long spells[c]
Employment grade				
Unified grades				
1–6	1.0 –	1.0 –	1.0 –	1.0 –
Unified grade 7	1.96 (1.81–2.14)	2.03 (1.56–2.67)	1.51 (1.20–1.89)	1.11 (0.60–2.05)
Senior Executive Officer	2.30 (2.11–2.51)	2.25 (1.70–2.97)	2.09 (1.67–2.63)	1.08 (0.58–2.04)
Higher Executive Officer	3.04 (2.80–3.30)	3.27 (2.50–4.25)	3.13 (2.54–3.87)	2.13 (1.23–3.69)
Executive Officer	5.33 (4.91–5.79)	4.49 (3.43–5.88)	3.57 (2.89–4.41)	2.47 (1.43–4.27)
Clerical Officer/ Office Support	6.85 (6.28–7.47)	6.33 (4.79–8.36)	4.04 (3.27–4.97)	3.76 (2.22–6.45)
Educational level (years)				
≤16	1.0 –	1.0 –	1.0 –	1.0 –
17–18	1.17 (1.11–1.22)	0.90 (0.77–1.04)	1.03 (0.97–1.10)	0.83 (0.71–0.97)
>19	1.29 (1.23–1.35)	0.94 (0.82–1.08)	1.29 (1.22–1.36)	0.96 (0.83–1.13)

Notes:
(a) Rate ratios for employment grade are adjusted for age and level of education and those for education are adjusted for age and grade. All rate ratios 95% CI.
(b) Seven days or less.
(c) Over seven days.

Data from the Whitehall II study show that grade and education are independent predictors of sickness absence. Table 4.1 shows, however, that, when both predictors are put into the same predictive model, grade emerges as the stronger independent predictor. This is contrary to most investigators' findings with measures of education and occupation. It may be that, in the Whitehall II study, factors related to occupation are more important in the aetiology of socioeconomic differences in health than are factors related to education. Before reaching this conclusion, however, we should consider the relative precision of measurement. In Whitehall II, grade of employment is a precise measure of hierarchical position, whereas our measure of education is relatively imprecise. This may be one of the relatively few examples where an occupation-based measure of class is more precise than a measure based on education. This may be at least part of the explanation of the greater predictive power of grade.

Townsend proposed measures of socioeconomic deprivation. He developed an index for classifying areas that combines household access to a car, housing tenure (whether a dwelling is owned, rented from the local authority or privately rented), percentage unemployed and percentage living in

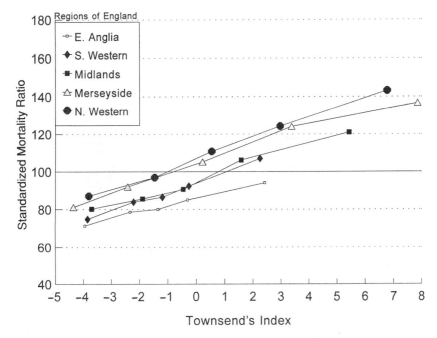

Figure 4.5 All-cause mortality in regions of England by degree of deprivation divided into fifths. (Eames *et al.* 1993)

crowded conditions (Townsend *et al.* 1988). Figure 4.5 contains analyses of mortality in small geographical areas (electoral wards) grouped according to scores on the Townsend index. It shows that the average mortality in each quintile of social deprivation is higher than in the quintile below it (Eames *et al.* 1993). One interpretation of this apparent gradient is that relative deprivation is an important predictor of mortality level. Alternatively, it is possible that there is a threshold of deprivation above which mortality is raised, and each quintile contains progressively greater proportions of deprived households.

Whether or not these measures predict mortality because they are indicators of material circumstances may be debated. What is not in doubt is that they are predictors. Figure 4.6 shows mortality data from the first Whitehall study with the population divided according to grade and car ownership. Within each grade, car owners have lower mortality than non-car owners. It is not suggested that there is anything especially healthy about owning a car. Rather, it is a further indicator of social position. Adding it to grade spreads the risks even further. There is here a four-fold mortality differential between the least favoured and the most favoured groups (Davey Smith *et al.* 1990).

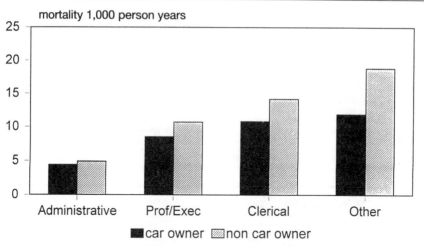

Figure 4.6 All-cause mortality by employment grade and car ownership among civil servants. (Davey Smith *et al.* 1990)

Quite apart from the meaning they may contain, indicators such as housing tenure or car ownership have further pragmatic value. Registrar General's social class cannot classify accurately people who have no occupation. This applies especially to retired persons and married women not employed outside the home. Household measures, such as access to a car, or housing tenure, predict just as well in these groups as among 'employed' people (Goldblatt 1990).

It is no doubt important to have a measure with appropriate precision that relates to an appropriate concept. Nevertheless, finding the appropriate measure of social position will not by itself solve the aetiological question. It will be necessary to explore the relevant links between social position and ill health.

SOCIAL PATTERNS OF DISEASE ARE NOT FIXED

One response to the demonstration of social variations in disease rates is that they exist everywhere and are therefore intrinsic to social organization. It is implied that, if social differentials in health are a consequence of the complex organization of society, there is little that can be done about them.

While it is true that social differentials in health have been observed widely, wherever they have been sought, the magnitude of the differentials, i.e. the slope of the gradient, is not fixed. It varies over time and place. Figure 4.7 shows percentage changes in mortality rates in Scotland between the early 1980s and 1990s by area classified according to degree

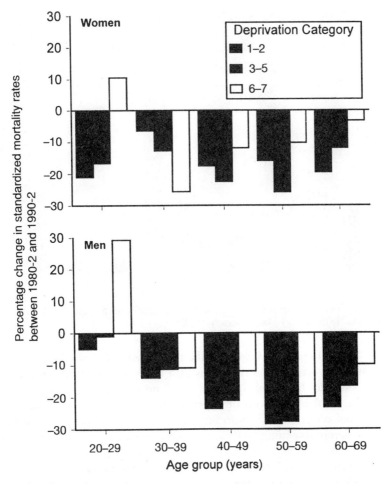

Figure 4.7 Mortality change in Scotland by social deprivation. (a) Women. (b) Men. (McLoone and Boddy 1994)

of deprivation. For men and for women, with the exception of one age group, the decline in mortality is least in the most deprived areas. At ages 20–29 mortality actually increased in the most deprived areas. This increase among young men and women was due largely to suicide (including deaths that were undetermined as to whether accidentally or purposely inflicted) (McLoone and Boddy 1994). Analyses confirm a widening differential in mortality between manual and non-manual groups for every region in Britain (Marmot and McDowall 1986). Similarly, in Finland, there has been a widening gap in mortality across social groups (Valkonen *et al.* 1990).

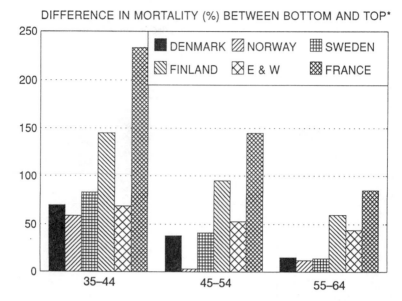

DIFFERENCE IN MORTALITY (%) BETWEEN BOTTOM AND TOP*

Figure 4.8 Inequality in mortality between occupational groups *E&W* England and Wales. (Kunst and Mackenbach 1992)

The data in Figure 4.5 show that the relation between social deprivation and mortality varies across regions within England. The slope of the relation appears to be somewhat shallower in East Anglia, for example. Further, at equivalent levels of deprivation on the Townsend score there are regional differences in mortality. This may result from the measures having different 'meaning' in different parts of the country. In other words, a given score may not indicate equal levels of deprivation in different geographical regions. These are, after all, indicators. A second interpretation is that the relation between deprivation and mortality actually varies in different geographical areas. There may be other factors determining geographical differences in mortality.

Comparing socioeconomic differences internationally also has methodological problems. Many of these were avoided in a study by Kunst and Mackenbach that used an occupational classification of social class in six European countries (Kunst and Mackenbach 1992). Figure 4.8 shows that the ratio of mortality between the lowest and the highest groups varies by age and by country.

If socioeconomic gradients in health change over relatively short periods of time, and are different in different countries and geographical settings, such gradients need not be inevitable. If the gradients vary there must be reasons why. Better understanding of the reasons may form the basis of action to alleviate them.

SOCIAL DETERMINANTS OF INTERNATIONAL DIFFERENCES

Comparison of disease patterns on a global scale leads to the obvious conclusion that social, economic and cultural forces are primary in determining the major differences in infant mortality, life expectancy and disease patterns that exist around the world. When informed that life expectancy at birth in 1992 in Guinea-Bissau and Afghanistan is 43 years, whereas life expectancy in Japan is 78.6 years, we have little difficulty in speculating that this fact may be related to the economic fortunes of the different countries. In fact the real gross domestic product *per capita* (expressed in purchasing power parities) is $19,400 in Japan and $700–$750 in Guinea-Bissau and Afghanistan (United Nations Development Programme 1994).

Although poverty, expressed as real income, is a major reason for these huge international differences in health status, there is no simple link between GDP and life expectancy. This is illustrated in Table 4.2, from the Human Development Report published by the United Nations Development Programme (1994). The report uses a Human Development Index which combines real GDP, life expectancy and education. It then ranks countries from 1 (Canada) to 173 (Guinea) on this index. Table 4.2 shows some exceptions to the link between income and life expectancy, for three groups of countries, within which the countries have similar levels of GNP. Guinea and Sri Lanka have similar levels of income *per capita*, but life expectancy in Guinea is 43.9 years and in Sri Lanka 71.2. As the table shows, within the income band, the higher the adult literacy rate the longer the life expectancy. There is a similar finding within each of the other two income bands.

The general conclusion from this example is that social factors are likely to exert a powerful influence on life expectancy. Level of education is a powerful predictor in addition to income. Caldwell speculated that countries such as Sri Lanka which achieve long life expectancies in spite of low incomes have certain features in common. These include 'a substantial degree of female autonomy, a dedication to education, an open political system, a largely civilian society without a rigid class structure, a history of egalitarianism and radicalism, and of national consensus' (Caldwell 1986). As a test of these notions, he showed that countries whose infant mortality was lower than would have been predicted from their GNP had a high female proportion at school (Caldwell 1986).

Similarly, Hobcraft showed, in twenty-five developing countries, that mother's education shows a linear relation to survival chances (Hobcraft 1993). Figure 4.9 shows the association between maternal education and child survival, adjusted for paternal occupation as well as paternal

Table 4.2 Similar income, different Human Development Index, 1991–2

Country	GNP per capita (US$)	HDP rank	Life expectancy (years)	Adult literacy (%)	Infant mortality (per 1,000 live births)
GNP per capita around $400 to $500					
Sri Lanka	500	90	71.2	89	24
Nicaragua	400	106	65.4	78	53
Pakistan	400	132	58.3	36	99
Guinea	500	173	43.9	27	135
GNP per capita around $1,000 to $1,100					
Ecuador	1,010	74	66.2	87	58
Jordan	1,060	98	67.3	82	37
El Salvador	1,090	112	65.2	75	46
Congo	1,040	123	51.7	59	83
GNP per capita around $2,300 to $2,600					
Chile	2,360	38	71.9	94	17
Malaysia	2,520	57	70.4	80	14
South Africa	2,540	93	62.2	80	53
Iraq	2,550	100	65.7	63	59

Note:
(a) Human Development Index, a composite measure of life expectancy, education and income as purchasing power parities (United Nations Development Programme 1994).

education and region. Similarly, the relation between paternal occupation and child survival is adjusted for the other variables. Adjustment attenuates the relation of father's occupation quite markedly. The odds ratio in the most favoured category is changed from 0.56 to 0.84. By contrast adjustment changes the odds ratio in the most favoured maternal education category only from 0.42 to 0.52. One interpretation of these data is that they support the direct causal link with mother's education. Possible explanations include: a shift in familial power structures permitting the educated woman to exert greater control over health choices; increased ability to manipulate the modern world; and a shift from fatalistic acceptance of health outcomes towards implementation of health knowledge (Hobcraft 1993). There needs, however, to be a caveat. Maternal education may simply be a more precise and more quantitative ranking of social position than father's occupation and occupational status. Greater measurement precision alone could account for the 'better performance' of maternal education in multivariate models.

In Chapter 7, Wilkinson shows another reason for the lack of a clear relation between income and life expectancy. Up to a level of GNP of about $5,000 *per capita*, there is a tight relation between income and life expectancy (World Bank 1993). Above that level of income the relation

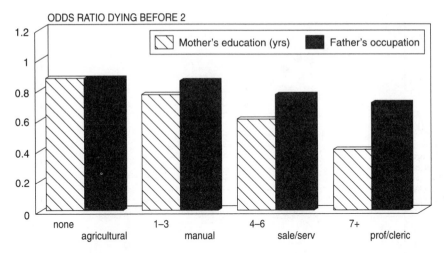

Figure 4.9 Adjusted odds ratios of dying before 2 years of age, according
to mother's education and father's occupation in twenty-five developing
countries. Each parent's ratio is adjusted for the other's, plus father's education and region. (Hobcraft 1993)

with life expectancy is shallow. Wilkinson shows that the relation is much
tighter with income inequalities (Wilkinson 1992).

The general point to emerge from Wilkinson's work is that social and
economic influences on health are not confined to developing countries,
nor are they encapsulated by measures of mean income alone. Similarly,
the message from the work of Caldwell (Caldwell 1986), Hobcraft
(Hobcraft 1993) and the Human Development Report (United Nations
Development Programme 1994) suggests that other factors related to
social organization are crucially important.

This may account for some of the differences we see in Europe. Figure
4.10 shows life expectancy at age 15, for 1970 and 1991, for countries in
Europe. There are dramatic differences in life expectancy across Europe
(Bobak and Marmot 1995), but this measure removes their effect from life
expectancy. For men, the countries of central and eastern Europe (the former Communist Bloc countries) had a decline in life expectancy during this
twenty-one-year period. This was in marked contrast to the improvements
in the countries of the European Union and the Nordic countries of Europe.
The differences are large. In 1991 life expectancy in Hungary for men was
52 years, compared with nearly 61 years in Iceland, Sweden, Greece and
Israel (which latter is included among WHO European countries). For
women, there were improvements in life expectancy in all parts of Europe
but, as with the men, the differences widened between east and west.

This widening east–west gap may be similar to the widening social variations seen within countries. Certainly, it represents a change. Throughout

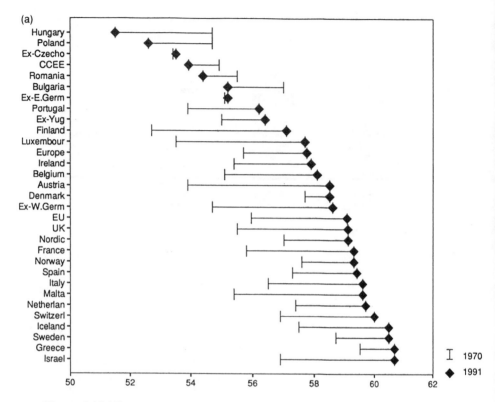

Figure 4.10 Life expectancy at age 15 in 1970 and 1991. (a) Men. (Bobak and Marmot 1995)

the post-war period, mortality in Czechoslovakia was similar to that of Austria and Germany (Bobak and Feachem 1992). Around 1970 there was a change. Life expectancy continued to improve in those western European countries but remained stagnant or declined in the countries of central and eastern Europe.

If we cast our eye farther afield we see further contrasts. Figure 4.11, for men, shows the decline in life expectancy in the former Soviet Union and Hungary, and an increase in the United States and Canada similar to that observed in western European countries. Japan shows an even more dramatic picture. Life expectancy in 1965 was less than in the UK and similar to Hungary. By 1992 Japan had the longest life expectancy in the world; 76 years for men and 82 years for women (World Bank 1992, 1994; United Nations 1993). Over the same period Singapore also increased life expectancy by seven years, to 72 in men and 77 in women.

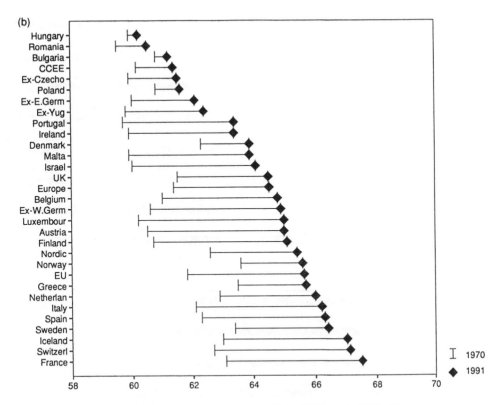

Figure 4.10 continued Life expectancy at age 15 in 1970 and 1991. (b) women. (Bobak and Marmot 1995)

If we ask how these two Asian countries achieved such a remarkable improvement in life expectancy, we must look at social and economic factors (Marmot and Davey Smith 1989). Japan now has one of the highest GNPs *per capita* in the world and Singapore's economy grew at 8.3 per cent annually through the 1970s and at 6.6 per cent through the 1980s. This compares favourably with the average annual growth rate of high-income economies of 3.2 per cent in the 1970s and 2.9 per cent in the 1980s (World Bank 1993). In addition, Japan has among the narrowest income distributions of any wealthy country.

The picture we are painting is that countries characterized by increasing wealth, a comparatively equitable distribution of income and high investment in education are countries with a better health record. How the social and economic forces are translated into better health is taken up in the rest of this book. A framework for approaching explanations is given in the next section.

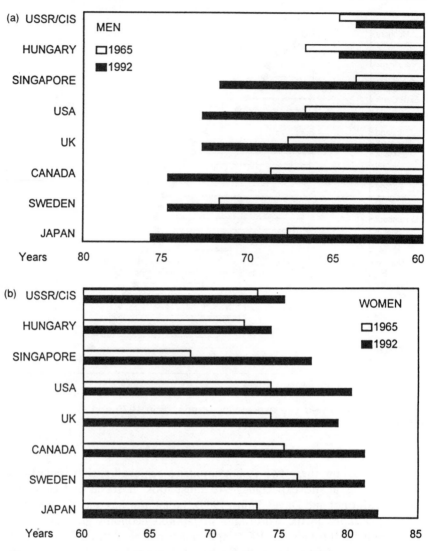

Figure 4.11 Life expectancy at birth, selected countries, 1965 and 1992. (a) Men. (b) Women. (World Bank 1992, 1994, United Nations 1993)

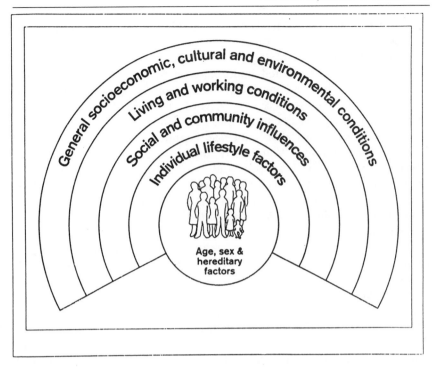

Figure 4.12 Factors influencing health. (Dahlgren and Whitehead 1991)

FRAMEWORK FOR EXPLAINING SOCIAL AND ECONOMIC DISEASE PATTERNS

The landmark Black Report (Black *et al.* 1988) posed four classes of explanation for inequalities in health: artefact, selection, culture and behaviour, and material conditions (Blane 1985). Research since the Black Report makes it clear that the first two explanations are unlikely (Goldblatt 1990; Power *et al.* 1991). Other factors are important (Marmot *et al.* 1995a).

Dahlgren and Whitehead have produced a general framework of the determinants of health, reproduced as Figure 4.12 (Dahlgren and Whitehead 1991). Much of research and policy to improve health focuses on biological factors in the innermost circle, or individual lifestyle factors in circle 4. This is perhaps a natural extension, both of the clinical approach to disease and of the revolution in biological understanding. The first emphasizes the primacy of the individual patient; the second the molecular and biochemical basis of pathogenesis. Research into prevention has, to a large extent, focused on individual risk factors for disease. These, in general, have resided in the inner two circles, i.e. individual biological characteristics or lifestyle factors. Approaches to prevention have tended to follow this research by emphasizing the manipulation of individual risks.

There is little in this book on diet, smoking, alcohol, physical activity or risk-taking sexual and other behaviours. This is not because they are unimportant. Each of them, viewed in the health field as part of 'life style' are of undoubted importance in the aetiology of the major causes of morbidity and mortality. We accept the importance of these lifestyle factors but then ask two types of question. To what extent are they influenced by social, cultural and economic factors? Are there other psychosocial pathways that influence health? This can be illustrated from the Whitehall and Whitehall II studies. Figure 4.2 shows the prevalence of smoking in these two studies of civil servants, according to grade of employment. It shows that although the prevalence of smoking declined over the twenty years separating the two studies, the social gradient in smoking prevalence persisted, i.e. higher smoking rates in lower grades.

It is not sufficient, therefore, to ask what contribution smoking makes to generating the social gradient in ill health, but we must ask, why is there a social gradient in smoking?

The importance of the second type of question was also illustrated in the Whitehall study (Marmot 1986: 21). The social gradient in mortality from coronary heart disease was similar among smokers and non-smokers. A combination of all the individual risk factors that were measured in the study accounted for a quarter of the mortality gradient (Marmot *et al.* 1984a). Even allowing for imprecision in the measurement of risk factors, at least half the social gradient had to be due to factors other than the risk factors measured: smoking, plasma total cholesterol level, blood pressure level, body mass index, physical inactivity, and height.

Some of the explanation for these unexplained parts of the social gradient presumably reside in circles 2 and 3 of Figure 4.12. They exert a strong influence on biology. If they do not operate through the risk factors listed, there must be other biological pathways through which they act. An important part of the research agenda is to trace the links between social and biological pathways that underlie a social patterning of disease. Figure 4.12 does not make it explicit that these factors may operate throughout the life course. The research reviewed in other chapters of this book are compatible with the view that there is a cumulation of advantage and disadvantage throughout the life course that determines patterns of disease in later life.

POLICY IMPLICATIONS

A framework that emphasizes the social determinants of health has important implications for health policy. To a large extent in political discussion health policy is usually equivalent to policies for the organization and funding of medical services. All societies spend a large proportion of their resources on medical care. It is therefore appropriate to have vigorous debate and research as to the extent to which it is meeting society's needs. It is not appropriate for the health debate to stop there. The framework emphasized here suggests that policies for health should focus on the wider inputs to health. Such inputs are beyond the sphere of influence of health departments and need to involve a variety of agencies, departments and settings both public and private. The details of such potential policies are taken up in the specific chapters of this book.

REFERENCES

Black, D., Morris, J.N., Smith, C., Townsend, P. and Whitehead, M. 1988 *Inequalities in Health: the Black Report; The Health Divide*, London: Penguin.

Blane, D. (1985) An assessment of the Black Report's explanation of health inequalities, *Sociology of Health and Illness*, 7: 421–445.

Bobak, M. and Feachem, R.G.A. (1992) Health status in the Czech and Slovak Federal Republic, *Health Policy and Planning* 7(3): 234–242.

Bobak, M. and Marmot, M.G. (1995) East–West health divide and potential explanations, in *Proceedings of the European Health Policy Conference*, Copenhagen, 1995 (submitted).

Brunner, E.J., Marmot, M.G., White, I.R., O'Brien, J.R., Etherington, M.D., Slavin, B.M., Kearney, E.M. and Davey Smith, G. (1993) Gender and employment grade differences in blood cholesterol, apolipoproteins and haemostatic factors in the Whitehall II study, *Atherosclerosis* 102: 195–207.

Caldwell, J.C. (1986) Routes to low mortality in poor countries, *Population and Development Review* 2: 171–220.

Dahlgren, G. and Whitehead, M. (1991) Tackling inequalities: a review of policy initiatives, in M. Benzeval, K. Judge and M. Whitehead (eds) *Tackling Inequalities in Health: an Agenda for Action*, London: Kings Fund Institute, 1995.

Davey Smith, G., Shipley, M.J. and Rose, G. (1990) Magnitude and causes of socioeconomic differentials in mortality: further evidence from the Whitehall study, *Journal of Epidemiology and Community Health* 44: 265–270.

Eames, M., Ben-Shlomo, Y. and Marmot, M.G. (1993) Social deprivation and premature mortality: regional comparison across England. *British Medical Journal* 307: 1097–1102.

Erikson, R. and Goldthorpe, J.H. (1992) *The Constant Flux*, Oxford: Clarendon.

Fox, A.J. and Goldblatt, P. (1982) *Socio-demographic Mortality Differentials*, OPCS Longitudinal Study 1, London: HMSO.

Goldblatt, P. (1990) Mortality and alternative social classifications, in P. Goldblatt (ed.) *Longitudinal Study: Mortality and Social Organisation*, London: HMSO.

Hobcraft, J. (1993) Women's education, child welfare and child survival: a review of the evidence, *Health Transition Review* 3(2): 159–175.

Joseph Rowntree Foundation (1995) *Inquiry into Income and Wealth*, York: Joseph Rowntree Foundation.

Kunst, A.E. and Mackenbach, J.P. (1992) *An International Comparison of Socioeconomic Inequalities in Mortality*, Rotterdam: Erasmus University.

McCord, C. (1990) Excess mortality in Harlem, *New England Journal of Medicine* 322: 173–177.

McLoone, P. and Boddy, F.A. (1994) Deprivation and mortality in Scotland, 1981 and 1991, *British Medical Journal* 309: 1465–1470.

Marmot, M.G. (1986) Social inequalities in mortality: the social environment, in R.G. Wilkinson (ed.) *Class and Health*, London: Tavistock.

Marmot, M.G. (1992) Coronary heart disease: rise and fall of a modern epidemic, in M.G. Marmot and P. Elliott (eds) *Coronary Heart Disease Epidemiology*, Oxford: Oxford University Press.

Marmot, M.G. and Davey Smith, G. (1989) Why are the Japanese living longer?, *British Medical Journal* 299: 1547–1551.

Marmot, M.G. and McDowall, M.E. (1986) Mortality decline and widening social inequalities, *Lancet* 1: 274–276.

Marmot, M.G., Syme, S.L., and Kagan, A. (1975) Epidemiologic studies of CHD and stroke in Japanese men living in Japan, Hawaii and California: prevalence of coronary and hypertensive heart disease and associated risk factors, *American Journal of Epidemiology* 102: 514–525.

Marmot, M.G., Shipley, M.J. and Rose, G. (1984a) Inequalities in death: specific explanations of a general pattern, *Lancet* 1: 1003–1006.

Marmot, M.G., Adelstein, A.M. and Bulusu, L. (1984b) Lessons from the study of immigrant mortality, *Lancet* 1: 1455–1458.

Marmot, M.G., Smith, G.D., Stansfeld, S., Patel, C., North, F., Head, J., White, I., Brunner, E. and Feeney, A. (1991) Health inequalities among British civil servants: the Whitehall II study, *Lancet* 337: 1387–1393.

Marmot, M.G., North, F., Feeney, A. and Head, J. (1993) Alcohol consumption and sickness absence: from the Whitehall II study, *Addiction* 88: 369–382.

Marmot, M.G., Bobak, M. and Davey Smith, G. (1995a) Explanations for social inequalities in health, in B. Amick, S. Levine, A. Tarlov and D. Walsh (eds) *Society and Health* (in press).

Marmot, M.G., Ryff, C.D., Bumpass, L., Shipley, M. and Marks, N. (1995b) Social inequalities in health: a major public health problem (submitted).

Marmot, M.G., Head, J.A. and Swerdlow, A.J. (1995c) Socio-economic circumstances and trends in immigrant mortality (submitted).

Morris, J.N. (1974) *Uses of Epidemiology*, third edition, London: Churchill Livingstone.

North, F., Syme, S.L., Feeney, A., Head, J., Shipley, M.J. and Marmot, M.G. (1993) Explaining socio-economic differences in sickness absence: the Whitehall II study, *British Medical Journal* 306: 361–366.

Office of Population Censuses and Surveys (1978) *Occupational Mortality 1970–72*, London: HMSO.

Pappas, G., Queen, S., Hadden, W. and Fisher, G. (1993) The increasing disparity in mortality between socio-economic groups in the United States, 1960 and 1986, *New England Journal of Medicine* 329: 103–109.

Pilgrim, J.A., Stansfeld, S.A. and Marmot, M.G. (1992) Low blood pressure, low mood? *British Medical Journal* 304: 75–78.

Power, C., Manor, O. and Fox, J. (1991) *Health and Class: the Early Years*, London: Chapman & Hall.

Roberts, R., Brunner, E., White, I. and Marmot, M. (1993) Gender differences in occupational mobility and structure of employment in the British civil service, *Social Science and Medicine* 37: 1415–1425.

Stansfeld, S.A. and Marmot, M.G. (1992a) Deriving a survey measure of social support: the reliability and validity of the Close Persons Questionnaire, *Social Science and Medicine* 35: 1027–1035.

Stansfeld, S.A. and Marmot, M.G. (1992b) Social class and minor psychiatric disorder in British civil servants: a validated screening survey using the General Health Questionnaire, *Psychological Medicine* 22: 739–749.

Stansfeld, S.A., Davey Smith, G. and Marmot, M.G. (1993) Association between physical and psychological morbidity in the Whitehall II study, *Journal of Psychosomatic Research* 37: 227–238.

Stansfeld, S.A., Feeney, A., Head, J., Canner, R., North, F. and Marmot, M.G. (1995a) Sickness absence for psychiatric illness, *Social Science and Medicine* 40: 189–197.

Stansfeld, S.A., North, F.M., White, I. and Marmot, M.G. (1995b) Work characteristics and psychiatric disorder in civil servants in London, *Journal of Epidemiology and Community Health* 49: 48–53.

Syme, S.L., Marmot, M.G., Kagan, H. and Rhoads, G. (1975) Epidemiologic studies of CHD and stroke in Japanese men living in Japan, Hawaii and California, *American Journal of Epidemiology* 102: 477–480.

Townsend, P., Phillimore, P. and Beattie, A. (1988) *Health and Deprivation: Inequality in the North*, London: Croom Helm.

United Nations (1993) *World Population Prospects*, 1992 revision, New York: Oxford University Press.

United Nations Development Programme (1994) *Human Development Report 1994*, New York: Oxford University Press.

Valkonen, T., Martelin, T. and Rimpela, A. (1990) *Socio-economic Mortality Differences in Finland 1971–85*, Helsinki: Central Statistical Office in Finland.

Virchow, R. (1958) Industrialism and the sanitary movement, in G. Rosen (ed.) *A History of Public Health*, New York: MD Publications.

Wilkinson, R.G. (1986) Socio-economic differences in mortality: interpreting the data on their size and trends, in R.G. Wilkinson (ed.) *Class and Health*, London: Tavistock.

Wilkinson, R.G. (1992) Income distribution and life expectancy, *British Medical Journal* 304: 165–168.

World Bank (1992) *World Development Report 1992*, New York: Oxford University Press.

World Bank (1993) *World Development Report 1993*, New York: Oxford University Press.

World Bank (1994) *World Development Report 1994*, New York: Oxford University Press.

ACKNOWLEDGEMENTS

I would like to thank Mandy Feeney for her help in the preparation of this chapter. The Whitehall II study is supported by the Medical Research Council, the Health and Safety Executive, the British Heart Foundation, the National Heart Lung and Blood Institute, the Agency for Health Care Policy Research, the New England Medical Centre Division of Health Improvement, the Institute for Work and Health, Toronto, the Volvo Foundation and the John D. and Catherine T. MacArthur Foundation Research Network on Successful Midlife Development.

Part II

Environment and economic growth

Chapter 5

Social determinants of health
The sociobiological translation

Alvin R. Tarlov

This chapter will provide a modern definition of health that emphasizes health's social context, summarize evidence for the view that the social determinants of health are paramount, and provide a conceptual framework for the production of health that accounts for differential vulnerability to disease according to the social hierarchy. A conjecture will be offered to explain how social characteristics are received as sensory stimuli by man and translated into biological signals that are antecedent to disease that becomes clinically manifest later in life. An emphasis on societal characteristics as powerful determinants of a population's health has important relevance to policy formulations if the goal is to improve health.

HEALTH NEWLY DEFINED

Health has been conventionally defined in terms of the prevalence of diseases, or the absence of disease. More recently, health has been redefined in terms that assess the level of functioning and well-being in every day living within the social context.

Good health is assigned the highest value in every society. It is considered the most precious of attributes. Definition of health as an operational concept, however, has been elusive. From antiquity health has been thought of as a physical or mental state. Most assessments of health have focused on the absence of major threats to society at that time, such as starvation, epidemics of infection and, in the past 100 years, chronic disease.

Departing from the prior definitions of health which emphasized the absence of disease, Henry E. Siegrist, MD, the William H. Welch Professor of History of Medicine at the Johns Hopkins University, wrote in 1941, 'Health is, therefore, not simply the absence of disease: it is something positive ...' (Siegrist 1941: 100). The World Health Organization's constitution stated in 1947, 'Health is a state of complete physical and social well-being and not merely the absence of disease or infirmity' (WHO 1947). The WHO statement forty-eight years ago established a watershed of ideas on the concept of health. The new emphasis on positive well-being and social interaction was introduced and accepted.

The endeavour to define health during the past half-century unveiled a remarkable consistency of three conceptual components (Dubos 1962; McDermott 1977: 136; Parsons 1979; Dwore and Kreuter 1980: 103–119; Kickbusch 1986; Nutbeam 1986: 113–127; de Leeuw 1989: 11–68). One, health is a *capacity* to perform, a relative state, a continuous variable. Two, the capacity to perform is used to achieve *individual fulfilment* such as the pursuit of values, tasks, needs, aspirations and potential. Three, since capacities and fulfilment operate in a social environment, good health provides the potential to effectively *negotiate the demands of the social environment*. Health is seen as a state of being required to pursue specified aspirations. Health is the capacity for individual fulfilment. The following definition is a synthesis of the concepts provided by others over the past half-century.

Health is the capacity, relative to potential and aspirations, for living fully in the social environment. The definition is applicable to a population as well as to an individual. Maintenance and enlargement of the capacity is the goal of all health improvement strategies. The definition emphasizes 'living fully'. Death and morbidity rates, the principal measures of health worldwide, are only indirect and perhaps not highly sensitive indicators of a population's health. The 3.7 years longer life expectancy of the Japanese, and the 2.1 years of the Swedish, compared with Americans may underestimate the true health differences if capacity for living fully in the social environment were measured.

DETERMINANTS OF HEALTH

There are four categories of determinants of the health of a population: genes and biology; medical care; health-related behaviours such as nutrition, tobacco use, physical fitness and alcohol excess; and the social characteristics within which living takes place. Of these, the social characteristics predominate.

Genes and biology

The modern era of genetics extends from the Watson–Crick discovery of the double-helix configuration of genes in 1953 to the present work of the Human Genome Project, an international collaborative attempt to identify the specific location and DNA sequence of each of the 100,000 genes on the twenty-three pairs of human chromosomes (Watson 1968). The medical relevance of modern genetics has an A phase and a B phase.

The A phase can be referred to as *single gene inheritance*. It began in 1956 with the discovery by Carson, Ickes, and Alving of x-linked glucose-

6-phosphate dehydrogenase deficiency as a cause of primaquine-induced haemolytic anaemia in black men (Carson 1956). The ensuing forty years have brought the discovery of thousands of single gene mutations that cause disease, including sickle cell haemoglobin, thalassaemia, cystic fibrosis, Huntington's disease, and 10 per cent of breast and colon cancers. Victor McKusick at Johns Hopkins University has created a growing catalogue of single mutant gene disorders in humans, a list that now contains over 3,000 known inherited diseases (McKusick 1994). The DNA sequences of genes related to dozens of diseases have been worked out and could possibly be therapeutically useful later. Although to my knowledge the fraction of the total disease burden of man attributable to single gene inheritance has not been estimated, it may be at the 1–5 per cent level.

The B phase can be referred to as *multiple gene inheritance* or *polygenic inheritance*, a phase in a steep growth period currently. Susceptibility to a specific chronic disease is conferred by a specific combination of normal genes, perhaps as few as two or as many as twelve. The specific combination does not include any mutant genes. The gene combination does not 'cause' a disease, but is permissive of or provides resistance to the disease developing. The gene combination when in association with individually adopted health habits and with specific external social influences determines which if any chronic disease develops. Even in the presence of a complete polygenic combination the disease will not develop or will be markedly attenuated unless the related health habits and social factors are present to create the permissive interaction. Only a fraction of persons having the gene combination will develop the disease. The disease expression will vary across a population, depending on the completeness of the permissive gene combination and the strength of the associated health habits and social influences. The clinical manifestation (phenotype) is the net result of the interaction of the three factors, i.e. gene combination, individual acquired behavioural characteristics, and the social environment.

Evidence is building for polygenic inheritance (Copeland *et al.* 1993). A major advance was made recently by Todd's group at Oxford University (Davies *et al.* 1994). They identified five genes in combination, and estimate that there may be as many as eighteen, that are responsible for the familial clustering of Type I diabetes.

Since the expression of the polygenes in a specific disease requires association with non-biological antecedents that are social, a separate prevalence attribution for polygenic inheritance has not been attempted. The best that can be done with the current state of knowledge is to assume tentatively that genes as a determinant of health account for 1–5 per cent of the total disease burden of man. This point is arguable. Further research will help to elucidate the point.

Medical care

The awesome advances in biomedical science and technology in the past 100 years have brought earlier diagnoses, more effective treatments, and merciful relief of pain and other disabling symptoms. But medical care is a late intervention in the disease development process, usually taking place twenty or more years after the start of the pathological disease process. Medical care can have only modest effects on morbidity and mortality rates, the data upon which health is conventionally measured. Bunker, Mosteller, and Frazier have estimated the separate contribution of medical care to the extension of life expectancy from forty-five to seventy-five years in the twentieth century in the United States (Bunker *et al.* 1994). For their estimates they used changes in condition-specific mortality data, treatment efficacy from randomized clinical trials, and evidence for the efficacy of preventive screening, immunization, and treatment services. They reported that, of the thirty-year gain in life expectancy, five years (17 per cent) could be attributed to medical care interventions known to be effective. (They also reported the potential of adding one to one and a half years to life expectancy if services were more perfectly applied to all people.)

Further evidence, albeit indirect, of the effect of medical care as a determinant of health is the lack of relationship between a nation's level of health care expenditure, either *per capita* or as a percentage of gross national product, and its life expectancy. A publication of the World Bank (1993: 53) comments, 'At any level of income and education, higher health spending should yield better health, all else being equal. But there is no evidence of such a relation.'

Health-related behavioural risk factors

Marmot has estimated the contribution of behavioural risk factors to health, using Whitehall II data (Marmot 1993: 35–49). Using the ideal (probably not achievable) assumption that the risk factors of the entire British population could be lowered to the bottom two quintiles of the civil servant population with respect to plasma cholesterol, blood pressure and having never smoked, coronary heart disease death rates would be lowered 60 per cent for the entire population, with reductions also in some other causes of death. Sixty per cent might be considered the maximum possible health improvement under idealized behavioural control circumstances. What accounts for the other 40 per cent?

Marmot showed that in the Whitehall population about 25 per cent of the stepwise gradient related to occupational class in coronary heart disease death rates could be accounted for by adjusting the data for age, tobacco smoking, blood pressure, plasma cholesterol, blood sugar, and height (Marmot 1993: 41). Seventy-five per cent of the social gradient must be accounted for by factors other than those risk factors.

In other analyses Marmot has examined the association between job class and the rates of work absence greater than seven days among Whitehall II men. The absence ratio was about seven to one between the lowest and the highest classes. Accounting for about a third of the work absence–job grade ratio were personal health behaviours, psychosocial work characteristics, and social circumstances outside of work, including lack of social support and difficulty paying bills (Marmot 1993: 38).

Social characteristics

To summarize the determinants of health, genetic inheritance may account for 5 per cent or less of the total disease burden. Medical services have contributed about 17 per cent to the gain in life expectancy in the twentieth century. Health-related behavioural risk factors accounted for between 25 per cent and 60 per cent of the gradient in health across social classes in the United Kingdom, but many of the behavioural risk factors have aetiological roots in the social environment. Assigning the risk factors exclusively to the behavioural risk factor determinants category obfuscates the effects of societal characteristics on cigarette smoking, excessive use of alcohol, imprudent diet, lack of exercise, sexual risk and so forth. Assigning a quantitative attribution to each of many determinants when they all interact and the dimensions of their measurements differ is not attainable. Looking at the data generally and making some coarse assumptions, it would appear that a substantial fraction of the variation in health from one population to another, or among various strata within a single population, is unexplained by variations in genetic inheritance, medical care, and behavioural risk factors. The substantial unexplained portion probably is related to social characteristics, the subject of the following section.

EVIDENCE FOR THE SOCIAL DETERMINANTS

The past 11,000 years of human experience illustrate the successive influence on health of unstable food supply, plagues and epidemics, and in the twentieth century chronic disease, all connected with social influences. In the late twentieth century differential vulnerability to disease of each distinctive strata in the social gradient has become the key determinant of a population's health. A population's health at any time in history is the net result of the interaction of people with their social and physical environment.

The information in Table 5.1 has been greatly oversimplified to make the point that health results from the interaction between man and the

Table 5.1 Changing threats to health over eleven millennia

Health era	Threats to health	Manifestation	Reference sources	Health goal	Strategies to produce health	Health measurement
Physical deprivation 9000 BC–present	Lack of food, shelter, and clothing	Starvation and exposure	Old Testament Archaeological and Anthropological literature	Survival of the tribe Reproduction	Grain and livestock domestication Shelter, fuel	Survivability over generations
Infectious diseases 2000 BC–present	Insanitary water and food, and crowding	Plagues and epidemics	Old Testament 1954 cholera epidemic at Broad St pump McNeill (1976)	Avoidance of the scourge	Sanitation, vaccination, antibiotics, symptomatic treatments for dehydration, fever	Deaths during epidemics
Chronic diseases 1900–present	Affluence Leisure Harmful life style	Heart disease, cancer and stroke	Health insurance actuarials and claims Epidemiological studies	Cure of the disease and control of the symptoms	Medical care: antisepsis, anaesthesiology, surgery, pharmaceuticals, organ substitution and replacement, gene manipulation Disease prevention	Morbidity and mortality rates and life expectancy
Socioecological determinants 1947–present	Differential vulnerability to disease based on social stratification: education, housing, job, income	Impaired functional capacity and well-being Premature death	WHO (1947) Doll (1950)[a] Surgeon General's Report 1964 and 1979[b] Breslow (1967) Lalonde (1974) Syme and Berkman (1976) Amler and Dull (1987)	Quality-of-life enhancement	Health production, develop the circumstances for living fully	Self-reported functioning and well-being Expected years of life without activity limitation

Notes: (a) Doll and Hill (1964).
(b) US Department of Health, Education and Welfare (1964, 1979).

social circumstances and physical environment in which living takes place. That is, the socioecology is a paramount determinant of the health of a population. The determinants of health, strategies to improve health, and appropriate measurements of the state of health change radically over time. Note that the table extends each era to the present; the eras overlap. Starvation continues as a mortal problem for a substantial fraction of the world's 5.5 billion people. While smallpox has been eradicated, cholera and measles epidemics continue as major problems even in some communities within nations having advanced economies. AIDS, a recently identified infectious disease, has achieved epidemic proportions worldwide. Among some nations, and among some sub-populations of nations, lung cancer, diabetes, and hypertension continue to rise as predominant causes of disability and death. Even within a nation or within a city, threats to health and health status vary greatly among different sub-populations. The following two points can be made with confidence. The interaction of man with the social and physical environment is a predominant determinant of health. Within a population micro-socioecological differences among groups are surgically precise in their imposition of distinctive conditions for health and distinctive patterns of disease on each group. That is why the rates of disease and impairment are unevenly distributed, not only among nations, but within nations, states, counties, cities, and neighbourhoods (McCord 1990).

When the most recent ice age receded about 11 millennia ago, nomadic man was given wider range for hunting wild sheep and deer and foraging for nuts and seeds. There is lack of clarity as to what came first, farming wild grain or domestication of wild boar, or other livestock (Wilford 1994). Perhaps the sequence was different in different climates, with the development of cereal production first in the warmer valleys and more temperate climates of the Middle East, while husbandry of wild boar preceded grain production in the highlands of eastern Turkey, both occurring about 10,000 years ago. Nevertheless, there is general agreement that the development of farming, livestock husbandry, durable shelter, and sources of fuel ended nomadism in favour of a more stationary village existence. The gain in physical security provided a large boost to reproductive success and survivability.

In subsequent centuries the growth of manufacturing and commerce led to urban development and crowding and to a new disease era characterized by plagues and other infectious epidemics. The discovery was made, principally in Turkey, that smelting copper with tin yielded a very hard and forgeable material (bronze) that was ideal for tools. The Bronze Age (4000 BC to 2500 BC) and its production of tools permitted improved farming, manufacturing, mass production, long-distance trade and urban growth. Cities with populations in the hundreds of thousands arose. The first empire, the Akkadian empire, rose in Mesopotamia, between the Tigris and Euphrates rivers, about 2300 BC. Great prosperity was achieved through a strong economic base of wheat, barley and sheep. The empire suddenly collapsed in 2200 BC for reasons that remained unknown until recently. Archaeological evidence based on soil moisture analysis revealed that the region's collapse was occasioned by an abrupt climate change with a devastating drought that lasted 300 years and led to the decimation of a prosperous civilization (Weiss *et al.* 1993). Large numbers of Akkadians, scores of thousands, headed to cities in the south, overwhelmed the water and food supplies and created urban catastrophe. A good example of the interaction of socioecology with the health of populations.

There is ample documentation of the era in which infections predominated (2000 BC to the present). The Bible refers often to epidemics in antiquity. Plague, or 'Black Death', caused by the simple bacterium *yersinia pestis* carried by fleas and rodents, killed 27 million people, or one-third of the world's population, in the Middle Ages, from AD 1345 to 1350 (McGraw 1993). Smallpox killed one-third of the Amerindian population in Mexico and other Central American areas from 1518 to 1526, accounting for the ease of conquest of millions of Aztec and other Indians by a few hundred Spaniards at that time (McNeill 1976: 207–209). Tuberculosis claimed one billion lives in the nineteenth and twentieth centuries (Ryan 1993). The worldwide influenza pandemic of 1918–19 claimed 20 million lives (McNeill 1976: 288). The determinate influence of epidemics on the course of civilization is illuminatingly described by William H. McNeill (1976).

In 1989 the Smithsonian Institution held a symposium titled 'Disease and Demography in the Americas: Changing Patterns before and after 1492' as part of the celebration of the quincentenary of Columbus. There is controversy over the size of the pre-Columbian New World population, but it may have been near 100 million. Pre-Columbian disease in the New World was highly prevalent and related to problems of diet, over population, social organization and sanitation. Tuberculosis and treponemal disease were common. There is evidence for large regional variability in disease prevalence, related in part to the climatic preferences of pathogens, differences in the nutritional value of food and other factors (Verano and Ubelaker 1992).

There is consensus on the devastating impact on the Indian populations after contact with the Europeans. Some estimate the size of the Indian population that had contact with the Europeans to have been reduced to one-twentieth its pre-contact size. Among the infectious diseases imported by the Europeans and to which the non-immune endemic Americans were exposed were measles, diphtheria and smallpox as well as high prevalence of the more chronic infectious diseases such as tuberculosis and syphilis. Other factors contributed to the appalling decline of the Indian population, including warfare, social and cultural disruption, population concentration, soil depletion, diminished nutritional quality, and poor sanitation (Veranos and Ubelaker 1992).

The Smithsonian volume documents, using modern techniques of anthropology, archaeology, palaeopathology, and historical demography that the expression of health and disease resulted powerfully from the interaction of man with his social and physical environments. Health and disease are not due to random circumstances. This was true in the Americas pre- as well as post-Columbus and is equally valid today to explain variations in health status.

The infection era, although extending into modern life in some populations and still the predominant albeit declining cause of death overall in the entire world, is no longer the predominant health threat in industrialized societies. For 1990, using disability-adjusted life years (DALY), a combined measure of both mortality and disability, the distribution of DALY loss for the entire world population of 5.3 billion was 45.8 per cent for communicable diseases, 42.2 per cent for non-communicable diseases and 11.9 per cent for injuries. Parallel figures for the 0.8 billion people residing in nations having established market economies were 9.7 per cent, 78.4 per cent, and 11.9 per cent, respectively (World Bank 1993: 27).

The waning of infections on a global basis has been too simply ascribed to the development of vaccines and antibiotics, improved sanitation, and to better treatments such as rehydration and medications to lower body temperature. There is ample evidence that the closing of the infection era was primarily the effect of improved agricultural production, beginning with the second agricultural revolution (eighteenth century) and of improved social circumstances such as economic growth and higher standards of living, including improved nutrition and housing. Thomas McKeown made this point in his book *The Modern Rise of Population* (McKeown 1976). Leonard Sagan added cogently to this subject (Sagan 1987).

The decline of infectious disease mortality in modern times has been accompanied by a remarkable prolongation of life expectancy from birth: for the United States 49 years in 1900 (Sagan 1987: 19) to 75.4 years in 1990 (US Bureau of the Census 1993: table 115). Over this same period of infectious disease decline, however, there has been an equally dramatic reciprocal rise in death rates from chronic disease (Figure 5.1).

The chronic diseases that now account for 75 per cent of the deaths in the United States are, in descending order of prevalence, cardiovascular disease, cancers, obstructive lung disease, diabetes, and liver disease. Reiterating a point made above, there is large heterogeneity of disease profiles among the nations of the world. In some nations, South Africa as an example, malnutrition remains a principal cause of death among black infants and children. In others, such as Bangladesh, epidemic death

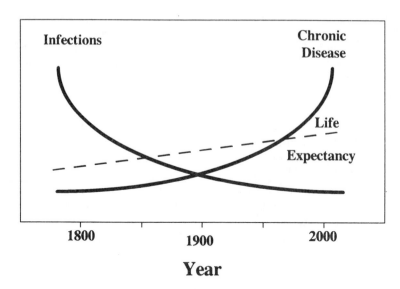

Figure 5.1 Mortality rates and life expectancy. During the past 200 years there has been a dramatic fall in US death rates from infectious diseases and a reciprocal rise in deaths from chronic diseases. Over the same period life expectancy nearly doubled

through cholera infection remains a major problem. Infectious epidemics and inadequate nutrition go hand in hand (McKeown 1976). But in the advanced economies of the world in North America, Europe and some parts of the Far East, transition to the chronic disease era has been complete.

Among nations, patterns of physical deprivation, infection, chronic disease, and life expectancy are strongly associated with standard of living or *per capita* income (World Bank 1993: 34–35). The developing countries continue to struggle with insufficient food supplies and unsanitary conditions, while the developed countries have achieved standards of living from which the basic necessities of living are available in plentiful supply for most of the people and high standards of sanitation have been adopted. But why in societies wherein the standards of living have successfully eliminated physical deprivation and infectious disease does rising prevalence of chronic disease supervene?

The standard of living, efficiency of production, and effective systems for redistribution of income achieved in advanced economies have not only provided the minimum necessities of life but have provided incomes that allow wide access in those societies to surplus income. Overeating, diets high in the more costly and fattier foods from meats, obesity, high

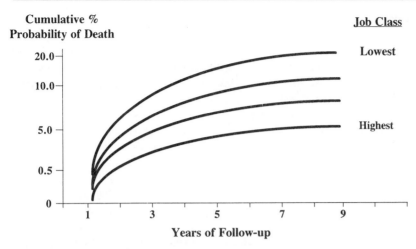

Figure 5.2 Death rates associated with job class. A study of 17,000 civil servants in the United Kingdom shows that the death rate of those in the lowest job class was four times that of employees in the highest job class, with a continuous gradient among the job strata at each period in time

purchase rates and use of tobacco and alcohol, and diminished physical requirements of most employment have resulted. Chronic disease patterns emerge from affluence.

During the past 100 years of chronic disease predominance and biomedical science and technology advancement, progress in health has been measured using conventional epidemiological methods, chiefly changes in morbidity and mortality rates from specific disorders, and lengthening of life expectancy. There have been notable improvements. Death rates from cardiovascular disease have declined 30 per cent over the past thirty years (National Center for Health Statistics 1986; Kawachi *et al.* 1991). Life expectancy continues to lengthen. There is evidence that these improvements, although partly attributable to medical care, are largely related to socioecological changes such as a shift towards the healthier in tobacco use, diet, and physical fitness. Disease origin is rarely simply a biological affair, only its manifestations are. The major fundamental determinants of the health of populations are external to man's biology.

Powerful evidence for the role of social circumstances as paramount determinants of population health has been provided by studies *within* populations that demonstrate high correlations between the twin gradients of social strata and health. The correlation and associated work have been moved forward notably by Michael Marmot, his graduate mentor Leonard Syme at Berkeley, and their legions of disciples. Since the twin gradients are the subject of this book, discussion of the research findings in this chapter will be limited to one study (Marmot *et al.* 1984).

Marmot and colleagues studied 17,000 civil employees in the United Kingdom over a ten-year period. Prevalence of disease and death rates were recorded and analysed according to four broad job classes (related to educational attainment and income). The results (Figure 5.2) show that the employees in the lowest job classes had disease and death rates that were four times greater than the rates in the highest job class, with a continuous gradient in between. The interlinked gradients of employment class and health status were verified for each chronic disease analysed separately. Underlying pervasive social influences exert common detrimental effects for all disease categories.

Studies generally similar to that of Marmot *et al.* verify the tight connection between the gradients of social classification and health in every society in which class and health have been studied. In addition to the present book, four recent book-length publications provide highly useful reference and data sources on the relationship between social characteristics and health (Honda 1993; Evans *et al.* 1994; *Daedalus* 1994; Amick *et al.* 1995). Any endeavour to substantially improve the health of populations should be based on an understanding that health is the net result of the interaction of people with their social and physical surroundings, the social ecology of health.

A SOCIOECOLOGICAL FRAMEWORK FOR THE PRODUCTION OF HEALTH

Each population of people is immersed in a social milieu that is as variable as the number of different populations or the number of subgroups within a population. The social milieu has dozens of features that are important to health, but the features fall into three categories: personal; community; societal. The health of a population is predominantly the net result of the interaction of people with their social milieu, the socioecology of health. The socioecology is a major determinant of the health of a population, and explains why there is so much variation in health across different populations, or among subgroups within a population.

In previous sections of this chapter the four major classes of determinants of health were discussed and evidence was reviewed that points powerfully towards social characteristics being a paramount determinant. In this section a conceptual framework for considering how the social determinants work, the socioecological framework, will be described. This framework, although not widely known or accepted, is not new but is an attempt to provide a simple visual image from which strategies for research, analyses and policy formulations can be developed.

Population health can be conceptualized as three concentric rings of health determinants surrounding a central core that contains the population of people of concern.[1] The inner or proximal ring refers to the immediate surrounding influences such as family, friends, home, neighbourhood, norms of behaviour, expectations and sense of opportunity for fulfilment. The second or intermediate ring refers to community or area influences such as schools, churches, work sites, the local economy and availability of jobs, natural resources, cleanliness of air, water and soil, effectiveness of local government and services, and a sense of meaning, participation and pride in those local affairs that affect the quality of living. The third or distal ring refers to macrosocial influences, including the characteristics of the economic and government system, national priorities, laws and regulations, business and employment standards, tax and monetary policies, public and private investment in the infrastructure of an effective society, the population's sense of security, fairness and justice, and the evenness or unevenness of the distribution of resources and opportunity.

Within a ring the various features are highly interactive. Moreover, the rings are porous, allowing features of one ring to interact with features in another ring. Sometimes features of an inner ring interact with and influence features of an outer ring, although the predominant direction of influence is probably inward.

Sorting out the specific contribution of each individual feature in the rings to the health of a population would be a major accomplishment. It would provide direction for policies and other interventions to improve health. That research objective has been elusive, probably for four reasons. First, all or most of the features within each ring and between the rings are interactive. It is not like a game of pool wherein a ball in the outer ring strikes a stationary ball in the intermediate ring which in turn collides with a resting ball in the inner ring which once activated falls into the core pocket. All of the balls are in motion most of the time and have wide spheres of simultaneous influence, so that the net direction and force of the final movement have multifactorial contributing influences of varying valence. The capacity of the currently most often applied multivariate analyses, including regression methodologies, are inadequate for the empirical needs of sound policy formulations to improve health. New hypotheses, and the development of new theories on the determinants of health, require the development of new methodologies.

Second, the mechanisms are unknown by which social characteristics are received/perceived by humans, processed into biological signals, and converted into disease. This sociobiological translation will be discussed in a subsequent part of this chapter.

Third, the interactions and effects among the four principal categories of health determinants have not been elucidated or even studied to any significant extent.

Fourth, the principal measures of health currently in use, morbidity and mortality, are crude and late stage indicators of health. Sickness absence from work as used by Marmot, disability-adjusted life years as introduced by Christopher Murray (World Bank 1993) and functional health and well-being measures developed by Ware, Bergner, Kaplan, Patrick and others will likely provide more sensitive and discerning indicators of health, but these measures have not yet been widely introduced into health surveillance databases (Stewart and Ware 1992; Patrick and Erickson 1993).

The socioecological conceptualization of health provides a framework for a research agenda. Progress on the research agenda is required before progress can begin on revision of specified societal characteristics to achieve improved population health.

SOCIOBIOLOGICAL TRANSLATION

A great new frontier for science is to gain an understanding of the mechanisms by which the social characteristics that are responsible for creating differential vulnerability to disease across different social groups are translated into biological processes that are forerunners of disease.

How do gradient variations in societal characteristics result in gradient variations in health? Returning to the visualized image of the socioecological framework, by what mechanisms is the health of the population in the central core affected by features of the social order in the concentric rings? What are the sensory mechanisms by which human beings receive messages regarding their social circumstances, convert the information into perceptions, and then translate the perceptions into biological signals that are antecedents to disease that may take decades before becoming clinically apparent? How is the process of sociobiological translation affected by other determinants of health, especially specific gene combinations? And if details of the entire process from social characteristics to early disease onset became known could interventions be crafted that would significantly improve health? The possibilities intrinsic to these questions generate the energy and inspiration for the International Centre for Health and Society and for others around the globe working on the social determinants of health.

There should be little doubt that a sociobiological translation takes place. The conceptualization of the process offered in the following paragraphs cannot be elevated to the status of theory or hypothesis. It is offered as a speculation to help move the research agenda forward (Figure 5.3).

Identity is a personality trait that informs an individual who he is and where he belongs within the social structure.[2] It provides a context for the development of social affiliations. Who am I similar to and with whom should I associate? It helps youth formulate their expectations of the future, both the possibilities and the limitations. Identity can place bounds

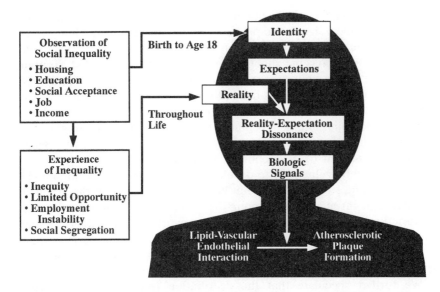

Figure 5.3 Sociobiological translation is proposed as a mechanism by which human beings receive messages about the social environment and convert the messages to biological signals that trigger the processes of disease development

on opportunities, or can provide an almost limitless expectation of the future.

Identity begins to take shape early in life, perhaps at age 2 or 3, and is completely formed by around age 18. Once formed it is one of the most stable and durable of all personality traits. Identity is constructed from observations and experiences, prominently early in life in the home with parents and siblings, later in school with other students and teachers, in the neighbourhood with friends, and in work circumstances. In the context of the socioecology of health, inequality in housing, education, social acceptance, job type and income are observed and experienced by a child at an early age. The effect of television viewing on identity formation must be significant.

Later in development (Figure 5.3), perhaps when youths start to make specific plans for their own future, but also throughout the life course, the stark reality of inequality becomes appreciated. Observations and experiences of inequity, limitations in opportunities for jobs, housing, and income, employment instability, and social segregation intersect with expectations derived from identity. When expectations and reality clash, we speculate, the chronic, persistent, inescapable dissonance between what a person would like to do or become and what seems accomplishable triggers biological signals that are antecedent of chronic disease development.

The disease becomes clinically manifest only after decades of persistent signals. The biological signals are probably subtle, but steady and long-term.

The transduction of the signal to specific disease may receive its specificity from polygenic inheritance. Within any one social stratum the reality–expectation dissonance and resulting biological signal may be of similar strength among the individuals within the stratum. Some individuals will have the multiple gene combination that permits a lipid-vascular endothelial interaction that is the forerunner of atherosclerosis. Others will have inherited a gene combination that permits the signal transduction related to development of cell-surface insulin insensitivity. Still others will be vulnerable to development of arteriolar smooth muscle constriction, and so forth. The point being made here is that the gradient prevalence of chronic disease among the distinctive social strata is related to variations in the strength of the dissonance that results from the identity–expectations–reality interplay. The specific chronic disease that develops in any one individual is determined by that individual's specific polygenic inheritance.

We further speculate that the distribution (prevalence) of specific predisposing polygenic combinations is roughly similar among the various social strata. The gradient of chronic disease prevalence among the strata is related largely to variations in the social characteristics within which the lives of the participants in each strata are played out.

Experiments are under way with high-school students in Boston to test the relationship between specific social strata identity and patterns of physiological and behavioural responsiveness. The work is being carried out under controlled conditions in the psychology laboratories of Professor Jerome Kagan at Harvard University. Social group identity is a principal variable. Maureen Menendez is conducting the actual experimental work in the laboratory. Dr Ben Amick, Dr Elizabeth Goodman, Professor Sol Levine, and Professor Alvin Tarlov are collaborating. The results from the experiments may provide some evidence, albeit general, on the veracity of the concept of sociobiological translation as presented in Figure 5.3. Funds for the research are provided by the Functional Outcomes Program of the Henry J. Kaiser Family Foundation at the New England Medical Center.

INTEGRATED POLICIES NEEDED

Social evolution has brought modern man into circumstances of living that often are contrary to attainment of good health. The socioecological framework for the production of health postulates that substantively improved population health will be achieved only if public, business, and personal policies, practices, and norms across a broad front are reshaped towards a society that intrinsically fosters better health. The following paragraphs stem from the perspective of an American commenting about America. The ideas might not be transferable to other societies.

The need to improve the health of the American people is evident in comparisons of the health of the twenty-five member nations of the Organization for Economic Co-operation and Development (OECD) as recently published (World Bank 1993). The United States ranks in the bottom tertile in life expectancy at birth, babies with low birth rate, peri-natal mortality, infant mortality, probability of dying by the age of 5, DPT immunization rates, communicable disease prevalence, non-communicable disease prevalence, injuries, and years of life lost per 100,000 population. The contribution of genetic differences to the low US ranking must be very small considering that the genetic stock of Americans has been derived relatively recently in genetic or evolutionary terms and predom-inantly from the nations with which the health comparisons are made. Some fraction of the explanation must be attributable to failure of the medical care system to serve the entire population. Although the US spends 50 per cent more for health care *per capita* than any other nation of the world, there is very little correlation between *per capita* health care expenditures and health among the OECD nations (World Bank 1993). Some fraction of the differences could be due to variations in habits of living such as tobacco use, alcohol abuse, nutritional differences, and lack of physical conditioning but these attributions must be small when compar-isons are limited to the industrialized or wealthy nations of the world.

Support for the idea that social characteristics comprise the predomi-nant explanation for Americans' low health status may be derived from some signs of social pathology which activate in harmful ways the concen-tric rings of the socioecological framework for the production of health. The signs include high rates of drug abuse, crime, violence, family dysfunc-tion, divorce, and homelessness, pervasive employment instability, lack of health insurance, and low rates of participation in voting processes for elected officials. It appears, then, that policies directed to achieving greater levels of social well-being within the socioecological framework are called for if improving overall population health is a goal.

Surely the United States should press on to adopt a universal health insurance system. Surely we should continue the efforts led by the federal government to reduce tobacco use, diminish the rates of alcoholism, prevent injuries, adopt more healthy diets, and improve physical fitness. More substantive and durable-over-time health improvement, however, will require macrosocial and community policies that adjust fundamental societal characteristics towards the more healthy.

Adjustments of the features in the three concentric rings will be made difficult by politics and conflicts with established values. Beyond those hurdles the challenge is complicated by interactions among most of the features in the rings and the bidirectionality of some interactions.

Unintended side effects also will be a problem. The following suggestions are general and intended to provide a simple framework for a modest beginning. General aims will be offered, rather than specific interventions or strategies. The general aims selected for attention are derivative of the empirical evidence cited in the chapter. The aims reflect the themes presented in this chapter. The general aims can be classified as *corrective* and *ameliorative*.

Corrective

Corrective aims are intended to make adjustments to broad features of the social structure that appear to be exerting harmful influences on population health. The aims are intended to: reduce material deprivation; invest in infrastructure; lower social gradients; and enhance security.

Reduction of the prevalence of deprivation of food, clothing, housing, medical care and the opportunity to earn these essentials should be a priority of the nation. Of the four corrective aims, this is the only one directed primarily towards one specific segment of the population, namely low-income and the poor. The nation has been working earnestly for sixty years or more on this subject and with some notable successes. The social security and Medicare systems are two of the most remarkable and enduring. The present structure of the welfare system, although expressing laudable American values, has demonstrated some long-term negative consequences that command fundamental revision. We should retain the values and objectives, revise the incentive structure, and strengthen the national commitment and priority. A clear national commitment in itself, apart from specific programme implementation to solve and prevent poverty, is likely to result in a small gain in the health of the poor.

Larger and sustained investment in the infrastructure for a healthy society is key to the health and well-being of the entire population, not just one segment. These investments should be in education, transport, communication, job creation and training, improved conditions of work, environmental cleanliness, and health care.

The degree of unevenness of the distribution of wealth, income and opportunity are robust correlates of population health in many societies (Wilkinson 1992). This unevenness is likely to be a major factor in the relatively poor health of Americans because the steepness of the gradient in wealth and income in the United States is at the extreme among the OECD nations (World Bank 1993). Corrective action to attain a less skewed distribution of income, wealth and opportunity is likely to be the most difficult of all the aims to achieve. Yet we and many other nations have had vast experience in various tax and income transfer policies. Lowering the gradient should be a core national priority. Social gradients are inevitable, but there must be a threshold of steepness beyond which serious health effects occur. Since steep social gradients seriously affect the health of all segments of the social hierarchy, gaining a national consensus to reduce the income gradient should attract a broad constituency if presented to the public as a health issue.

The sense of security and stability in America may have been reduced to levels that perturb physiological homeostasis to levels that over years or decades favour the development of disease. Twentieth-century changes in some key features of American life have increased the levels of insecurity in four domains: economic; physical; health care; and confidence in government.

Regarding economic insecurity, the social security 'trust' fund alternates from near bankruptcy at one moment to an attractive capital source to help balance the budget at another. Reduction of social security benefits has become a continual threat. Pension funds operated by employers appear unprotected when management declares that the pension need of employees is overfunded and the corporation elects to use the capital for other purposes. At the same time American patterns of ever-increasing levels of consumption have resulted in levels of savings that have become so low as to be inadequate to finance the nation's economic development needs or individual needs during periods of unemployment or retirement.

Another dimension of economic insecurity relates to employment instability. Over the past fifty years many changes have had a negative effect on a family's confidence that paid employment can provide for its needs uninterruptedly. Working women have increased the labour pool substantially in the past fifty years. Labour unions or alternative forms of protection of the interests of workers have been weakened. The skills of labour have not been sufficiently upgraded to meet the demands of a service and information-based economy. Large fractions of manufacturing jobs have been transferred overseas to lower-cost labour markets. The concept of the 'company town' has practically disappeared as corporate consolidation and locally invisible employment decision-making have been transferred to distal headquarters. US companies, to meet the challenges of global competition, have remarkably increased production efficiency and downsized work force numbers. Real wages of the middle class have declined. This has led to two or multiple job families, with some consequences for family function and stability. Monetary policy has evolved to an exclusive focus on inflation control that completely subverts the activation of monetary policies that could decrease unemployment rates.

Regarding physical insecurity the high rates of crime, violence, and homicide in the everyday American experience can be postulated to have a disease-promoting effect via sociobiological translation across the entire population, independent of the direct health affects on the victims themselves.

Insecurity with respect to health care is felt by a large fraction of the US population, including the poor, single-parent families, workers in low-paying or part-time jobs, the unemployed, and some who are employed in small businesses that do not provide health insurance. The elderly are chronically insecure relative to long-term care, and feel a heightened sense of insecurity currently because the US Congress is deliberating cuts in Medicare benefits.

Insecurity may also be generated by the general cynicism with which Americans view their elected officials and government processes. There is a pervasive lack of confidence in the ability of the government to solve many large problems that face the country. The public perceive political haggling on lowering the deficit. Many citizens feel that elected officials demonstrate lack of concern for the unemployed and programmes to lower unemployment. Collective security is endangered when the populace believes that the government cannot assure greater fairness in the distribution of resources, bring violence under control, provide universal health insurance, or provide leadership and direction for higher quality and well-being in American life.

Ameliorative

Ameliorative aims are designed to provide relief for those individuals who today have a health problem or an imminent threat to their health. Ameliorative strategies seldom aim for fundamental social remodelling. Ameliorative programme interventions in population health are the analogues of symptom treatment in medical practice, i.e. they are very useful but do not strike at the basic cause.

Lisbeth Schorr provided a useful analysis of a wide variety of programmes designed to break the cycle of disadvantage in children (Schorr 1988). Programmes that have worked successfully include more uniformly accessible prenatal care, early pre-school programmes, school-based health clinics, adolescent counselling and mentoring services, family support services, nutrition support and others. For adults, job training, job corps, substance abuse treatment programmes and many other programmes have been shown to be effective.

For maximum benefit to society both ameliorative and corrective interventions should be implemented in an integrated and comprehensive programme to provide both contemporary opportunities for improvement and longer-term corrections of macrosocial characteristics that influence population health in fundamental ways.

The four problems that have been selected for corrective action in this chapter include material deprivation, inadequate national investment in infrastructure, steep social gradients in education and income, and a pervasive sense of insecurity. All four of these problems can disturb the socioecology of health. All four can be expected to exert quantitative effects that differ across the socioeconomic gradient. The higher a group's position in the hierarchical structure the less exposure it will have to the problem, the greater the resources it has to withstand or cope with the problem and, with respect to sociobiological translation, the lower will be the level of dissonance between reality and expectations. In this formulation the health consequences across the social strata should follow a continuous gradient, affecting the health of all members of society but to different quantitative degrees depending on their social level. For this reason all Americans could share a common personal motivation for advocating programmes to improve the health of the nation. If the formulations of health determinants in this chapter are validated, and if the low health status of Americans relative to other economic counterpart nations becomes popular knowledge, national will on a broad popular base could develop that would make it politically feasible to take these and other corrective actions to improve health. Patient research, patient planning, patient politics, patient resources, and patient programming are required.

NOTES

1 The concentric ring concept was devised by Peter L. Berger for a sociological perspective of an individual's position in control by society (Berger 1963: 73–78). I am indebted to Kathryn Lasch, Ph.D., for calling my attention to the concentric ring idea.
2 The author was introduced to the concept of identity in psychology by Professor Jerome Kagan of Harvard University.

REFERENCES

Amick, B.C., III, Levine, S., Tarlov, A.R. and Walsh, D.C. (1995) *Society and Health*, New York and Oxford: Oxford University Press.

Amler, R.W. and Dull, H.B. (eds) (1987) *Closing the Gap: the Burden of Unnecessary Illness*, New York: Oxford University Press.

Berger, Peter L. (1963) *Invitation to Sociology: a Humanistic Perspective*, Garden City, New York: Anchor Books.

Bunker, J.P., Frazier, H.S. and Mosteller, F. (1994) Improving health: measuring effects of medical care, *Milbank Quarterly* 72: 225–258.

Carson, P.E., Flanagan, C.L., Ickes, C.E. and Alving, A.S. (1956) Enzymatic deficiency in primaquine-sensitive erythrocytes, *Science* 124: 484–485.

Copeland, N.G., Jenkins, N.A., Gilbert, D.J. (1993) Genetic linkage map of the mouse: current applications and future prospects, *Science* 262: 57–82.

Daedalus, Journal of the American Academy of Arts and Sciences (1994) *Health and Wealth*, Cambridge, Mass.: American Academy of Arts and Sciences.

Davies, J.L., Kawaguchi, Y., Bennett, S.T. and Todd, J.A. (1994) A genome-wide search for human Type I diabetes susceptibility genes, *Nature* 371: 130–136.

de Leeuw, E.J.J. (1989) *The Sane Revolution – Health Promotion: Backgrounds, Scope, Prospects*, Assen: Van Gorcum.

Doll, R. and Hill, A. (1964) Mortality in relation to smoking: ten years' observation of British doctors, *British Medical Journal* I: 1399–1410.

Dubos, R. (1962) *Torch of Life*, New York: Simon & Schuster.

Dwore, R.B. and Kreuter, M.W. (1980) Update: reinforcing the case for health promotion, *Family and Community Health* 2: 103–119.

Evans, R.G., Barer, M.L. and Marmor, T.R. (eds) (1994) *Why are some People Healthy and others not? The Determinants of Health of Populations*, Hawthorne, N.Y.: Aldine de Gruyter.

Honda Foundation (1993) *Proceedings, 11th Discoveries Symposium*, Prosperity, Health and Well-being, Toronto: Canadian Institute for Advanced Research.

Kawachi, I., Marshall, S. and Pearce, N. (1991) Social class inequalities in the decline of coronary heart disease among New Zealand men, 1975–1977 to 1985–1987, *International Journal of Epidemiology* 20: 393–398.

Kickbusch, I. (1986) Health promotion: A global perspective, *Canadian Journal of Public Health* 77: 321–326.

Lalonde, M. (1974) *A New Perspective on the Health of Canadians*, Ottawa: Government of Canada.

McCord, C. (1990) Excess mortality in Harlem, *New Engand Journal of Medicine* 322: 173–177.

McDermott, W. (1977) Evaluating the physician and his technology, *Daedalus* 106: 136.

McGraw, D. (1993) The plague: it's not just history, *Boston Globe*, 6 September 1993, p. 33.

McKeown, T. (1976) *The Modern Rise of Population*, London: Edward Arnold.

McKusick, V.A. (1994) *Mendelian Inheritance in Man: a Catalog of Human Genes and Genetic Disorders*, eleventh edition, Baltimore and London: Johns Hopkins University Press.

McNeill, W.H. (1976) *Plagues and Peoples*, Garden City, New York: Anchor Press/Doubleday.

Marmot, M.G. (1993) Social differentials in health within and between populations, in *Proceedings of the 11th Honda Foundation Discoveries Symposium, Prosperity, Health and Well-being*, Toronto: Canadian Institute for Advanced Research.

Marmot, M.G., Shipley, M.J. and Rose, G. (1984) Inequalities in death-specific explanations of a general pattern, *Lancet* 1: 1003–1006.

National Center for Health Statistics (1986) Vital Statistics Report, Final Mortality Statistics.

Nutbeam, D. (1986) Health promotion glossary, *Health Promotion* 1: 113–127.

Parsons, T. (1979) Definitions of health and illness in the light of American values and social structures, in E.G. Jaco (ed.) *Patients, Physicians, and Illness*, third edition, New York: Free Press.

Patrick, D.L. and Erickson, P. (1993) *Health Status and Health Policy: Quality of Life in Health Care Evaluation and Resource Allocation*, New York and Oxford: Oxford University Press.

Ryan, F. (1993) *The Forgotten Plague: How the Battle against Tuberculosis was Won – and Lost*, Boston, Mass.: Little Brown.

Sagan, L. (1987) *The Health of Nations*, New York: Basic Books.

Schorr, L.B. with Schorr, D. (1988) *Within our Reach: Breaking the Cycle of Poverty*, New York: Anchor Press/Doubleday.

Siegrist, H.E. (1941) *Medicine and Human Welfare*, New Haven: Yale University Press.

Stewart, A.L. and Ware, J.E., Jr (1992) *Measuring Functioning and Well-being: the Medical Outcomes Study Approach*, Durham, N.C. and London: Duke University Press.

Syme, S.L. and Berkman, L.F. (1976) Social class, susceptability and sickness, *American Journal of Epidemiology* 104: 1–8.

US Bureau of the Census (1993) *Statistical Abstract of the United States 1993*, Washington, D.C.: US Government Printing Office.

US Department of Health, Education and Welfare (1964) *Smoking and Health: Report of the Advisory Committee to the Surgeon General of the Public Health Service*, Washington, D.C.: US Government Printing Office.

US Department of Health, Education and Welfare (1979) *Healthy People: The Surgeon General's Report on Health Promotion and Disease Prevention*, Washington, D.C.: US Government Printing Office.

Verano, J.W. and Ubelaker, D.H. (eds) (1992) *Disease and Demography in the Americas*, Washington, D.C., and London: Smithsonian Institution Press.

Watson, J.D. (1968) *The Double Helix*, New York: Atheneum.

Weiss, H., Cowity, M.A., Wetterstrom, W., Gruchard, F., Senior, L., Meadow, R. and Curnow, A. (1993) The genesis and collapse of third millenium north Mesopotamian civilization, *Science* 261: 995–1004.

Wilford, J.N. (1994) *New York Times*, 31 May, p. C1.

Wilkinson, R.G. (1992) Income distribution and life expectancy, *British Medical Journal* 304: 165–168.

World Bank (1993) *World Development Report 1993, Investing in Health*, New York: Oxford University Press.

World Health Organization (1947) *World Health Organization Constitution*, Geneva: World Health Organization.

Chapter 6

What's been said and what's been hid

Population health, global consumption and the role of national health data systems

Clyde Hertzman

It is well known that differences in *per capita* income among the countries of the world correlate with differences in longevity between them. Early in this century the relationship was simple: life was longer in countries with higher *per capita* incomes, and it increased in a monotonic, if not wholly linear, fashion. But in recent decades the relationship between health and wealth has become more complex as rich nations have grown richer.

By 1970 the world's richest nations had reached unprecedented levels of national wealth and a distinct 'flat of the curve' had begun to emerge, such that increasing increments of income among those countries with *per capita* incomes greater than US $10,000 (in 1991 dollars) were no longer associated with further increases in life expectancy. By 1990 all of the countries of the Organization of Economic Co-operation and Development, the world's wealthiest nations, found themselves on this 'flat of the curve' (World Bank 1993: 34). At the same time, the traditional monotonic relationship between health and wealth persisted among the world's poorer countries – a pattern referred to here as the 'steep incline,' to distinguish it from the 'flat of the curve'.

There are many interpretations of these relationships, but one of the simplest is that the material factors which limit health status can be marginalized when national income reaches a certain level. This interpretation is powerful because it gives a common perspective to different elements of the international development community which have very different understandings of how to create economic growth, based upon a common observation that economic growth, traditionally defined, is a laudable objective regardless of how it is achieved. From the standpoint of economic development and health, reaching the flat of the curve means matching the world's 'most advanced' societies in a way which is essentially benign. The underlying message is that the relationship between the healthy and wealthy countries and the poor and unhealthy countries ought to be one of imitation of the former by the latter.

This view is not going unchallenged because it is vulnerable to new insights emerging from the worldwide movement for sustainable development

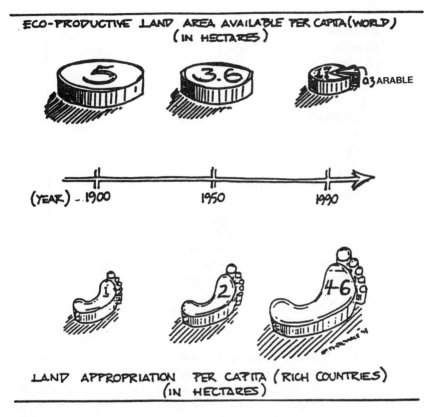

ECO-PRODUCTIVE LAND AREA AVAILABLE PER CAPITA (WORLD)
(IN HECTARES)

5

3.6

.03 ARABLE

(YEAR) - 1900   1950   1990

1   2   4-6

LAND APPROPRIATION PER CAPITA (RICH COUNTRIES)
(IN HECTARES)

Figure 6.1 Availability and use of ecoproductive land. (Boothroyd *et al.* 1994:
116)

about how rich and poor nations appropriate global resources. One such
insight is found in the calculation of the 'ecological footprint', which is
a measure of the area of the Earth's surface appropriated for its use by a
given population in a given year (Boothroyd *et al.* 1994: 114).

When land appropriated for energy, agriculture, and forest products is
added to the area of the built environment, it turns out that as the rich
nations grew richer their levels of consumption of ecologically productive
land grew rapidly. Between 1950 and 1990 the appropriation of ecologically productive land by the world's richest countries increased from
approximately 2 ha to 4–6 ha *per capita*. Over the same time period the
global supply of ecoproductive land declined from approximately 3.6 ha to
1.7 ha *per capita* (Figure 6.1), primarily as a result of population growth.
In other words, over the last forty-five years the fraction of the world's ecoproductive resources appropriated by the richest countries has, for the first

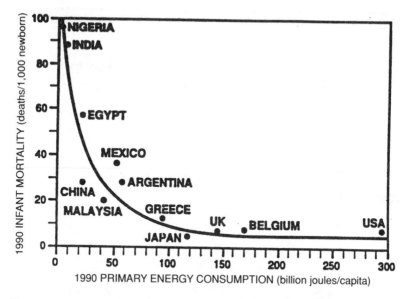

Figure 6.2 Infant mortality and energy consumption around the world. (Smil 1993: 127)

time in history, exceeded a level that everyone can share. The richest are leaving the world's poorest nations with little room to increase consumption, at least of those goods and services which derive from ecologically productive land. In order to allow the rest of the world to reach the mean consumption levels of the world's richest countries, the planet Earth would need to appropriate at least two more planets'-worth of ecoproductive land. Despite the marginal efficiencies which could be achieved through technological innovation, this is clearly an impossible dream.

If this perspective is valid, the relationship between the health and the wealth of nations takes on a new character. The benign and abstract construct of *per capita* income can be replaced in the international comparisons by more hard-edged measures of appropriation of ecologically productive land. This has been tried with respect to energy consumption, and demonstrates that, for international comparisons of both infant mortality and life expectancy, the shape of the curve is the same as it is for national income (Smil 1993: 127–128). Up to a certain level of energy consumption the health outcome improves rapidly, but, once again, there is a flat of the curve wherein the vast differences in energy consumption among the world's richest countries do not correlate with differences in either measure. For instance, Figure 6.2 shows no improvements in national infant mortality rates across a range of energy consumption of 120 billion J to 300 billion J *per capita*.

When this observation is considered alongside the evidence of scarcity of global resources, the relationship between countries on the steep incline and those on the flat of the curve is transformed. The flat of the curve no longer seems benign, but begins to look as though it exists at the expense of the steep incline. This, in turn, transforms the definition of success in national development and health. The most successful group of countries turn out to be those which maximize their health status while limiting increases in consumption. From the standpoint of global citizenship, these are the countries found at the left end of the flat of the curve, where the world's best health status coexists with the minimum necessary levels of consumption. Those countries found further to the right are increasingly inefficient producers of health which also, through competition for global resources, may well be limiting the health chances of the countries on the steep incline.

If success were measured by the ratio of life years produced to ecoproductive land consumed, the world's healthiest country is not on the flat of the curve at all. It is Costa Rica. By 1991 that country delivered a life expectancy of 76 years to its citizens, compared with an average of 77 years for the world's twenty-two richest countries. It did this on a national income of $1,850 *per capita*, compared with an average of $21,050 for the twenty-two richest nations. (From here on, national income levels will be used as a surrogate measure of the size of their ecological footprint. This is because we have insufficient data to measure it in any other way. Although income and consumption are not equivalent, the consuming capacity of poor societies is, generally, much lower than that of the rich, so that broad comparisons between rich and poor will retain their validity.) As in the richest nations, malnutrition among the Costa Rican population under 5 years of age is reported by international sources to be zero (World Bank 1993: 293). Costa Rica is not the only poor low-consuming society with world-class longevity, and recognition of this group of societies is not new. In general, they are characterized by a high level of literacy and independence among the female population and high levels of spending on education and welfare compared with other countries in their income bracket (Caldwell 1986).

The characteristics of poor but healthy societies may be useful to other developing countries striving to make the best use of scarce resources, but this knowledge provides little help to wealthy societies which, over time, will be pressured to reduce their current appropriation of global ecoproductive resources to make room for others. What will happen if the developing world decides that the products of ecoproductive land which are currently being exported to the developed world for cash ought to stay where they are? This circumstance raises an important question: can wealthy societies maintain their health status while consuming less of the world's ecologically productive resources? The question is fundamentally about pathways, not endpoints. The endpoints were already known. The flat of the curve, and the existence of countries like Costa Rica, already demonstrate that lower levels of consumption are compatible with high levels of health status. What is still at issue is this: can the highest-consuming societies successfully 'become more like Costa Rica', in terms of consumption patterns, without undermining social stability and sharply increasing inequality in the socioeconomic domain?

CAN WE LIVE AS WELL ON LESS?

A very indirect answer to the question may be extracted under duress from studies of the relationship between economic growth, income equity, and gains in life expectancy in wealthy societies (Wilkinson 1992a, b) and from studies comparing the magnitude of socioeconomic gradients in mortality between a wealthy country with high mortality (Britain), and another with low mortality (Sweden) (Vagero and Lundberg 1989). Wilkinson's work suggests that equality of income distribution in wealthy societies is a predictor of relatively high life expectancy among them. Preservation of relative equality over time in the face of economic pressures towards increasing income inequality is a positive predictor of the rate of increase in life expectancy. On the other hand, differing rates of economic growth *per se* over the past twenty years have not been predictive of growth rates in life expectancy in wealthy countries. Vagero's work suggests that societies which can keep the magnitude of the socioeconomic gradient in life expectancy to a minimum can maintain better health status for each social class than societies with large socioeconomic gradients in life expectancy.

An optimist may see in these findings evidence to promote the view that wealthy societies can maintain or improve their health status irrespective of income level (and, presumably, level of consumption) by addressing equity issues. But that would be a premature conclusion. Even those who detest the researcher's plea for ever more data would have to agree that an adequate answer requires a much more careful and detailed understanding of the determinants of health in whole societies than has been achieved so far.

Consider, for example, some rough calculations which have been made of the size of the ecological footprint of different classes of citizens in Canada (still, at this writing, a wealthy society). It turns out that the rich leave a much larger footprint than the poor. Members of professional couples with two cars and no children leave a footprint which is approximately three times as large as the members of an average-income Canadian family, and four times as large as members of a family living on social assistance. Indeed, consumption among those on social assistance approaches a level which is globally sustainable.

Unfortunately, the health status of such families is nowhere near as good as that of those who consume more. The life expectancy gradient in Canada across quintiles of family income is approximately six years for men and two years for women (Wilkins *et al.* 1989: 137), but increases to approximately ten years for both sexes when disability-free life years are considered (Wilkins 1992). Although it may be unlikely that these differences are tied to the material advantages of consumption *per se*, differences in consumption patterns are nevertheless an integral part of social class differences in wealthy societies. In the absence of further evidence, one would have to seriously consider the prospect that making the wealthy consume at the same level as those who are already at global sustainability would drive the health status of the population down.

CENTRAL AND EASTERN EUROPE: A CAUTIONARY TALE

Are there natural experiments available to us which might be informative about the pitfalls of planned reductions in consumption across whole societies? It is true that acute reductions in consumption during famine are a threat to life and limb, but no one would suggest that episodes of starvation share essential similarities to the problem at hand. More relevant are the experiences of middle-income societies where purchasing power has been sharply curtailed but where outright starvation has not resulted.

The best documented of these is the experience of central and eastern Europe since 1989. Within three years of the sudden political and economic changes of that year, real wages in every country of the former Warsaw Pact had fallen significantly: between 15 per cent and 35 per cent (UNICEF 1993: 78). These changes were accompanied by increases in the proportion of household income being spent on food in some countries in the region, especially Russia, Ukraine, Bulgaria, and Romania. Average *per capita* consumption of meat, fish, and dairy products declined in these countries, with an accompanying decline in the size of the ecological footprint. At the same time there was marked disruption of the social environment, as demonstrated by 19–35 per cent declines in crude marriage rates and more modest reductions in pre-primary school enrolment. But the most significant change was that, by 1993, death rates had risen dramatically in all of the former Warsaw Pact countries except Hungary (UNICEF 1993: 21). This is a startling finding, which could not have been predicted by those who believe that socioeconomic influences on health status are essentially cohort effects with decades-long latent periods, or by those who believe that individual choices regarding smoking and fatty diet have been the principal determinants of east–west differences in health status across Europe.

The abrupt increase in mortality raises yet another question: was increased mortality an inevitable concomitant of sharp declines in disposable income, or could the outcome have been buffered somehow? In particular, was the disruption of the social environment a significant intermediate step? So far only the dilemmas have compounded and not the evidence. A different approach is needed.

AN ANIMAL MODEL OF THE DETERMINANTS OF HEALTH IN WHOLE SOCIETIES

Perhaps it would be better to start with a preliminary model of the determinants of health in whole societies and try to improve upon it. At the very least it would create a framework for organizing the vast and fragmented base of literature which already exists. Over time it would provide a starting point for new investigations, which, through testing the underlying assumptions of the model, would improve its validity.

There are significant barriers to creating a comprehensive model of the determinants of health in whole populations. Human societies are complex, and the study of the determinants of health is limited by money, time, and the supply of useful natural experiments. But these limitations do not apply as much to studies of certain other primate populations which, nevertheless, show remarkable similarities to humans. Most useful among these are the studies of free-ranging baboon populations of the Serengeti (Sapolsky 1993). Their usefulness derives from the fact that the investigators were able to juxtapose measurements of the well-being of individual baboons with a detailed understanding of their individual identities, and the social dynamics and living conditions of the entire baboon community 'in the wild'.

The term 'in the wild' suggests that, somehow, Sapolsky's investigations avoided the Heisenberg uncertainty principle, and did not change the community through the process of investigation. This assumption can be questioned, both in terms of the studies' manipulation of the food supply and in terms of the role of blood collection in influencing the response to stress that it was meant to detect. Still, they are as close to natural observations as any human longitudinal study. There is no point here in letting the best be the enemy of the good; better, instead, to use Sapolsky's studies as a hypothesis base for the determinants of health in human societies.

(The outcome measure of interest was resting serum cortisol. There is an extensive rationale for the claim that it serves as both a measure of perceived chronic stress and a predictor of future well-being and survival. Low resting serum cortisols correlate with low cortisol levels during periods of low acute stress, and short, sharp bursts of cortisol secretion in relation to acute stress. High resting cortisol levels correlate with high cortisol levels during periods of low acute stress, and prolonged increases during periods of acute stress. Low resting cortisol is the favourable pattern from the standpoint of perception of stress, well-being, and survival.)

The model of the determinants of well-being in baboon society which emerges from these studies is adopted here as a preliminary model of the determinants of health in human societies. It has four elements, which are as follows:

1   *Rank.* When all other factors are held constant, higher rank in the baboon community means lower serum cortisols (i.e. greater well-being). Among the male population, rank tends to be unstable, and subject to constant attempts by young baboons or outsiders to rise in the hierarchy. Among female populations rank is more stable. It is taught by mother to daughter and follows orderly changes throughout the life cycle.

2   *Social stability and its enforcement.* When baboon societies are stable those in dominant positions have higher levels of well-being than they do during periods of instability. Instability usually comes in the form of a challenge to the dominance hierarchy by young males 'on the way up' or outsiders trying to establish themselves in the troop. When stability is imposed by high levels of violence and coercion the non-dominant baboons have lower levels of well-being than when it is maintained with low levels of violence and coercion.

3   *The experience of rank, stability, and enforcement.* When social instability occurs, some non-dominant baboons will actually experience increases in well-being. This is because their relations with those higher in the hierarchy are traditionally stressful. These relationships may be interrupted by the preoccupations the more dominant baboons have with each other during fights for supremacy. Other low-ranked baboons, however, will do worse if they become the victims of displaced aggression from the losers in the fight for social dominance.

4   *Personality and coping styles.* Individual characteristics matter, too. The ability to distinguish seriously threatening situations from ruses, to distinguish winning a fight from losing it, to relieve stress by displacing aggression, and to develop friendships and strategic alliances, all lead to increased well-being. Each of these characteristics has a component which is related to circumstances of upbringing and mentorship.

With one eye on this primate model, and the other on people, it is possible to identify the analogous elements of human society and deem them to be candidates for the principal determinants of health and well-being. It also becomes easier than it was, in the absence of the primate model, to create a preliminary model of the relationships between these elements. For instance, in contrast to the models of the determinants of

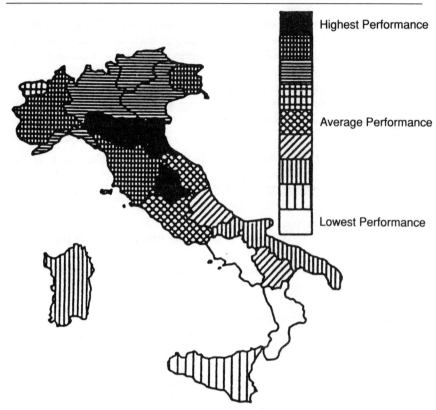

Figure 6.3 Institutional performance in the Italian regions, 1978–85. (Putnam *et al.* 1993: 84)

health which underlie most of our existing research in human societies, the primate model suggests that *all* levels of societal aggregation need to be considered simultaneously in research, in order to fully explain inequalities in health and well-being. Rank and social stability are, fundamentally, characteristics of whole societies, although they may be encrypted either in society as a whole (social stability) or in the individual (rank). Rank, stability, and enforcement are experienced, to a greater degree at the individual and local level. Personality and coping styles are primarily individual, but have a social network aspect. Analogous human models would have to take simultaneous account of individuals, voluntary social networks, and local and national communities. Moreover, each relevant factor has both a cross-sectional and a longitudinal dimension to it, so that both time frames would need to be included, too.

At the highest level of aggregation, it does not take a great deal of imagination to see the relationship with various aspects of human society. For instance, the role of rank in baboon societies translates into the role of

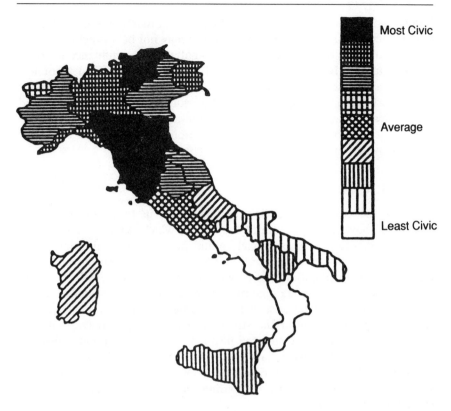

Figure 6.4 The civic community in the Italian regions. (Putnam *et al.* 1993: 97)

socioeconomic status as a determinant of health in human societies. After all, social class gradients in health status closely parallel the findings of rank and well-being in baboon societies. The individual experience of rank, stability, and enforcement translates into the day-to-day stresses of good times (e.g. work-life/home-life conflicts) and bad times (e.g. loss of control at work, lay-offs, long-term unemployment). Personality and coping styles need little translation, and speak to the role of social support, the value of good beginnings, the role of personality styles (e.g. type A and type B personalities), and coping skills in dealing with an increasingly complex and difficult world.

Not all of the analogies between the determinants of health in baboon society and human society are so unforced. For instance, it is possible to see a parallel between the pattern of increased well-being in baboon communities with low levels of violence and coercion, and the findings, described earlier, which show that relative income equality (Wilkinson 1992a, b) and shallow social class gradients in health (Vagero and

Lundberg 1989) are determinants of longevity in human societies. But, in reality, income and health gradients may or may not be a function of how society maintains order. A more careful analysis of the influence of social stability and methods of enforcing it would have to take into account a wider array of factors, including government programmes (i.e. the social safety net), historical/cultural factors (i.e. social capital formation), and the political/economic situation (e.g. the political transformation of central and eastern Europe, the rise of ethnic nationalism, recession, or abrupt changes in the terms of trade).

SOCIAL CAPITAL

Consider the concept of social capital, which, in terms of the model described above, is a measure of the way in which stable societies function on a day-to-day basis. Social capital has been formally defined as those 'features of social organization, such as networks, norms, and trust, that facilitate coordination and cooperation for mutual benefit' (Putnam 1993: 35–36). From the standpoint of population health, social capital is an attractive concept because it has potential to serve as a measure of society's capacity to buffer the stressors of modern life. It is feasible to use because it has been translated into a series of measurable constructs which are calculable using data routinely available at the regional and national level in many countries. Furthermore, its use is illustrated in a series of worked examples comparing northern with southern Italy (Putnam *et al.* 1993).

The main objective of this work was to understand why regional government, introduced to Italy in 1970, seemed to function much better in the north of Italy than in the south. To this end, measurable constructs were defined which, collectively, represent social capital. The most useful of these are institutional performance and civic community. Institutional performance is defined as how responsive representative government is to its constituents and its efficiency in conducting the public's business. In practice, it is composed of measures of the policy process and internal operations, the content of policy decisions, and the capacity to carry out policy. Civic communities are defined as those which value solidarity, civic participation, and integrity; and where social and political networks are organized horizontally, not hierarchically (Putnam 1993: 36). It is composed of measures of civic engagement, political equality, social structures of co-operation, and, finally, qualities of solidarity, trust, and tolerance.

Figures 6.3 and 6.4 show how the regions of Italy score on the indexes of institutional performance and civic community. They show that the northern regions such as Tuscany and Lombardy, which have a thousand-year tradition of civic society, score higher than the southern regions. The

Table 6.1 Proportion of regional variation in mortality explained (r^2) by social capital formation in Italy

Mortality variable	Life expectancy (1986–90)	Infant mortality (1987)	Infant mortality (1951)	% of mortality 1–14 (1991)	% of mortality 15–24 (1991)	% of male mortality 45–64 (1991)
Institutional performance	0.07	0.45**	0.56***	0.49**	0.15	0.01
Civic community	0.11	0.49**	0.67***	0.36*	0.11	0.02

Notes: *p < 0.01, **p < 0.005, ***p < 0.0005.

Source: Putnam *et al.* (1993); Istituto Nazionale di Statistica (1994).

southern regions have a much weaker civic tradition but a stronger tradition of family loyalty, which has served as a sanctuary against forces of political and economic control which were seen as being alien, hostile, and threatening.

Table 6.1 summarizes available data on mortality and social capital formation in Italy. For each mortality variable, it presents the proportion of the variation in rates across the regions of Italy which is 'explained' by the indices of civic community and institutional performance. The table shows that there is a strong association between increasing social capital formation and decreasing infant mortality rates, but no association with overall life expectancy. This association is stronger for infant mortality from the past (1951) than for infant mortality from the present (1987). Child mortality (ages 1–14), as a proportion of total mortality, is also lower in regions with higher levels of social capital formation. At older ages the effect disappears. In particular, premature male mortality in mid-life (age 45–64) is not associated with social capital formation.

These outcomes are only partially consistent with what might be expected by analogy with the baboon model. This may be because the construct of social capital, whatever the analogy, is irrelevant to human health. More likely, it is because the attributes tapped by measures of social capital are only a small part of the underlying multilevel process of interest. In other words, the full importance of social capital may only be adequately tested when its effects are considered simultaneously with other levels of social and temporal aggregation, as has been suggested above. Social capital should not be considered in isolation from the other characteristics of human society raised by the baboon model.

For instance, it may be that the protective effects of greater social capital in northern Italy are matched in later life by the healthful effects of the Mediterranean diet in the south. But any evaluation of this prospect

Table 6.2 Explanatory power of smoking, high blood pressure and high cholesterol (r^2) in the MONICA study (%)

Type of mortality	Men	Women
Ischaemic heart disease	23*	14*
All-causes	40	34

Note: *95% confidence intervals include 0.0.

Source: World Health Organization MONICA Project (1994).

would quickly run into a large obstacle: the lack of data which simultaneously account for individual habits and social capital. To be sure, sample surveys and international comparison studies exist for the relevant factors, but they have not been studied together, using multilevel models as would be appropriate.

Consider the second half of the equation: Mediterranean diet and other health behaviours. The World Health Organization's MONICA study evaluated the power of smoking, high blood pressure, and high cholesterol to explain international differences in ischaemic heart disease and all-cause mortality. The results were disappointing. Table 6.2 shows that the explanatory power of these three risk factors is weaker in relation to ischaemic heart disease mortality than all-cause mortality (WHO 1994: 513). These data, ironically, reduce the validity of both associations, since on biological grounds the respective strengths of association should be reversed. But they do not negate the role of smoking, high blood pressure, or cholesterol as health risks in any given community. They simply challenge the notion that individual health behaviours within a society, by themselves, can explain differences in health status between societies. This is not a surprising finding on the basis of the baboon model. The simplest explanation of the reversal is that reductions in smoking, high blood pressure, and cholesterol levels are characteristic of societies which are able to collectively mobilize the energy to address health issues. This 'ability to mobilize' would be the real protective factor, which, of course, sounds suspiciously like a construct similar to social capital.

SUMMING UP

This chapter was motivated by the question 'Can wealthy societies maintain their health status while consuming less of the world's ecologically productive resources?' In reality, it is a litmus test of the current state of understanding of the determinants of population health. Although it is only one of many litmus tests that could have been posed, it is attractive because it is realistic; it raises a challenge wealthy societies may actually face in the not-too-distant future.

The results of the litmus test are disappointing. They reveal the need for a more coherent model of the determinants of health than currently exists. The search for a preliminary model initially led away from the original question, into the realm of studies of the well-being of primates in the wild. Despite this, the model which emerged looked surprisingly like an organized collection of variables which have already been studied in large human populations, but, unfortunately, not simultaneously. This is a helpful observation, because it leads to a feasible set of priorities for the next generation of national health data gathering.

Specifically, this inquiry supports the development of a network of data systems and surveys that have a longitudinal as well as a serial cross-sectional capability, and that can simultaneously account for individual, local, regional, and national characteristics. Commonly measured constructs, such as social networks and social class, need to be supplemented by other dimensions suggested by the baboon model, such as cognitive development and competence, and, also, measures of the buffering capacity of society. The social capital construct is a good start for this, but may need some refinement by the population health community before it will be suitable. Measures of work-life versus home-life conflicts and work strain need to be incorporated into more general population samples than they have been so far. Finally, new national health data systems will need to be readily comparable among the wealthy societies if international comparison studies of the future are going to answer complex questions in population health like those posed here.

REFERENCES

Boothroyd, P., Green, L., Hertzman, C., Lynam, J., Manson-Singer, S., McIntosh, J., Rees, B., Wackernagel, M. and Woolard, R. (1994) Tools for sustainability: iteration and implementation, in C. Cordia and R. Simpson (eds) *The Ecological Public Health*, Griffith University, Nathan, Australia: Institute of Applied Environmental Health.

Caldwell, J.C. (1986) Routes to low mortality in poor countries, *Population and Development Review* 12: 171–220.

Instituto Nazionale di Statistica (1994) Selected tables of mortality, Rome, Italy.

Putnam, R.D. (1993) The prosperous community: social capital and public life, *American Prospect* 13: 35–42.

Putnam, R.D., Leonardi, R. and Nanetti, R.Y. (1993) *Making Democracy Work: Civic Traditions in Modern Italy*, Princeton: Princeton University Press.

Sapolsky, R.M. (1993) Endocrinology al fresco: psychoendocrine studies of wild baboons, *Recent Progress in Hormone Research* 48: 437–468.

Smil, V. (1993) *Global Ecology: Environmental Change and Social Flexibility*, New York: Routledge.

UNICEF (1993) *Central and Eastern Europe in Transition: Public Policy and Social Conditions*, Regional Monitoring Report No. 1, Florence: International Child Development Centre.

Vagero, D. and Lundberg, O. (1989) Health inequalities in Britain and Sweden, *Lancet* 2: 35–36.

Wilkins, R. (1992) Personal communication.

Wilkins, R., Adams, O. and Brancker, A. (1989) Changes in mortality by income in urban Canada from 1971 to 1986, *Health Reports* 1(2): 137–174.

Wilkinson, R.G. (1992a) Income distribution and life expectancy, *British Medical Journal* 304: 165–168.

Wilkinson, R.G. (1992b) National mortality rates: the impact of inequality, *American Journal of Public Health* 82(8): 1082–1084.

World Bank (1993) *World Development Report. Investing in Health: World Development Indicators*, New York: Oxford University Press.

World Health Organization MONICA Project (1994) Ecological analysis of the association between mortality and major risk factors of cardiovascular disease, *International Journal of Epidemiology* 23(3): 505–516.

Chapter 7

How can secular improvements in life expectancy be explained?

Richard Wilkinson

Perhaps the most important challenge facing those interested in population health is our ignorance of why life expectancy continues to rise in most countries. This chapter starts with a discussion of why it is difficult to understand what is driving the long-term rise in life expectancy. After discussing the nature and weakness of the relationship with economic growth in the developed world, an attempt is made to identify the kinds of factors which may explain why similar levels of real income are associated with ever higher levels of life expectancy as time goes by.

Most of the world continues to enjoy a long-term decline in death rates which adds several years to life expectancy with every decade that passes. Yet, despite the overwhelming importance of this process, its causes are largely unknown. As often as not, discussion of the subject still starts from McKeown and Lowe's (1974) analysis of the decline in mortality in Britain from the late nineteenth century to the middle of the twentieth. This is a poor basis to start a discussion of present trends because in the developed world the decline in mortality is no longer governed, as it was, by the decline in childhood infections. The relevance of McKeown's thesis to the Third World today is also limited by the fact that the potential contribution of medicine in the fight against infections was much smaller before the middle of the twentieth century than it has been since. For what it is worth, McKeown and Lowe's historical analysis of mortality trends in Britain showed that much of the decline in infections came too early to be attributed to medical advances – that is to say, before effective treatment or immunization was usually available. They also pointed out that most of the decline in mortality was from airborne infections and so could not be attributed to cleaner water supplies or to the building of sewers. Having denied the primary role to medical care or to public health measures, McKeown and Lowe fell back on the increasing standard of living as the only remaining possibility. However, they gave no direct empirical evidence of a relationship between rising living standards and falling mortality rates.

More recently attempts have been made to measure the relationship between rising gross national product *per capita* and increasing life

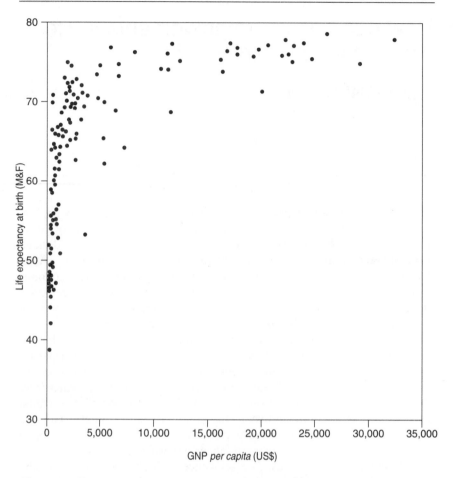

Figure 7.1 The changing relationship between GNP *per capita* and life expectancy

Note: Dots represent individual countries with corresponding GNP

expectancy. On the basis of cross-sectional and time trend analysis, Preston (1976) concluded that no more than 10 per cent of the rise in life expectancy is associated with increases in gross national product *per capita* (GNPpc). This is particularly surprising because even the contributions which come from the application of modern medical advances and preventive knowledge are likely to be at least loosely related to economic growth. However, looking at the basic data almost twenty years later produces much the same picture.

The shape of the cross-sectional relationship between GNPpc and life expectancy is well known (Figure 7.1). Life expectancy rises steeply as

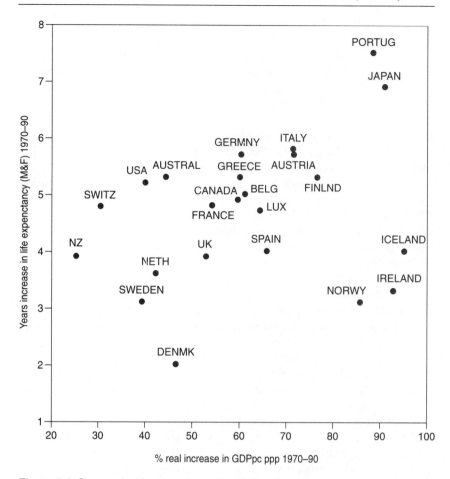

Figure 7.2 Change in life expectancy in relation to percentage change in real GDP *per capita*, 1970–90, at purchasing power parities; *r* = 0.30 (n.s.)

one moves from the poorer to the less poor developing nations. When one reaches countries with the higher living standards of the developed world, the increase in life expectancy begins to level out until, among the richest nations, it appears that even big differences in GNPpc make little or no difference to life expectancy: the curve becomes almost completely flat. On the basis of this cross-sectional picture one is tempted to say that after nations have reached a certain threshold level of income further increases in living standards make no substantial difference to life expectancy. However, putting exactly the same data for GNPpc on a log. scale suggests that there remains a rough relationship among both rich and poor nations between any proportional increase (say a doubling) of GNPpc and a given absolute increase in life expectancy. The flattening we saw in Figure 7.1 simply reflects the fact that in a country which is perhaps twenty times as rich as another it takes twenty times the absolute increase in its standard of living (and in its resource consumption) to double national income as it does to double the income of the poorer country – all for the same number of additional years' life expectancy.

Yet if we look at the relationship between GNPpc and changes in life expectancy over time the evidence of a relationship becomes even more tenuous. The size of the absolute increase in average incomes (as measured by a change in GNPpc) over the twenty-year period 1970–90 is quite unrelated to concurrent increases in life expectancy. Even when the changes in life expectancy are expressed as percentage increases (analogous to the effect of using the log. scale earlier), the relationship fails to reach statistical significance. In case the problem is related to the inaccuracy of the measurement of GNPpc, or the arbitrary nature of the exchange rates used to convert national currencies, we can look just at the rich market economies belonging to the OECD (see Figure 7.2). For these countries the measurement is probably better than in poorer countries where a smaller part of life is monetized. In addition, it is possible to convert the currencies using 'purchasing power parities' which are calculated to reflect the cost of a standard basket of goods in different countries. Even here the correlation coefficient which measures the strength of the relationship between percentage increases in GNPpc and life expectancy is only 0.3 and fails to reach statistical significance. It suggests (much as Preston did) that no more than 10 per cent of the increase in life expectancy is associated with increases in average incomes.

What happens is that life expectancy improves not by countries moving out along a given curve relating life expectancy to GNPpc, but by their moving on to a curve which is higher and to the left of the earlier one (Figure 7.3). This process of the curve moving upwards has been going on throughout the twentieth century. In effect, a given standard of living buys (or is associated with) better and better life expectancy as time goes by. If money has anything to do with it, the evidence suggests that income is becoming increasingly effective over time in purchasing health. If 10 per cent of the improvement in mortality is directly associated with improvements in income, then 90 per cent is associated with something which improves the gearing between any given income level and health. The search is then for one or more income gearing factors which have become increasingly powerful during the course of this century. Let us call this factor (or collection of factors) factor x.

The difficulty of accepting that there is such a weak relationship between economic growth and the simultaneous improvements in health is that almost all the processes that one might suggest are driving the health improvements are in an important sense supported, enabled, paid for, or produced by the rise in incomes which economic growth brings.

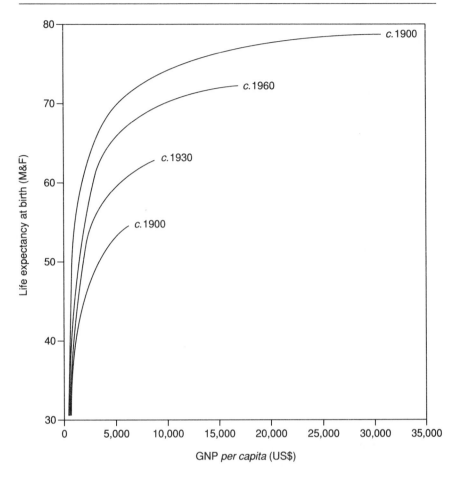

Figure 7.3 The changing gearing of GNP *per capita* to life expectancy. (After World Bank 1993)

Even if the long-term decline in mortality turned out to be due to factors such as education or medical care, to provide high standards across a population is beyond the means of poor countries: higher standards of provision are made possible by economic growth. Not only that, but it seems common sense to assume that some aspects of the higher living standards achieved through economic growth will benefit health. To try to explain the 'unexplained' 90 per cent of the rise in life expectancy by reference to environmental factors which are not fundamentally a product of economic growth seems an impossible task. Indeed, the fact that the *shape* of the relationship between life expectancy and GNPpc remains the same over time suggests that there are powerful links between them somewhere – even if health does improve more by moving on to new, higher, curves than by moving out along an existing curve (Figure 7.3). Hence my assertion that what we are looking for is an income gearing factor, not measured by monetary measures of real income, but which is nevertheless likely to be a product of economic growth.

Before going further let us first get the issue of medical care out of the way. Although there is a widespread assumption that standards of health in the developed world are largely a product of medical care, such a view is not supported by the evidence. Both within and between developed countries there is no clear relationship between medical provision – such as doctors per head or expenditure – and mortality rates. Although deaths from diseases which are regarded as 'amenable' to medical treatment are falling faster than deaths from all other causes, deaths from amenable causes account for only a small proportion of all deaths. In addition, variations in death rates from such causes are related more closely to social and economic factors than to variations in the provision of medical care (Mackenbach *et al.* 1990). The explanation for this situation is not that medical treatment is ineffective but that its benefits are completely overshadowed by the power of environmental factors. More important than small improvements in survival from cancers or cardiovascular conditions are the factors which determine the *incidence* of these conditions among the population. Even if medicine doubled the survival time of people with these conditions (which would be a very major achievement), the impact of that on life expectancy would be dwarfed by a doubling – or halving – of the incidence of the same conditions.

Nor is an expansion of healthy life styles the main cause of the long-term decline in mortality. Mortality has declined in countries and in periods when smoking was increasing, and the decline extends to diseases where we know of little or no effective preventive action which individuals can take. Our present knowledge of behavioural risk factors does little to explain international variations or trends in health.

Let us return, then, to factor x. One of the obstacles to understanding the impact of economic growth is the way it is measured. That we tend to talk about economic growth rather than economic development hints at the problem. In reality economic development is a complex process of qualitative change which transforms societies of largely independent agricultural producers into largely interdependent urban societies using sophisticated mechanical, chemical and electronic technologies to produce goods and services. That is to say, it is fundamentally a process of qualitative change. Yet its measurement – in terms of growth rates – depends on subsuming these qualitative changes in an index of quantitative change. From the point of view of indices of economic growth, it is as if people in the developed industrial societies simply had more of the same set of things that people in pre-industrial societies have.

It may be thought that the role of qualitative change is important only in the long term. However, if in some sense qualitative change is the weightier component of change in the long term, then on average this will also be true within any short term. Indeed, one of the best ways of showing the importance of qualitative change is in understanding the poor predictive power of input–output analysis over periods as short as five years. The basis of input–output analysis is a table in which every industry (including the various service sectors and usually including households as a sector supplying labour in exchange for goods and services) is both a row and a column in the table. Each cell in the table shows what an industry in any row sold to the industries in each column. Thus the column for the motor industry shows how much it bought from the steel industry, from chemicals, paints, plastics, from office machinery makers, etc. The point of such tables is that they appear to allow you to examine the impact on each sector of changes in output elsewhere in the system. Rather than showing the overall annual transactions between sectors, the cells in the table (in practice a vast computer data bank) can be converted to show what each sector needs to buy from every other per unit of output. The coefficients in the table are then a reflection of the current technology. Innovation will change the use of different materials and components which go into making a car, just as fax machines – and telephones before them – must have changed the amount of postal services which offices need to buy. As often as not innovations are resource-saving. What soon became clear from attempts to use input–output tables was that they did not do much to improve the accuracy of economic forecasting. The problem was, that rather than the coefficients in the table remaining constant, the *most important source of change* was of course the way the coefficients changed in response to technical innovation.

The point of this story is merely to emphasize that economic growth – whether in the long or in the short term – is basically a process of *qualitative* change. Inevitably, the attempt to produce indices of a 'growth' process made up of qualitative changes of every imaginable kind, as if it were a process of quantitative increase, is bound to fail. Indices of 'real' or 'physical' output can never take account of changes in the quality of any product. From their point of view a 1936 car is the same as a 1996 car and a 1986 computer the same as a 1996 computer. They can measure the fact that we produce more cars and computers now but not that they have become quite different machines. This is important because the tendency for innovation to lead to changes in the quality of goods, and indeed to new types of goods, goes unrecorded in economic indices. So if, as most people would guess, the improvements in quality resulting from innovation heavily outweigh the deteriorations, there are unrecorded increases in real income from technical change in addition to the recorded increases from quantitative growth. This might lead to a tendency for the curve relating life expectancy and GNPpc to move upwards. It would, for instance, include all the advantages that refrigeration has brought to food supplies, to fresh storage, to food transport and to the ability to supply fresh fruit and vegetables out of season – all of which are likely to benefit health but none of which will be adequately reflected in figures of real income. The same is true of the development of paints or petrol without lead in them, or of the change to gas central heating which reduced fire risks and pollution from coal smoke. One would expect such innovations to change the gearing of income to health.

However, what we have discussed so far is only the effect it would have if qualitative *material* change was put back into the equation. What may be equally important are the qualitative changes in *social* life which economic development brings in its wake. I will not attempt to summarize here the changes in family and urban life which have accompanied industrialization. Instead I want to draw attention to reasons for thinking that there may have been a change in the relative power of material and psychosocial factors driving health improvements in developed countries. Although we can get rid of the levelling of the curve of life expectancy against GNPpc among the rich countries by putting GNPpc on a log. scale, one cannot escape the implication that it is becoming increasingly expensive to gain improvements in health through the relationship with income – despite the fact that over time even the countries on the horizontal part of the curve continue to move to ever higher curves. What is more, the point at which the curve levels out roughly corresponds with the period when countries pass through the so-called 'epidemiological transition'. Here we must make a brief digression.

The epidemiological transition is when infectious diseases cease to be the main causes of death, leaving cancers and degenerative diseases (usually including rising rates of heart disease) as the main causes of death. But what is particularly interesting is another kind of change which typically takes place during the same time span. Several of the diseases of affluence, so named because they were more common among the rich in the richer countries, changed their social distribution to become more common among the poor in affluent societies. This type of change not only included heart disease, stroke, hypertension, and duodenal ulcers, but most significantly, it included a change in the social distribution of obesity. For centuries the rich had been fat and the poor had been thin. Because being fat was an indication that you lived a life well above minimum subsistence, it was associated with status and affected people's judgements of physical attractiveness. The epidemiological transition seems to mark the point at which living standards among the majority of the population have risen to a level where basic subsistence is no longer in question (Wilkinson 1994a). Above that, infections, which are associated with poverty the world over, cease to be a major threat. The majority have enough to become fat and they develop the diseases previously associated with affluence. As a result, obesity loses its connotations of social status, aesthetics change, and the slimming industry is born. Another piece of this jigsaw is that the decline in the proportion of babies born weighing less than 2,500 g ceases. Every year since the 1950s between 6 and 7 per cent of all babies born in Britain have weighed less than 2,500 g despite major increases in living standards.

The impression from this group of events is that the epidemiological transition marks the point – or rather the period – when the absolute standard of living ceases to be the main limitation on the population's health. Living standards have risen enough for the bulk of the population to have regular access to basic necessities. The infectious diseases associated with absolute poverty fade away and, as the curve in Figure 7.1 shows, further increases in GNP *per capita* yield diminishing health returns.

What does not change, however, is that income distribution remains an important determinant of national mortality levels. Although income differences between developed countries make little difference to health, income differences *within* countries relate very closely to health. Throughout the developed world there is a health gradient from the rich, with the best health, to the poor, with the worst. Initially, the fact that mortality rates are related closely to income differences within developed countries, but only weakly to differences between them, appears to be a paradox. The solution is that what is affecting health within countries is relative income. That has now been demonstrated on a number of different data sets (Wilkinson 1994b). They show that countries with narrower income differences tend to have longer average life expectancy. Even as income differentials change within countries – increasing or decreasing the scale of relative poverty – it is possible to see the effect on the rate of improvement in average life expectancy.

It looks, then, as if prior to the epidemiological transition it is the absolute standard of living which most affects health, but that later on its importance declines, leaving the scale of relative income differences as one of the most powerful influences on national mortality rates. Although changes in income distribution do affect the rate at which life expectancy improves, it is important to recognize that there is a steady background rate of improvement – usually an increase of two to three years per decade – even when there is no change in income distribution. It is, of course, this background rate of improvement we would like to understand. Knowing that relative income has a powerful impact on national mortality rates does not, of course, tell us what is driving the long-term improvement, but it does tell us about the kind of things to which national mortality rates are sensitive. The distinction between absolute and relative income is, of course, the comparative element: with relative income it is not someone's absolute standard of living that matters, but where they stand in relation to others. It is hard (but not impossible) to explain this link except through inherently social – or, more accurately, psycho-social – pathways.

As well as considering qualitative material change as a contributor to factor x as it changes the gearing between GNPpc and life expectancy, the importance of income distribution means we need to consider whether there could also be a psychosocial component. Could economic growth have social implications which could contribute to the necessary gearing factor between GNPpc and life expectancy? Could some of the psycho-social pathways involved in the health effects of income distribution also be driven by economic growth?

There are, of course, a number of obvious similarities between the effects of absolute and relative poverty. Evidence from studies of unem-ployment and job insecurity suggests that financial insecurity is a health hazard (Bartley 1994). Insecurity can come in relation to the need for basic essentials as well as in relation to the need to cover current commit-ments. Financial worries and debt are a common source of stress and are often implicated in domestic conflict. A sense of hopelessness, despera-tion, depression and lack of a sense of control have all been associated with higher mortality rates and are all likely to be affected by both rela-tive and absolute poverty. So to feel that the 'absolute' wolf is a little further from the door brings some of the same increased peace of mind as feeling that the 'relative' wolf is further from the door. However, there is little reason to think that these benefits will play any income gearing role over time in relation to rising real income as currently measured. Unless we can explain how the same level of material security can be bought for less and less as time goes by (thus fitting the relationship between health and GNPpc), these issues are unlikely to be a component of factor x.

It is likely that one of the benefits of a rising standard of living is that a less physically perilous and demanding existence will lead to a softening of the quality of social and emotional life. Certainly there have been very major changes in this direction during recent history. Many developed countries have abolished corporal punishment of children at school and many have also ended the death penalty as part of the criminal code. The latter is obviously more important symbolically than directly. However, both are part of a larger change towards a less intolerant culture. Changes such as the legalisation of homosexuality and abortion which have taken place in most developed countries could be seen as part of the same phenomenon. But none of this captures what one might call the post-Freudian recognition of the emotional and psychological world which has changed everything from beliefs about child-rearing to the recognition of post-traumatic stress disorder in the emergency services and elsewhere. There is also a widespread move in European languages towards more familiar forms of address, not only dropping titles but assuming that strangers use first names immediately, and towards abandoning the most obvious signs of deference between social classes.

Lest anyone doubt the reality of the vast improvements which have taken place in the nature of psychosocial life, a glance at de Mause's *History of Childhood* (1974) will be reassuring. His opening sentences are 'The history of childhood is a nightmare from which we have only recently begun to awaken. The further back in history one goes, the lower the level of child care, and the more likely children are to be killed, abandoned, beaten, terrorized and sexually abused.' He suggests that if we go back far enough 'most children were what we would now consider abused' (p. 3). So confident is he of the processes of change which he describes that he goes as far as to suggest that 'the central force for change in history is neither technology nor economics, but the psychogenic changes in personality occurring because of successive generations of parent–child interactions'. On the wider importance of such changes, de Mause believed that 'because psychic structure must always be passed from generation to generation through the funnel of childhood, a society's child-rearing practices . . . are the very condition for the transmission and development of all other cultural elements, and place definite limits on what could be achieved in all other spheres of history' (p. 3). Although de Mause describes these changes as 'independent of social and technological change' (p. 3), I would prefer to see them as made possible, at least loosely, by the decreasing harshness of material life. Likewise, although children's emotional formation will affect their psychosocial life when they in turn become adults, child-rearing practices and the character of adult social life will both be directly influenced by the material conditions in which people live.

Whether related to these changes or not, another social process which may perhaps provide an income gearing function of a kind which might also be related to income distribution is the strength of community life. In an important study of the strength of community life in the twenty regions of Italy, Putnam (1993) identifies a social variable which he calls 'civic community', measured by such things as the number of local associations (sports, cultural, charitable, special interest groups, etc.), electoral turnout and newspaper readership. He is trying to measure people's involvement in the life of the community beyond immediate self-interest. His claim that this is an important variable is based on the fact that it is a powerful predictor of how well the institutions of the regional governments (set up in 1970) function. He summarizes his results as follows:

> Some regions of Italy have many choral societies and soccer teams and bird-watching clubs and Rotary clubs. Most citizens in these regions read eagerly about community affairs in the daily press. They are engaged by public issues . . . Inhabitants trust one another to act fairly

and to obey the law. Leaders in these regions are relatively honest. They believe in popular government, and they are predisposed to compromise with their political adversaries. Both citizens and leaders here find equality congenial. Social and political networks are organised horizontally, not hierarchically. The community values solidarity, civic engagement, co-operation, and honesty. Government works. Small wonder that people in these regions are content!

At the other pole are the 'uncivic' regions, aptly characterised by the French term *incivisme*. Public life in these regions is organised hierarchically, rather than horizontally. The very concept of 'citizen' here is stunted. From the point of view of the individual inhabitant, public affairs is the business of somebody else – *i notabili*, 'the bosses', 'the politicians' – but not me. Few people aspire to partake in deliberations about the commonweal, and few such opportunities present themselves. Political participation is triggered by personal dependence and private greed, not by collective purpose. Engagement in social and cultural associations is meagre. Private piety stands in for public purpose. Corruption is widely regarded as the norm, even by politicians themselves, and they are cynical about democratic principles. 'Compromise' has only negative overtones. Laws (almost everyone agrees) are made to be broken, but fearing others' lawlessness, people demand sterner discipline. Trapped in these interlocking vicious circles, nearly everyone feels powerless, exploited and unhappy. All things considered, it is hardly surprising that representative government here is less effective than in more civic communities.

(Putnam 1993: 115)

Some of Putnam's description seems particularly Italian and no doubt some of the characteristics which distinguish civic from less civic communities will differ from one society to another. His evidence does, however, establish a strong case for thinking that the strength of community life is an important variable which differs from one place to another. Although he was not concerned with health, he does say that civic community is a stronger predictor of infant mortality than regional differences in prosperity. As well as mentioning the more egalitarian ethos of places with a stronger civic life, he mentions in a footnote that his measure of civic community is highly correlated with income distribution ($r = 0.81$, $p < 0.001$). It seems possible that the quality of the social fabric and the strength of community life may be part of the explanation of why income distribution is related to average mortality rates. Epidemiological evidence suggests not only that close social relations are important to health, but that the same is true of social affiliations in the community more widely (Berkman and Syme 1979). Putnam's evidence that people are happier or more satisfied in more highly civic societies is another reason for thinking that they will have better health.

The lack of research into the relationship of civic society to health makes it impossible to do more than suggest that it is a variable which may be worth exploring. If the strength of the civic community is related to health, its relationship with economic development is such that it could plausibly contribute to the income gearing factor x. Although closely associated with economic development in modern Italy, Putnam's analysis of historical data suggests to him that rather than economic development strengthening civic community, stronger civic communities provide a more favourable basis for economic growth. But whichever way they are linked, community development could contribute to the income gearing effect. In conjunction with the other psychosocial changes we have mentioned, there is room for a sizeable psychosocial contribution related to, or at least accompanying, economic growth.

The failure of mortality rates to improve in most eastern European countries during the 1970s and 1980s shows that we cannot take the rise in life expectancy for granted. I have argued for the need to identify processes which change the gearing between income and health. There are two main sources of change which would fit the specification. The first is the continuous stream of technical innovations which yield qualitative improvements in material life, and the second is an amorphous series of changes in the nature of psychological and social life. Though invisible to indices of economic growth, both may be inextricably bound up with the process of qualitative change which we know as economic development. Given the probable environmental consequences of economic growth and the desirability of increased life expectancy, the question arises as to whether the qualitative progress associated with economic and social development can be separated from quantitative economic growth. Maybe we can continue to enjoy 90 per cent of the increases in life expectancy by pursuing innovation and change without growth. It seems likely that it will not be long before some of the consequences of the environmental damage associated with economic growth start to have health effects which negate the 10 per cent of the increase in life expectancy attributable to quantitative growth. If so, then the optimum course may be to pursue qualitative change and the processes of material and social innovation which probably lie behind the bulk of the increase in life expectancy over time. The qualitative social and material changes taking place over time seem much the most plausible source of the changing relationship between income and health over time from which most of our health gain is derived.

We are unable to identify with any precision the cultural, social and psychosocial improvements in life which are likely to have contributed to health during the long course of economic development. Nor is it possible to distinguish them clearly from the direct material benefits of economic growth which have nurtured them. However, the concept of 'civilization' comes to our rescue. It is a concept which is both universally recognized and yet suitably vaguely defined. While clearly distinguished from economic growth itself it is, in everyone's mind, loosely enough associated with economic development to provide the income gearing processes we need. In addition, it contains in the root of the word the reference to civility, citizenship and the nature of social development while not ignoring important aspects of material advance. Intuitively we recognize that although the level of civilization is only loosely related to economic growth, the nature of civil life is where we should hope to reap the most important benefits of growth. Perhaps we should think of civilization with its wealth of human connotations as the intermediary between economic growth and rising life expectancy. We should certainly think of it – rather than economic growth – as the ultimate objective.

REFERENCES

Bartley, M. (1994) Unemployment and ill-health: understanding the relationship, *Journal of Epidemiology and Community Health* 48(4): 333–337.

Berkman, L.F. and Syme, S.L. (1979) Social networks, host resistance and mortality: a nine-year follow-up study of Alameda County residents, *American Journal of Epidemiology* 109: 186.

de Mause, L. (1974) The evolution of childhood, in L. de Mause (ed.) *The History of Childhood*, London: Condor.

Mackenbach, J.P., Bouvier-Colle, M.H. and Jougla, E. (1990) 'Avoidable' mortality and health services: a review of aggregate data studies, *Journal of Epidemiology and Community Health* 44: 106–111.

McKeown, T. and Lowe, C.R. (1974) *An Introduction to Social Medicine*, second edition, Oxford: Blackwell.

Preston, S. (1976) *Mortality Patterns in National Populations*, London: Academic Press.

Putnam R.D., Leonardi, R. and Nanetti, R.Y. (1993) *Making Democracy Work: Civic Traditions in Modern Italy*, Princeton: Princeton University Press.

Wilkinson, R.G. (1994a) The epidemiological transition: from material scarcity to social disadvantage? *Daedalus* 123(4): 61–77.

Wilkinson, R.G. (1994b) Health, redistribution and growth, in A. Glyn and D. Miliband (eds) *Paying for Inequality: the Economic Cost of Social Injustice*, London: Rivers Oram Press.

Part III

The family and life course

Chapter 8

Patterns of attachment, interpersonal relationships and health

Peter Fonagy

PARENTING, THE FAMILY AND STRESS

Modern Western society is unusual in seeing the family as an institution defined by a marriage and which has at its core the benefit of children. In contrast to such child-centred models of the family, other cultures emphasize the family and kinship as the transmission of wealth and power, as well as of cultural tradition. Leach (1994) points to a curious and complex anomaly. Whereas in non-Western societies children are 'needed as apprentice people' (to validate the marriage, to work, to broaden kinships, etc.), in our culture children are 'wanted', not to meet practical social needs, but rather to fulfil perhaps biologically rooted, and certainly deeply felt, personal desire. Society's ambivalence about children may well be linked with this exclusively personal emotional (rather than, say, economic) investment in the next generation.

Western democracies tend to spend less on children than on adults. In the United States less than 5 per cent of the federal budget is devoted to programmes supporting families and children and 24 per cent on people over retirement age. The situation is similar in Canada and the United Kingdom. While families are delegated the responsibility for child-rearing by the state, little economic allowance is made for it in most countries. Individuals with parental responsibilities have to compete in the market place with those who have no child care responsibilities, as if there was no economic or social disadvantage associated with child care.

The strain, however, shows on the family. There are few epidemiological facts which are as accurately represented in the media, and therefore in popular culture, as the sad fate of the family in late twentieth-century Western society. It is generally known that almost 50 per cent of children born in the United States between 1980 and 1989 will experience divorce of their parents. The figure in the United Kingdom is likely to be close to this in the 1990s; the number of children involved in divorce and custodial parent's remarriage increased from 145,000 in 1981 to over 160,000 in 1991 (NCH, 1994: 10). The proportion of children in Britain in single-parent care was less then 10 per cent twenty years ago but is over 20 per cent now (NCH 1994: 10). The vast majority of these, over 90 per cent, are living with single mothers, who are likely to be at work or be highly deprived economically.

The social structure of work commitment and that of family life are poorly aligned in most Western cultures. A number of, again relatively well publicized, observations speak eloquently to this (for detailed reports see Galinsky *et al.* 1993; Fuchs 1988; Hochschild 1989). For example, 30 per cent of men and 40 per cent of women claim to feel 'used up' at the end of a working day. Downsizing, common across many industries in the 1980s and 1990s, has increased work loads further. Unemployment, or at least the threat of it, is likely to increase pressure even more. Mothers are still the primary providers of child care, yet their role in the work-place has become increasingly central since the 1960s. The average mother's 'second shift' is at least fifteen hours of housework and child care. According to one report, working men spend, on average five hours in 'primary child care' per week, whereas non-working mothers spend on average twelve hours (Robinson 1989). Employment halves the time mothers make available solely to their child but fathers not working increase the time they give to their child only marginally (about an extra thirty minutes per week). Because of the increased proportion of women in the work force, the time that parents have for primary child care has decreased substantially over recent years.

The impact of this set of social changes depends entirely on the quality of alternative child care offered to working families. The provision is far from ideal. Two major studies in the United States provide substantial grounds for concern (Whitebrook *et al.*, 1989; Galinsky *et al.*, 1994). Observation of nursery-type day care facilities reveals that infants and toddlers spend 50 per cent of their time wandering aimlessly and even older toddlers are occupied for only 33 per cent of their time. It is not surprising that only 30 per cent are regularly engaged in, and are perhaps capable of, co-operative pretend play. Children placed with relatives or childminders are little better off. Only 40 per cent of care providers plan activities for the child. Only 20 per cent of relatives looking after a child (usually grandmothers) appear to give consideration to the child's daytime activity. Independent ratings suggest that only 9 per cent provide 'good care' and over one-third are rated as providing inadequate care. For children looked after in a relative's home the latter figure goes up to 69 per cent.

This generally unfavourable picture is shown at its bleakest in the problem of unplanned adolescent pregnancies. The risks of such pregnancies are well known: (1) low-quality antenatal care, (2) lower likelihood of reducing nicotine intake, (3) less compliance with immunization schedules, (4) increased risk of child abuse and neglect, (5) lower birth weight,

(6) higher infant mortality (PHS Expert Panel 1989: 25; Zuravin 1987; Institute of Medicine 1985). Teenage pregnancy has a high cost to society. Teenage mothers face financial deprivation and long-term dependence on social security, which undoubtedly contribute to adverse sequelae such as increased risk of poor health and emotional and behavioural problems in the child, and a repetition of the pattern of early pregnancy in the next generation (Guttmacher Institute 1993; Sawhill 1992; Adams and Williams 1990; Hofferth 1987).

All this could be taken as moral panicmongering. Alternatively, it may be seen as a nostalgic harping back for times long gone when men were men, women were women, parents were parents and political correctness referred to not belonging and never having belonged to the Communist Party. There is little evidence to substantiate the assumption of any recent worsening of parenting. One of the most interesting findings of the Carnegie Task Force on Young Children (1994) is precisely how little the situation has changed. For example, in 1950, 45 per cent of parents regularly read to their children; in 1990 the figure was more or less unchanged at 47 per cent.

Nevertheless figures produced by UNICEF on the social health of children 1970–89 do indicate some worrying trends. When figures for the best ever level of infant mortality, spending on education, teenage suicide and income distribution are combined and contrasted with 1970, 1980 and 1989 levels in order to provide a single index of change of the social health of children across all industrialized countries, most countries are able to show improvements or at least no deterioration over the period. Unfortunately the notable exceptions are the United Kingdom and the United States, both of whose current levels of social health are at about 33 per cent of best ever levels and seem to have deteriorated significantly since 1980. Thus, while parents probably continue to behave as they have always done, society around them has changed to make the task of child-rearing more challenging.

THE IMPACT OF PARENTING ON HEALTH

All this would be of little concern if parenting was unrelated to, or perhaps only loosely coupled with, the child's current well-being and, even more important, his or her future functioning. There is an accumulation of empirical data on the importance of parenting for personality development and psychopathology. Witness to this interest is the series of papers recently published on the relationship between perceptions of parenting and characteristics of personality development and levels of morbidity. (See, for example, *Journal of Nervous and Mental Disease* 7–8, 1982; *American Journal of Psychiatry* 7, 1992; *Psychological Medicine*, 1992; *Psychiatrica Scandinavica*, 1992.)

Research using a wide range of methodologies uniformly reports that negative parental rearing is a major contributing factor to the development of individual vulnerability and thus the possible development of physical and psychiatric disorders. Some have argued that undue emphasis is placed upon the early experiences of the child in the process of socialization. This argument has, since the 1960s, been subject to both conceptual (Swanson 1961) and empirical (e.g. Maccoby and Martin 1983) scrutiny. The balance of evidence, however, now points to the pervasive and apparently irreversible impact of less than adequate early social relationships (e.g. Hodges and Tizard 1989a, b). The widespread adoption of a theoretical frame of reference emphasizing the centrality of developmental processes in child psychiatry (e.g. Cicchetti and Cohen 1995) has further served to focus scientific interest on parenting.

Family life and its vicissitudes are part of many causal models of social aspects of health. The need for relatedness is recognized as a basic human need (Baumeister and Leary 1995). Breaks in human relationships are triggers for health problems, both physical and psychological (Goodwin et al. 1987). The absence of family (social) support increases vulnerability, including immune competence (Kiecolt-Glaser, Garner et al. 1984; Kiecolt-Glaser, Ricker et al. 1984; Kiecolt-Glaser et al. 1987) and the availability of strong relationships increases resilience against illness (Hobfall and London 1986; Solomon et al. 1990).

By contrast, there is evidence that family dysfunction impacts on both educational attainment and psychological well-being. In the British National Child Development Study (Cherlin et al. 1991) both parent and teacher-rated behavioural problems were elevated in children of the divorced sample even when pre-divorce performance and family difficulties were controlled for. Similarly, reading and mathematics achievement were reduced relative to the children in the cohort whose lives were not touched by divorce. The major US study by Hetherington and Clingempeel (1992) on 'Coping with marital transitions' also showed behavioural and educational problems in children of divorce. Interestingly the problems appear to become, if anything, worse, for boys at least, if the mother remarried; following remarriage, mother's parenting became worse, with increased negativity and conflict in interactions with the child.

Four main implications may be drawn from the above. First, there is evidence that social, particularly work, pressures on the family are increasing. Second, the family, the major agent of parenting and the transmission of relationship skills to children, is less able to fulfil this function now than traditionally, as is manifested by the increasing rates of teenage pregnancies, family break-up, single-parent families and the decreasing time spent in primary child care even in two-parent families. Third, alternatives to family-based care of young children are currently less than satisfactory. Fourth, dysfunctional families in general, and the circumstance of divorce in particular, create emotional and educational problems for the child and increase parenting difficulties for the mother. All these facts are well known. What may be missing is a theoretical framework which might help translate these social trends into epidemiological observations concerning the variability of health in the population.

ATTACHMENT THEORY AS AN ORGANIZING FRAMEWORK

The focus of this chapter, attachment theory, aims to draw together a number of themes, explicitly or implicitly, present in many chapters of this book. Attachment theory concerns the nature of children's early experiences and the impact of these experiences on aspects of later functioning of particular relevance to health. Variables often regarded as critical in explanations of variations in health, such as mastery and control, anxiety, the interconnectedness of individuals and groups, as well as the different attitudes societies have to children, may all be approached from the viewpoint of attachment theory in terms of patterns of child-rearing. Patterns of child-rearing may be more or less conducive to the development of secure attachments. Attachment patterns may lead to the development of capacities conducive to 'healthy' attitudes and life styles and thus physical well-being.

The question we attempt to address here is how deprivation, in particular early deprivation, comes to affect the individual's health. As part of this question we are naturally also concerned to understand how such adverse consequences may be avoided. The key assumption made by the invoking of attachment theory is that individual social behaviour may be understood in terms of generic mental models of social relationships constructed by the individual. These models, although constantly evolving and subject to modification, are strongly influenced by the child's experiences with the primary caregivers. Let us now turn to the details of the theory.

THE NATURE OF THE ATTACHMENT SYSTEM

Attachment theory, developed by John Bowlby (1969, 1973, 1980), postulates a universal human need to form close affectional bonds. It is a normative theory of how the 'attachment system' functions in all humans. Bowlby described attachment as a special type of social relationship, paradigmatically between infant and caregiver, involving an affective bond. More significantly, it may also be seen as the context within which the human infant learns to regulate emotion (Sroufe 1990).

Reciprocity of early relationships, independent of other biological needs such as feeding and sexuality, appears to be one of the preconditions of normal development in primates. For example, normal development in macaques is observed only when relationships provide a sufficient level of reciprocity (Mason and Kenney 1974; Ruppenthal *et al.* 1976). In human infancy, attachment behaviours such as proximity seeking, orienting, smiling, crying, clinging, signalling, etc., are reciprocated by adult attachment behaviours such as smiling, touching, holding, rocking, which are triggered by the infant's behaviour and in turn strengthen attachment behaviours towards that adult in the child (Bowlby 1969). In most environments, infants organize attachment behaviours around one caregiving figure (a primary caregiver) and one or more secondary figures (Ainsworth 1982; Rutter 1981).

The activation of attachment behaviours in the infants are not, however, automatic. They depend on the infant's evaluation of a range of environmental signals which result in a subjective experience of security or insecurity (Bischof 1975; Sroufe 1979). The latter is determined by the immediate context, the history of care, the child's developmental level, all of which influence the infant's emotional experience. The attachment system is not co-terminus with the frequency or intensity of any particular attachment behaviour such as proximity seeking. It represents the integration of actions directed towards the primary caretaker with other behaviours in particular contexts. The experience of security is seen as the set goal of the attachment system and affect as mediating the relevant adaptive behaviours (Sroufe and Waters 1977). The attachment system is thus first and foremost a regulator of the small child's emotional experience.

The emotional quality of the relationship with the caregiver underpins the stability of the attachment organization both across situations and over time. The emotional quality of the relationship is clearly indicated by the manner in which the infant uses the caregiver when under stress. Most commonly infants are threatened by strange environments or following periods of separation. Infants normally respond to very prolonged separation by protest, despair and detachment (Bowlby, 1973). Reunions are often characterized by avoidance, anger and ambivalence (Heinicke and Westheimer 1966). Similar experiences, over relatively brief periods, give evidence of the strength of the attachment relationship.

THE DEVELOPMENT OF ATTACHMENT AND THE REGULATION OF AROUSAL

It is generally recognized that the human infant alone is as incapable of developing capacities for self-regulation as it is to ensure its own survival (Breger 1974; Emde 1989). The environment through caregiver interaction provides the necessary support for the steady progress of maturational processes. It is also recognized that in particular during the early months, when growth and maturation are most rapid, the degree and quality of caregiver assistance may be critical for the long-term biological organization of the child (Cicchetti *et al.* 1991; Collins and Depue 1992; Greenough and Black 1992; Greenough *et al.* 1987; Kraemer 1992). Regulatory experiences with the caregiver may strengthen or eliminate synapses which are over-produced in the infant's brain. The competition of neurobiological systems establishes enduring regulatory patterns, including patterns of emotional regulation which reinforce or weaken 'experience expectant neural processes'. These biological structures are thought to evolve because of the highly predictable occurrence of specific environmental contexts in the lives of young members of all species (Collins and Depue 1992: 68).

The infant's emotional experience in the relationship with the caregiver provides the context for the development of these neurobiologically based regulatory patterns (Emde 1989). The evolution of this relationship has been demonstrated to go through a number of predictable phases (for a more detailed review see Sroufe 1989, 1990). The first three months are marked by the caregiver's gradually increasing capacity to respond discriminatively to the infant's reflexive signals. In the second three months chained interaction sequences develop and apparently give-and-take interactions between the caregiver and infant may be observed which help the infant maintain organized behaviour in the face of increasing levels of arousal (Stern 1985). Throughout, the caregiver's responses to the infant's signals of moment-to-moment changes in their subjective experience give the infant's behaviours meaning and these become incorporated into a diadic regulatory system. The infant develops the experience that arousal in the presence of the caregiver will not lead to disorganization because, when threats are beyond the infant's coping capacity, the caregiver will be present to re-establish equilibrium. As development progresses the infant will increasingly identify his or her own role in eliciting assistance from the caregiver in the management of arousal.

During the second six months of life the infant takes an increasingly active role in initiating and maintaining and co-ordinating these exchanges (Sroufe 1989). Gradually, with increased motility, the infant actively seeks the physical proximity of the caregiver to perform the arousal regulatory function. In the final months of the first year the caregiver assumes the role of home base around which the infant can centre his or her expanding exploratory activities (Ainsworth 1973; Mahler *et al.* 1975). By this stage the infant's behaviour is intentional, purposeful, goal-directed, and apparently based on specific expectations. The evolution of these expectations about the availability and responsiveness of the caregiver lies at the core of attachment theory. The infant's reactions to new situations occur in the light of past experience, biasing its responses to the caregiver in the light of these expectations. Bowlby (1973) referred to the organization of these expectations of the caregiver and self in the relationship as an 'internal working model'.

PATTERNS OF ATTACHMENT IN INFANCY

The stability of early childhood attachment patterns is well demonstrated. Mary Ainsworth and her colleagues (Ainsworth 1969, 1985; Ainsworth *et al.* 1978) developed a procedure commonly known as the 'Strange Situation' which classifies infants and toddlers into one of four attachment categories. *Secure* infants explore readily in the presence of the primary caregiver, are anxious in the presence of a stranger and avoid him/her, are distressed by their caregiver's departure and brief absence, rapidly seek contact with the caregiver following a brief period of separation, and are reassured by renewed contact. The recovery from an overly aroused disorganized state is smooth and carried to completion in the sense that the infant returns to exploration and play.

Some infants, who are usually made less anxious by separation, do not automatically seek proximity with the caregiver on her return following separation and may show no preference for the caregiver over the stranger; these infants are designated *Anxious/Avoidant*. A third category, the *Anxious/Resistant* infant, manifests impoverished exploration and play, tends to be highly distressed by separation from the caregiver, but has great difficulty in settling after reunion, showing struggling, stiffness, or continued crying, or fuss in a passive way. The caregiver's presence or attempts at comforting fail to reassure, and the child's anxiety and anger appear to interfere with its attempts to derive comfort through proximity. Both these insecure groups appear to be coping with arousal and ambivalence through a precautious over-control of affect because they appear to be uncertain in their expectation that the caregiver will do his or her part to modulate their emotional arousal (Main 1981; Sroufe 1990).

A fourth group of infants appear to exhibit a range of seemingly undirected behavioural responses, giving the impression of disorganization and disorientation (Main and Solomon 1990). Infants who manifest freezing, handclapping, head banging, the wish to escape from the situation even in the presence of the caregiver, are referred to as *Disorganised/Disoriented*. It is generally held that for such infants the caregiver has served both as a source of fear and as a source of reassurance, hence the arousal of the attachment behavioural system produces strong conflicting motivations. Not surprisingly, a history of severe neglect or physical or sexual abuse is often associated with the manifestation of this pattern (Cicchetti and Beeghly 1987; Main and Hesse 1990).

It is generally held that the patterning of attachment-related behaviour is underpinned by different strategies adopted by children to regulate their

Packing Slip for Order ID: 058-2205975-7389918

Thank you for buying from nmciano on Amazon marketplace.

Shipping Address:
James Teufel
1013 Roberta Dr
Murphysboro, IL 62966-2916

Order Date: Feb 12, 2008
Shipping Service: Standard
Seller Name: nmciano
Contact Seller: nmciano@yahoo.com

Quantity	Product Details
1	Health and Social Organization: Towards a Health Policy for the 21st Century... **ASIN:** 0415130700 **Listing ID:** 0107B645857 **Condition:** Used - Good **Comments:** Cover worn. No marks in text.

Thanks for buying on Amazon Marketplace. Please be sure to rate your experience with this seller by visiting www.amazon.com/feedback. View more information about this seller at www.amazon.com/seller/nmciano.

emotional reactions. As affect regulation is acquired with the help of the child's primary caregiver, the child's strategy will be inevitably a reflection of the caregiver's behaviour towards him/her. Secure infants' behaviour is based on the experience of well co-ordinated, positive interactions where the caregiver is rarely over-arousing and is able to restabilize the child's spontaneously emerging disorganising emotional responses. Therefore, they remain relatively organized in stressful situations. Negative emotions are not seen as threatening in and of themselves but are regarded by the infant as serving a communicative function (Grossman *et al.* 1986; Sroufe 1979).

By contrast, *Anxious/Avoidantly* attached children are presumed to have experiences when their emotional arousal was not restabilized by the caregiver because of personal or social pressures on the caregiver and an associated mild neglect or even resentment of the child. The same expectations may arise in children who were over aroused through intrusive parenting, therefore they *over-regulate* their affect and steer away from situations that are likely to be emotionally arousing. *Anxious/Resistantly* attached children *under-regulate*, heightening their expression of distress possibly in an effort to elicit the expectable response of the caregiver. These children have low thresholds for threat and may become preoccupied with having contact with the caregiver, but show signs of frustration regarding this contact even when it is available (Sroufe 1979).

THE CONTINUITY OF PATTERNS OF ATTACHMENT

Bowlby proposed that the quality of childhood relationship with the caregivers results in internal representations or working models of the self and others that provide prototypes for later social relations. Internal working models are mental schemata, where expectations about the behaviour of a particular individual towards the self are aggregated. The expectations are themselves abstractions based on repeated interactions of specific types with that individual. If the child's physical injury is quickly dealt with, sources of unhappiness are rapidly addressed, the child will develop the legitimate expectation that, with that person at least, his distress is likely to be met by reassurance and comforting. The internal working model is the result of a natural process of abstraction of the invariant features from diverse social situations with a particular individual (Stern 1994). It is illustrated in a schematic form in Figure 8.1.

Such internal models of attachment remain relatively stable across the lifespan (Collins and Read 1994). Secure children, with the benefit of well-regulated caregiver-infant relationships behind them, are expected to evolve positive expectations concerning their exploratory competence, to achieve a reliable capacity for modulation of arousal, a good capacity for communication within relationships and, above all, confidence in

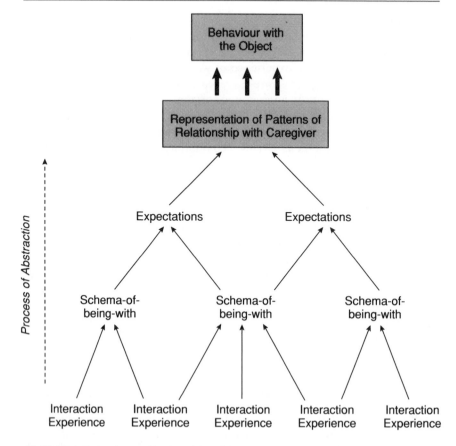

Figure 8.1 Behaviour with the object: the attachment theory formulation of interpersonal behaviour. Expectations regarding the behaviour of others are derived from schemata based on interaction experiences. The expectations are integrated into singular representations of patterns of relationship with the caregiver or 'internal working models'. In this way behaviour with others is based on interaction experiences with the original caregiving figure

the ongoing availability of the caregiver. Early experiences of flexible access to feelings is regarded as formative by attachment theorists, enabling secure children both to maximize the opportunities presented to them by the environment and draw on socially supportive relationships. The autonomous sense of self emerges fully from secure parent–infant relationships (Emde and Buchsbaum 1990; Lieberman and Pawl 1990; Fonagy *et al.* 1995). The increased control of the secure child permits it to move towards the ownership of inner experience and come to recognize the self as competent in eliciting regulatory assistance, to develop metacognitive control and to achieve an understanding of self and others as intentional agents whose behaviour is organized by mental states, thoughts, feelings, beliefs and desires (Sroufe 1990; Fonagy *et al.* 1995).

There is a substantial body of empirical work which confirms the relationship between early attachment experiences and later adaptation. In 4 to 8-year-old children, for example, infancy assessments are found to predict self-regulation (Sroufe 1989, 1990), self-esteem, self-reliance, self-efficacy, and the development of autonomy (Bates *et al.* 1985; Londerville and Main 1981; Matas *et al.* 1978). Prospective longitudinal research has also demonstrated that children with a history of secure attachment are rated (by independent raters, blind to their history) as more resilient, self-reliant, and self-efficacious (Sroufe 1983; Waters *et al.* 1979). The same children are shown to be rated by both their peers and their teachers to be more competent and to form deeper relationships (Sroufe 1983; Sroufe *et al.* 1990). Children with a history of secure attachment are also more socially oriented, frequently imitated, and empathic when observing distress in other children (Kestenbaum *et al.* 1989). These differences persist into middle childhood and early adolescence (see, for example, Urban *et al.* 1991).

Children with anxious attachment histories are rated as more dependent on adults and spend more of their time interacting with them than with children (Elicker *et al.* 1992). In the German longitudinal study (Grossman and Grossman, 1991) early attachment history was found to predict response to stressful situations. Children with secure histories more often reported seeking help or comfort from another individual. Most of these findings also hold up to adolescence, for example, 15-year-old children with a history of secure attachment are still seen to be more effective with peers, less dependent on counsellors in a camp setting, and generally more socially competent (Sroufe *et al.* 1993).

THE MEASUREMENT OF ATTACHMENT IN ADULTS

In contrast to attachment relationships in infancy, adult attachment relationships tend to be reciprocal. The relationship functions may cover sexual bonds, companionship, sense of competence, and shared purpose or experience (Ainsworth 1985). Measurement of attachment in adults is both possible and relatively fruitful. Adults do show a desire for proximity to the attachment figure, especially when stressed, and increasing comfort in the presence, and anxiety in the absence, of this figure (Weiss 1982).

Studies of adult attachment are broadly of two types: some studies have focused on patterns of attachment as revealed in the individual's cognitive working models of relationships (e.g. Bartholomew and Horowitz 1991; Cohn *et al.* 1992; Crowell and Feldman 1988; Hazan and Shaver

1987; Kobak *et al.* 1991; Main *et al.* 1985; Owens *et al.* in press). Other studies examined dimensions of attachment such as security or availability and other behaviours which they were found to predict (Collins and Read 1990; Feeney and Noller 1990; Kobak *et al.* 1991; Simpson 1990; West and Sheldon-Keller 1992).

There are at least six relatively high-quality measures available. Arguably the best of these is the *Adult Attachment Interview* (George *et al.* 1985), which asks subjects about childhood attachment relationships and the meaning which an individual currently gives to attachment experiences. The instrument is rated according to the scoring system developed by Main and Goldwyn (1994) which classifies individuals into Secure/ Autonomous, Insecure/Dismissing, and Insecure/Preoccupied categories. While *autonomous* individuals clearly value attachment relationships and regard them as formative, insecure individuals are poor at integrating memories of experience with their assessment of the meaning of that experience. Those *dismissing* of attachment deny or devalue early relationships. *Preoccupied* individuals tend to be confused, and angry or passive in their current relationships with their parents and others.

Kobak and Hazan (1991) provided an alternative method of scoring the interview using a Q-sort method with descriptors in two dimensions, security/anxiety and deactivation/hyperactivation. The psychometric properties of the interview are strong, with good test–retest reliability and discriminant validity (Bakermans-Kranenburg and van IJzendoorn 1993).

Bartholomew and Horowitz (1991) designed an attachment interview to assess prototypes of adult attachment. The interview is in two parts, one enquiring about friendships and romantic involvements and ideas about the significance of close relationships, whilst the second part asks for family background, child–parent relations and an overview of childhood experiences. The interview yields a four-way categorization: the *secure* individual is comfortable with the self in relationships and values relationships, and can be both intimate and autonomous; the *preoccupied* prototype is characterized by anxiety and emotionality and over-involvement in dependence relationships; the *dismissing* prototype values independence but denies the desire for intimacy; the *fearful* individual is anxious, distrustful and fearful of rejection. Bartholomew and Horowitz also developed a questionnaire which relates relatively well to the interview (Bartholomew and Horowitz 1991).

Hazan and Shaver (1987) developed a three-item self-selection measure aimed at assessing attachment styles in terms of feeling about the self in relationships. The secure style is comfortable with intimacy, dependence and reciprocity, and is not fearful of loss, while the avoidant style emphasizes lack of trust and discomfort with both intimacy and dependence; a third style is represented by ambivalent individuals who wish to be close, are anxious about rejection, and are aware that their need for intimacy is greater than that of other people. Simpson (1990) developed a more complex measure with thirteen items based on the Hazan and Shaver (1987) instrument. Collins and Read (1994) expanded the descriptions. A final improvement of this strategy of assessment was provided by Feeney and colleagues (1994), who provided a forty-item scale which yields subscale scores on confidence, discomfort with closeness, need for approval, preoccupation with relationships, and seeing relationships as secondary.

A somewhat different strategy was followed by Crowell in 1990 (see Crowell and Waters 1994), who offers an assessment of current relationships in a form parallel to the Main and Goldwyn instrument. The classification described by Owens and Crowell (1992) yields a classification of individuals who are secure, those who are dismissing about relationships, and those who are preoccupied with them. Whilst the first of these is optimistic about the way the relationship may develop, dismissing individuals provide little evidence that their partner is loving, supportive, or comforting, even when they idealize these relationships. In the preoccupied pattern, dependence, the need for control of the partner, and dissatisfaction and anxiety about the partner's ability to fulfil needs may be dominant.

There are other questionnaire measures such as the reciprocal attachment questionnaire (West and Sheldon-Keller 1992) which have had less work done on them, or the marital Q-sort designed by Kobak and Hazan (1991).

PREDICTION FROM ADULT ATTACHMENT MEASURES

The stability of these attachment assessments is dramatically illustrated by longitudinal studies of infants assessed with the Strange Situation and followed up in adolescence or young adulthood with the Adult Attachment Interview. Two studies (Hamilton 1994; Waters *et al.* 1995) have shown a 68–75 per cent correspondence between attachment classifications in infancy and classifications in adulthood. This work speaks to the remarkable stability of attachment classifications across the life span. Similar findings are beginning to emerge using other instruments (Hazan and Seifman 1994).

There are predictable differences related to the adult functioning of individuals, classified according to one or other of the attachment classifications listed above. On the whole, secure individuals are reliably shown to have superior interpersonal relationships and more social support (Kobac and Sceery 1988; Smith and George 1993; Levine *et al.* 1991; Horowitz *et al.* 1993).

Adult attachment patterns also link with self-esteem, which in most studies is shown to be significantly higher in secure young adults (Benoit *et al.* 1989; Treboux *et al.* 1992; Bartholomew and Horowitz 1991; Collins and Read 1990). These results are consistent with the assumption that attachment relationships contribute to self-esteem and the self-perception of the individual is in active control of his or her destiny.

On physiological measures, a number of interesting findings have been reported. Dozier and Kobac (1992) found that individuals using dismissing strategies showed increased skin conductance during a stressful interview, indicating that despite subjects' efforts to minimize the importance of such experiences they nevertheless show signs of physiological distress and arousal. These findings confirm those reported by Grossman and colleagues (Spangler and Grossman 1993), who show that recovery in cortisol level is delayed in insecurely attached children during the Strange Situation as well as lower base cortisol levels in insecurely attached infants. Such findings are consistent with Sapolsky's observations on primates, where stress responses were shown to be associated with the individual's experience of rank, friendship network, and the regulation of aggression, depending on the quality of early interactions experienced by the individual (Sapolsky 1993).

THE TRANSGENERATIONAL TRANSMISSION OF ATTACHMENT PATTERNS

There is further important evidence that attachment relationships may play a key role in the transgenerational transmission of hardship and deprivation. Individuals categorized as secure are three or four times more likely to have children who are securely attached to them (van IJzendoorn 1995). This turns out to be true even in prospective studies where parental attachment is assessed before the birth of the child (Benoit and Parker 1994; Fonagy et al. 1991; Radojevic 1992; Steele et al. in press; Ward and Carlson in press). These findings also emphasize the importance of quality of parenting in determining the child's attachment classification.

DETERMINANTS OF ATTACHMENT SECURITY

It is beyond the scope of this chapter to consider in detail the rich literature on determinants of infant security. There are many excellent reviews available, notably by Belsky (Belsky et al. 1995). Clearly genetic transmission may account for some component of the prediction from parental attachment status to the child's security of attachment (van IJzendoorn 1992). The influence of temperament on attachment security is controversial, but the balance of the evidence is now against the appropriateness of a temperamental account (Kagan 1982; Lamb 1984). There is little evidence that distress-prone infants become anxious-resistant babies (van den Boom 1990). Temperament changes in the first year of life (Belsky *et al.* 1991) and the attachment pattern of a child to his two parents is often inconsistent (Fox, *et al.* 1991) and appears to be dependent on the internal working model of each parent (Steele *et al.* in press).

The quality of maternal care has been repeatedly shown to predict infant security. The sensitive responsiveness of the parent is traditionally regarded as the most important determinant of attachment security in the infant (Isabella 1993; Isabella and Belsky 1991). The parameters assessed include: ratings of maternal sensitivity (e.g. Cox *et al.* 1992; Isabella 1993), prompt responsiveness to distress (Del Carmen *et al.* 1993), moderate stimulation (Belsky *et al.* 1984), non-intrusiveness (Malatesta *et al.* 1986), interactional synchrony (Isabella *et al.* 1989), warmth, involvement and responsiveness (O'Connor *et al.* 1992). These associations have been strengthened by findings from experimental studies, where the enhancement of maternal sensitivity has been shown to increase the proportion of secure infants in high-risk populations (van den Boom 1994). Similar parameters have been predictive for fathers (Cox *et al.* 1992) and for professional caregivers (Goosens and van IJzendoorn 1990).

Negative parental personality traits are associated with insecurity in many studies, although by no means all (Zeanah, *et al.* 1993). This has been shown for anxiety (Del Carmen *et al.* 1993), aggression (Maslin and Bates 1983) and suspicion (Egeland and Farber 1984). Parental psychopathology is also found to be a risk factor in some studies (Campbell *et al.* 1993). Of the contextual factors, support from the partner (Goldberg and Easterbrooks 1984) and from others in the mother's environment (Crnic *et al.* 1983) appear important. The strength of these associations is reinforced by experimental studies where social support was systematically manipulated (Lyons-Ruth *et al.* 1990; Jacobson and Frye, 1991; Lieberman *et al.* 1991).

These predictors of infant security are correlated with one another and are all likely to be unequally distributed across socioeconomic groups. It is known that socioeconomic status and other indicators of social deprivation are linked with both infant and adult classifications (e.g. Ward and Carlson in press; van IJzendoorn and Kroonenberg 1988; Crittenden *et al.* 1991; Zeanah *et al.* 1993). Poor parenting skills and the maltreatment of children are more common in families suffering economic hardship (Gabarino 1992). Insecure classification is more common in deprived groups. Maltreatment of children, strongly associated with economic deprivation (Belsky 1993), is most likely to be associated with the disorganized/disoriented pattern of infant attachment.

BRINGING THE EVIDENCE TOGETHER

Let us summarize the evidence presented thus far:

1 Early experience with the caregiver gives rise to stable patterns of responses in situations of distress based on the child's expectations about the caregiver's likely reactions.
2 The child's developing capacity for the regulation of arousal will be dependent on the nature of the early caregiving relationship.
3 Patterns of attachment are relatively stable across the life span.
4 Insecure attachment may be associated with long-term dysfunction in the modulation of arousal under stress.
5 Patterns of attachment are predictive of both social competence and the quality of relationships formed by the individual, including the capacity to use interpersonal relationships which may provide social support when facing stressful life experiences.
6 Patterns of attachment are determined by parental behaviour, and the quality of caregiving received by the child may be significantly improved using relatively brief and structured interventions.
7 The known determinants of attachment are likely to be currently unevenly distributed across social groups, with children born in the most disadvantaged environments receiving the lowest quality of parenting and manifesting the highest rates of insecure patterns of attachment.

The model that is tentatively proposed is outlined in Figure 8.2. The model links social deprivation, dysfunctional marital relations, and the parent's childhood history as a related set of causal factors which come to bear on the parent's capacity to relate to the child in a sensitive, prompt, and moderate way. According to the theory, stability is maintained through an active process of construction; people process information and elicit feedback which confirms their internal models of themselves and others (Main *et al.* 1985). Although attachment representations may change in response to life experiences which disconfirm existing models, a high rate of stability is expected in the absence of major life events. We assume therefore that the early relationship with the caregiver may be formative in two ways. Principally we assume that, in the case of insecure parent–child relations, the child may develop maladaptive internal representations of interpersonal relationships. As a consequence, it may experience a lack of control and understanding of others. Our own work on the relationship of attachment classifications to social development has demonstrated that sensitivity to the mental state of others, at least until 6 years of age, is clearly and strongly linked with the mother–infant relationship (Fonagy, Steele, Steele and Holder, in preparation). A securely attached individual will thus be more resilient in the face of psychosocial stress (Fonagy *et al.* 1994).

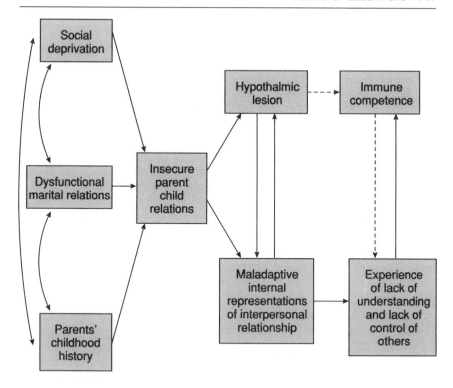

Figure 8.2 Attachment and health. The relationship of attachment and health is conceptualized as mediated through the creation of more or less adaptive internal representations of interpersonal relationships based on experience with the caregiver leading to experiences of lack of control and lack of appropriate understanding in subsequent social situations. It is not yet well demonstrated, but may well be possible, that early experience of stress in the context of less than adequate parenting may cause direct neurobiological deficits leading to reduced immune competence or other manifestations of a physiological deficit in dealing with stressful experiences. Attachment is thus seen as a pathway by which deprivation in early childhood may make itself felt in long-term health outcomes

Secondly, it may be argued that insecure individuals are psycho-physiologically vulnerable. Although further evidence will be needed, current studies point to inherent limits upon the insecure individual's ability to respond appropriately to stress. In particular, they may experience specific problems in modulating arousal and in the recovery phase of their stress response. Both these limitations upon their functioning are likely to act in ways which make them more vulnerable to physical and psychological disorder. As insecure attachment is unevenly distributed across social groups, it may be an important factor in explanations of the social variability of disease.

IMPLICATIONS

Among the major advantages of the model proposed here is the clear implication for effective remedial action which may well go some way towards addressing the inequalities issue. Early childhood prevention works (Carnegie Task Force 1994). Some of the critical components of possible action are outlined below, with the intention of providing an illustration of the kinds of action which may be taken which are likely to impact on health inequalities.

Responsible parenthood may be promoted by: (1) planning for parenthood; (2) delaying adolescent pregnancy; (3) expanding education about parenthood e.g. non-violent conflict resolution; (4) community-based parent support. In particular, parent training programmes have been tried, evaluated and found to be relatively successful: in Oregon, the 'Birth to Three Program'; in Texas, the 'Advance Program'; in Missouri, the 'Parents as Teachers Program'; in Minnesota, the 'Early Childhood Family Education Program'; in Kentucky, 'Family Resource Centres'; in Maryland, the 'Friends of the Family Program' (Carnegie Task Force, 1994: 38–41). The key elements of such programmes appear to be: (1) establishing on-going relationships with parents; (2) adapting the intervention to the styles and needs of individual families; (3) increasing understanding of child development and child relationships; (4) providing models of parenting; (5) teaching new parenting skills; (6) providing a network of social support and other parents; (7) facilitating access to community resources. Information on such programmes is summarized in Heinicke (1991, 1995).

Moving to a community level, much could be achieved by establishing community-based strategic planning processes through experimentation with family-centred communities and expanding head-start-type programmes. Additional changes would need social interventions with a global aim of improving the range and quality of child care choices. This could be achieved by: (1) more family-friendly workplace policies; (2) the State provision of high-quality child care; (3) the better monitoring of existing child care resources; (4) the establishment of community-based networks which link child care programmes.

Children are the future work force. Early experiences impact on educational achievement and the skill base of society (Okun et al. 1994). The importance of human capital to society's economic performance is undoubtedly increasing as technology becomes more and more sophisticated. Thus underinvestment in childhood is economically an increasingly risky strategy.

Transgenerational studies such as have been considered in this chapter demonstrate that inadequate parenting impacts on the capacity of individuals to parent their own children. Concern for children cannot thus be simply conceived of as humanitarian. Although children are vulnerable individuals, early experiences are increasingly seen as important determinants of later functioning, and the development and testing of effective strategies for ensuring that the maximum number of individuals will receive the benefit of the best available quality of child care must therefore be considered critical components of an effective social health strategy.

REFERENCES

Adams, G.C. and Williams, R.C. (1990) *Sources of Support for Adolescent Mothers*, Washington, D.C.: Congressional Budget Office.

Ainsworth, M.D.S. (1969) Object relations, dependence, and attachment: a theoretical review of the infant–mother relationship, *Child Development* 40: 969–1025.

Ainsworth, M.D.S. (1973) The development of infant–mother attachment, in B. Caldwell and H. Ricciati (eds) *Review of Child Development Research*, Chicago: University of Chicago Press.

Ainsworth, M.D.S. (1982) Attachment: retrospect and prospect, in C.M. Parkes and J. Stevenson-Hinde (eds) *The Place of Attachment in Human Behavior*, New York: Basic Books.

Ainsworth, M.D.S. (1985) Attachments across the lifespan, *Bulletin of the New York Academy of Medicine* 61: 792–812.

Ainsworth, M.D.S. (1989) Attachments beyond infancy, *American Psychologist* 44: 709–716.

Ainsworth, M.D.S., Blehar, M.C., Waters, E. and Wall, S. (1978) *Patterns of Attachment*, Hillside, N.J.: Erlbaum.

Bakermans-Kranenburg, M. and van IJzendoorn, M. (1993) A psychometric study of the Adult Attachment Interview: reliability and discriminant validity, *Developmental Psychology* 29: 870–879.

Bartholomew, K. and Horowitz, L. (1991) Attachment styles among young adults: a test of a four category model, *Journal of Personality and Social Psychology* 61: 226–244.

Bates, J., Maslin, C. and Frankel, K. (1985) Attachment security, mother–child interactions, and temperament as predictors of behavior problem ratings at age three years, in I. Bretherton and E. Waters (eds) *Growing Points in Attachment Theory and Research*, Monographs of the Society for Research in Child Development 50 (1–2, Serial No. 209).

Baumeister, R.F. and Leary, M.R. (1995) The need to belong: desire for interpersonal attachments as a fundamental human motivation, *Psychological Bulletin* 117: 497–529.

Belsky, J. (1993) Etiology of child maltreatment: a developmental-ecological analysis, *Psychological Bulletin* 114: 413–434.

Belsky, J. and Cassidy, J. (1994) Attachment: theory and evidence, in M. Rutter and D. Hay (eds) *Development through Life: a Handbook for Clinicians*, Oxford: Blackwell.

Belsky, J., Rovine, M. and Taylor, D.G. (1984) The Pennsylvania Infant and Family Development Project III: The origins of individual differences in infant–mother attachment: maternal and infant contributions, *Child Development* 55: 718–728.

Belsky, J., Fish, M. and Isabella, R. (1991) Continuity and discontinuity in infant negative and positive emotionality: family antecedent and attachment consequences, *Developmental Psychology* 27: 421–431.

Belsky, J., Rosenberger, K. and Crnic, C. (1995) The origins of attachment security: 'classical' and contextual determinants, in S. Goldberg, R. Muir and J. Kerr (eds) *John Bowlby's Attachment Theory: Historical, Clinical and Social Significance*, Hillsdale, N.J.: Analytic Press pp. 153–84.

Benoit, D. and Parker, K.C.H. (1994) Stability and transmission of attachment across three generations, *Child Development* 65: 1444–1457.

Benoit, D., Zeanah, C. and Barton, M. (1989) Maternal attachment disturbances in failure to thrive, *Infant Mental Health Journal* 10: 185–202.

Bischof, N. (1975) A systems approach toward the functional connections of attachment and fear, *Child Development* 46: 801–817.

Bowlby, J. (1969) *Attachment and Loss 1, Attachment*, New York: Basic Books, 1982.

Bowlby, J. (1973) *Attachment and Loss 2, Separation, Anxiety and Anger*, New York: Basic Books.

Bowlby, J. (1980) *Attachment and Loss 3, Sadness and Depression*, New York: Basic Books.

Breger, L. (1974) *From Instinct to Identity: the Development of Personality*, Englewood Cliffs, N.J.: Prentice-Hall.

Campbell, S.B., Cohn, J.F., Meyers, T.A., Ross, S. and Flanagan, C. (1993) Chronicity of Maternal Depression and Mother–Infant Interaction paper, presented at biennial meeting of the Society for Research in Child Development, New Orleans.

Carnegie Task Force on Meeting the Needs of Young Children (1994) *Starting Points: Meeting the Needs of our Youngest Children*, New York: Carnegie Corporation.

Cherlin, A.J., Chase-Lansdale, P.L., Furstenberg, F.F., Kiernan, K. and Robins, P.K. (1991) The Effects of Divorce on Children's Emotional Adjustment: Two Prospective Studies, paper presented at the meeting of the Society for Research in Child Development, Seattle.

Cicchetti, D. and Beeghly, M. (1987) Symbolic development in maltreated youngsters: an organizational perspective, in D. Cicchetti and M. Beeghly (eds) *Symbolic Development in Atypical Children*, San Francisco: Jossey-Bass, pp. 47–68.

Cicchetti, D. and Cohen, D.J. (1995) Perspectives on developmental psychopathology, in D. Cicchetti and D.J. Cohen (eds) *Developmental Psychopathology 1, Theory and Methods*, New York: Wiley.

Cicchetti, D., Ganiban, J. and Barnett, D. (1991) Contributions from the study of high-risk populations to understanding the development of emotion regulation, in K. Dodge and J. Garber (eds) *The Development of Emotion Regulation and Dysregulation*, New York: Cambridge University Press.

Cohn, D., Silver, D., Cowan, P., Cowan, C. and Pearson, J. (1992) Working models of childhood attachment and couples' relationships, *Journal of Family Issues* 13: 432–449.

Collins, N. and Read, S.J. (1990) Adult attachment relationships: working models and relationship quality in dating couples, *Journal of Personality and Social Psychology* 58: 644–683.

Collins, N.L. and Read, S.J. (1994) Representations of attachment: the structure and function of working models, in K. Bartholomew and D. Perlman (eds)

Advances in Personal Relationships 5, Attachment Process in Adulthood, London: Jessica Kingsley.

Collins, P. and Depue, R. (1992) A neurobehavioral systems approach to development psychopathology: implications for disorders of affect, in D. Cicchetti and S. Toth (eds) *Rochester Symposium on Developmental Psychopathology: 4, Developmental Perspectives on Depression,* Hillsdale, N.J.: Erlbaum.

Cox, M., Owen, T., Henderson, V. and Margand, N. (1992) Prediction of infant–father and infant–mother attachment, *Developmental Psychology* 28: 474–483.

Crittenden, P.M., Partridge, M.F. and Claussen, A.H. (1991) Family patterns of relationship in normative and dysfunctional families, *Development and Psychopathology* 3: 449–491.

Crnic, K.A., Greenberg, M.T., Ragozin, A.S., Robinson, N.M. and Basham, R.B. (1983) Effects of stress and social support on mothers and premature and full-term infants, *Child Development* 54: 209–217.

Crowell, J., and Feldman, S.S. (1988) Mothers' internal models of relationships and children's behavioral and developmental status: a study of mother–child interaction, *Child Development* 59: 1273–1285.

Crowell, J. and Waters, E. (1994) Bowlby's theory grown up: the role of attachment in adult love relations, *Psychological Inquiry* 5: 31–34.

Del Carmen, R., Pedersen, F., Huffman, L. and Bryan, Y. (1993) Dyadic distress management predicts security of attachment, *Infant Behaviour and Development* 16: 131–147.

Dozier, M. and Kobak, R.R. (1992) Psychophysiology in attachment interviews: converging evidence for deactivating strategies, *Child Development* 63: 1473–1480.

Egeland, B. and Farber, E.A. (1984) Infant–mother attachment: factors related to its development and change over time, *Child Development* 55: 753–771.

Egeland, B. and Sroufe, L.A. (1981) Attachment and early maltreatment, *Child Development* 52: 44–52.

Elicker, J., Englund, M. and Sroufe, L.A. (1992) Predicting peer competence and peer relationships in childhood from early parent–child relationships, in R. Parke and G. Ladd (eds) *Family–Peer Relationships: Modes of Linkage,* Hillsdale, N.J.: Erlbaum.

Emde, R. (1989) The infant's relationship experience: developmental and affective aspects, in A. Sameroff and R. Emde (eds) *Relationship Disturbances in Early Childhood,* New York: Basic Books.

Emde, R. and Buchsbaum, H. (1990) 'Didn't you hear my mommy?' Autonomy with connectedness in moral self-emergence, in D. Cicchetti and M. Beeghly (eds) *The Self in Transition,* Chicago: University of Chicago Press.

Feeney, J. and Noller, P. (1990) Attachment style as a predictor of adult romantic relationships, *Journal of Personality and Social Psychology* 58: 281–291.

Feeney, J., Noller, P. and Hanrahan, M. (1994) Assessing adult attachment, in M.B. Sperling and W.H. Berman (eds) *Attachment in Adults: Clinical and Developmental Perspectives,* New York: Guilford Press.

Fonagy, P., Steele, H. and Steele, M. (1991) Maternal representations of attachment during pregnancy predict the organization of infant–mother attachment at one year of age, *Child Development* 62: 891–905.

Fonagy, P., Steele, M., Steele, H. and Holder, J. (in preparation) Parent-child security of attachment facilitate acquisition of theory of mind.

Fonagy, P., Steele, M., Steele, H., Higgitt, A. and Target, M. (1994) The theory and practice of resilience, *Journal of Child Psychology and Psychiatry* 35: 231–257.

Fonagy, P., Steele, M., Steele, H., Leigh, T., Kennedy, R., Mattoon, G. and Target, M. (1995) Attachment, the reflective self, and borderline states: the predictive specificity of the Adult Attachment Interview and pathological emotional development, in S. Goldberg, R. Muir and J. Kerr (eds) *John Bowlby's Attachment Theory: Historical, Clinical and Social Significance*, New York: Analytic Press, pp. 233–78.

Fox, N.A., Kimmerly, N.L. and Schafer, W.D. (1991) Attachment to mother/attachment to father: a meta-analysis, *Child Development* 62: 210–225.

Fuchs, V. (1988) *Women's Quest for Economic Equality*, Cambridge, Mass.: Harvard University Press.

Gabarino, J. (1992) The meaning of poverty in the world of children, *American Behavioural Scientist* 35: 220–237.

Galinsky, E., Bond, J.T. and Friedman, D.E. (1993) *The Changing American Workforce: Highlights of the National Study*, New York: Families and Work Institute.

Galinsky, E., Howes, C., Kontos, S. and Shinn (1994) *The Study of Children in Family Child Care and Relative Care: Highlights of Findings*, New York: Families and Work Institute.

George, C., Kaplan, N. and Main, M. (1985) The Adult Attachment Interview, unpublished manuscript, University of California at Berkeley.

Goldberg, W.A. and Easterbrooks, M.A. (1984) The role of marital quality in toddler development, *Developmental Psychology* 20: 504–514.

Goodwin, J.S., Hunt, W.C., Key, C.R. and Samet, J.M. (1987) The effect of marital status on stage, treatment, and survival of cancer patients, *Journal of the American Medical Association* 258: 3125–3130.

Goosens, F. and van IJzendoorn, M. (1990) Quality of infants' attachment to professional caregivers, *Child Development* 61: 832–837.

Greenough, W. and Black, J. (1992) Induction of brain structure by experience: substrates for cognitive development, in M.R. Gunnar and C.A. Nelson (eds) *Minnesota Symposia on Child Psychology 24*, Hillsdale, N.J.: Erlbaum.

Greenough, W., Black, J. and Wallace, C. (1987) Experience and brain development, *Child Development* 58: 535–559.

Grossman, K.E. and Grossman, K. (1991) Attachment quality as an organizer of emotional and behavioral responses in a longitudinal perspective, in C.M. Parkes, J. Stevenson-Hinde and P. Marris (eds) *Attachment across the Life Cycle*, London: Tavistock/Routledge.

Grossman, K.E., Grossman, K. and Schwan, A. (1986) Capturing the wider view of attachment: a reanalysis of Ainsworth's Strange Situation, in C.E. Izard and P.B. Read (eds) *Measuring Emotions in Infants and Children 2*, New York: Cambridge University Press.

Guttmacher Institute, Alan (1993) *Facts in Brief: Teenage Sexual and Reproductive Behavior*, New York, 15 July.

Hamilton, C. (1994) Continuity and Discontinuity of Attachment from Infancy through Adolescence, unpublished doctoral dissertation, University of California at Los Angeles.

Hazan, C. and Seifman, D. (1994) Sex and the psychological tether, *Advances in Personal Relationships* 5: 151–177.

Hazan, C. and Shaver, P. (1987) Romantic love conceptualized as an attachment process, *Journal of Personality and Social Psychology* 52: 511–524.

Heinicke, C. (1991) Early family intervention: focussing on the mother's adaptation-competence and quality of partnership, in D.G. Unger and D.R. Powell (eds) *Families as Nurturing Systems: Support across the Life Span*, New York: Haworth.

Heinicke, C. (1995) Determinants of the transition to parenting, in M.H. Bornstein (ed.) *Handbook of Parenting 3*, Hillsdale, N.J.: Erlbaum.

Heinicke, C. and Westheimer, I. (1966) *Brief Separations*, New York: International Universities Press.

Hetherington, E.M. and Clingempeel, W.G. (1992) Coping with marital transitions: a family systems perspective, *Monographs of the Society for Research in Child Development*, Serial No. 227, vol. 57, Nos. 2–3.

Hobfall, S.E. and London, P. (1986) The relationship of self-concept and social support to emotional distress among women during the war, *Journal of Social and Clinical Psychology* 4: 189–203.

Hochschild, A. (1989) *The Second Shift: Working Parents and the Revolution at Home*, New York: Viking.

Hodges, J. and Tizard, B. (1989a) IQ and behavioral adjustment of ex-institutional adolescents, *Journal of Child Psychology and Psychiatry* 30: 53–75.

Hodges, J. and Tizard, B. (1989b) Social and family relationships of ex-institutional adolescents, *Journal of Child Psychology and Psychiatry* 30: 77–79.

Hofferth, S.L. (1987) Social and economic consequences of teenage childbearing, in S.L. Hofferth and C.D. Hayes (eds) *Risking the Future: Adolescent Sexuality, Pregnancy, and Childbearing 2*, Washington, D.C.: National Academy Press.

Horowitz, L., Rosenberg, S. and Bartholomew, K. (1993), Interpersonal problems, attachment styles, and outcome in brief psychotherapy, *Journal of Consulting and Clinical Psychology* 61: 549–560.

Institute of Medicine (1985) *Preventing Low Birth Weight*, Washington, D.C.: National Academy Press.

Isabella, R.A. (1993) Origins of attachment: maternal interactive behavior across the first year, *Child Development* 64: 605–621.

Isabella, R.A. and Belsky, J. (1991). Interactional synchrony and the origins of infant–mother attachment: a replication study, *Child Development* 62: 373–384.

Isabella, R. A., Belsky, J. and von Eye, A. (1989) Origins of infant–mother attachment: an examination of interactional synchrony during the infant's first year, *Developmental Psychology* 25: 12–21.

Jacobson, S.W. and Frye, K.F. (1991) Effect of maternal social support on attachment: experimental evidence, *Child Development* 62: 572–582.

Kagan, J. (1982) *Psychological Research on the Human Infant: an Evaluative Summary*, New York: Wiley.

Kestenbaum, R., Farber, E. and Sroufe, L.A. (1989) Individual differences in empathy among preschoolers' concurrent and predictive validity, in N. Eisenberg (ed.) *Empathy and Related Emotional Responses: New Directions for Child Development*, San Francisco: Jossey-Bass.

Kiecolt-Glaser, J.K., Garner, W., Speicher, C., Penn, G.M., Holliday, J. and Glaser, R. (1984a) Psychosocial modifiers of immunocompetence in medical students, *Psychosomatic Medicine* 46: 7–14.

Kiecolt-Glaser, J.K., Ricker, D., George, J., Messick, G., Speicher, C.E., Garner, W. and Glaser, R. (1984b) Urinary cortisol levels, cellular immunocompetency, and loneliness in psychiatric inpatients, *Psychosomatic Medicine* 46: 15–23.

Kiecolt-Glaser, J.K., Fischer, L.D., Ogrocki, P., Stout, J.C., Speicher, C.E. and Glaser, R. (1987) Marital quality, marital disruption, and immune function, *Psychosomatic Medicine* 49: 13–34.

Kobak, R.R. and Hazan, C. (1991) Attachment in marriage: effects of security and accuracy of working models, *Journal of Personality and Social Psychology* 60: 861–869.

Kobak, R.R. and Sceery, A. (1988) Attachment in late adolescence: working models, affect regulation and representations of self and others, *Child Development* 59: 135–146.

Kobak, R., Ferenz-Gillies, R., Everhart, E. and Seabrook, L. (1991) Maternal Attachment Strategies and Autonomy among Adolescent Offspring, paper presented at the biennial meeting of the Society for Research in Adolescence, Washington, D.C.

Kraemer, G.W. (1992) A psychobiological theory of attachment, *Behavioral and Brain Sciences* 15: 493–541.

Lamb, M.E., Thompson, R.A., Gardner, W.P., Charnov, E.L. and Estes, D. (1984) Security of infantile attachment as assessed in the 'strange situation': its study and biological interpretation, *Behavioral and Brain Sciences* 7: 127–147.

Leach, P. (1994) *Children First*, London: Michael Joseph.

Levine, L., Tuber, S., Slade, A. and Ward, M.J. (1991) Mothers' mental representations and their relationship to mother–infant attachment, *Bulletin of the Menninger Clinic* 55: 454–469.

Lieberman, A.F. and Pawl, J.H. (1990) Disorders of attachment and secure base behavior in the second year of life: conceptual issues and clinical intervention, in M.T. Greenberg, D. Cicchetti and E.M. Cummings (eds) *Attachment in the Preschool Years*, Chicago: University of Chicago Press.

Lieberman, A.F., Weston, D.R. and Pawl, J.H. (1991) Preventive intervention and outcome with anxiously attached dyads, *Child Development* 62: 199–209.

Londerville, S. and Main, M. (1981) Security of attachment, compliance, and maternal training methods in the second year of life, *Developmental Psychology* 17: 238–299.

Lyons-Ruth, K., Connell, D.B. and Grunebaum, H.U. (1990) Infants at social risk: maternal depression and family support services as mediators of infant development and security of attachment, *Child Development* 61: 85–98.

Maccoby, E. and Martin, J.A. (1983) Socialization in the context of the family: parent–child interaction, in E.M. Hetherington (ed.) *Handbook of Child Psychology: Socialization, Personality and Social Development* 4, New York: Wiley.

Mahler, M., Pine, R. and Bergman, A. (1975) *The Psychological Birth of Human Infants*, New York: Basic Books.

Main, M. (1981) Avoidance in the service of attachment: a working paper, in K. Immelmann, G. Barlow, L. Petrinovich and M. Main (eds) *Behavioral Development: The Bielefeld Interdisciplinary Project*, New York: Cambridge University Press.

Main, M. and Goldwyn, R. (1994) Adult Attachment Rating and Classification System, Manual in Draft: Version 6.0, unpublished manuscript, University of California at Berkeley.

Main, M. and Hesse, E. (1990) Parents' unresolved traumatic experiences are related to infant disorganized attachment status: is frightened and/or frightening parental behavior the linking mechanism? in M.T. Greenberg, D. Cicchetti and E.M. Cummings (eds) *Attachment in the Preschool Years*, Chicago: University of Chicago Press.

Main, M. and Solomon, J. (1990) Procedures for identifying infants as disorganized/disoriented during the Ainsworth strange situation, in M.T. Greenberg, D. Cicchetti and E.M. Cummings (eds) *Attachment in the Preschool Years*, Chicago: University of Chicago Press.

Main, M., Kaplan, N. and Cassidy, J. (1985) Security in infancy, childhood and adulthood: a move to the level of representation, in I. Bretherton and E. Waters (eds) *Growing Points of Attachment Theory and Research*, Monographs of the Society for Research in Child Development, Serial No. 209, 50(1–2).

Malatesta, C.Z., Grigoryev, P., Lamb, C., Albin, M. and Culver, C. (1986) Emotion, socialization and expressive development in pre-term and full-term infants, *Child Development* 57: 316–330.

Maslin, C.A. and Bates, J.E. (1983) Precursors of anxious and secure attachments: a multivariant model at age 6 months, paper presented at the biennial meeting of the Society for Research in Child Development, Detroit.

Mason, W. and Kenney, M. (1974) Redirection of filial attachments in rhesus monkeys: dogs as mother surrogates, *Science* 183: 1209–1211.

Matas, L., Arend, R.A. and Sroufe, L.A. (1978) Continuity of adaptation in the second year: the relationship between quality of attachment and later competence, *Child Development* 49: 547–556.

NCH Action for Children (1994) *Factfile*, London: NCH Action for Children.

O'Connor, M., Sigman, M. and Kassasi, C. (1992) Attachment behavior of infants exposed prenatally to alcohol, *Developmental Psychopathology* 4: 243–256.

Okun, A., Parker, J. and Levendosky, A.A. (1994) Distinct and interactive contributions of physical abuse, socioeconomic disadvantage, and negative life events to children's social, cognitive, and affective adjustment, *Development and Psychopathology* 6: 77–98.

Owens, G. and Crowell, J.A. (1992) Scoring Manual for the Current Relationship Interview, unpublished document, State University of New York at Stony Brook.

Owens, G., Crowell, J., Pan, H., Treboux, D., O'Connor, E. and Waters, E. (in press) The prototype hypothesis and the origins of attachment working models: child–parent and adult–adult romantic relationships, in E. Waters, B. Vaughn, G. Posada and K. Kondo-Ikemura (eds) *Constructs, Cultures and Caregiving: New Growing Points of Attachment Theory*, Chicago: University of Chicago Press.

Public Health Service Expert Panel on the Content of Prenatal Care (1989) *Caring for our Future: the Content of Prenatal Care*, Washington D.C.: US Public Health Service.

Radojevic, M. (1992) Predicting Quality of Infant Attachment to Father at 15 Months from Pre-natal Paternal Representations of Attachment: an Australian Contribution, paper presented at the twenty-fifth International Congress of Psychology, Brussels.

Robinson, J.P. (1989) Caring for kids, *American Demographics* 11: 52.

Ruppenthal, G.C., Arling, G.L., Harlow, H.F., Sackett, G.P. and Suomi, S.J. (1976) A 10-year perspective of motherless–mother monkey behavior, *Journal of Abnormal Psychology* 85: 341–349.

Rutter, M. (1981) Epidemiological-longitudinal approaches to the study of development, in W.A. Collins (ed.) *Minnesota Symposia on Child Psychology 15*, Hillsdale, N.J.: Erlbaum.

Rutter, M. (1995) Clinical implications of attachment concepts: retrospect and prospect, *Journal of Child Psychology and Psychiatry* 36: 549–572.

Sapolsky, R.M. (1993) *Why Zebras don't get Ulcers*, Oxford: Freeman.

Sawhill, I.V. (1992) Young children and families, in *Setting Domestic Priorities: What can Government do?* Washington, D.C.: Brookings Institution.

Simpson, J. (1990) Influence of attachment styles on romantic relationships, *Journal of Personality and Social Psychology* 59: 971–980.

Smith, J. and George, C. (1993) Working Models of Attachment and Adjustment to College: Parents, Peers and Romantic Partners as Attachment Figures, paper presented at the biennial meeting of the Society for Research in Child Development, New Orleans.

Solomon, Z., Waysman, M. and Mikulincer, M. (1990) Family functioning, perceived social support, and combat-related psychopathology: the moderating role of loneliness, *Journal of Social and Clinical Psychology* 9: 456–472.

Spangler, G. and Grossman, K.E. (1993) Biobehavioral organization in securely and insecurely attached infants, *Child Development* 64: 1439–1450.

Sroufe, L.A. (1979) Socioemotional development, in J. Osofsky (ed.) *Handbook of Infant Development*, New York: Wiley.

Sroufe, L.A. (1983) Infant–caregiver attachment and patterns of adaptation in pre-school: the roots of maladaptation and competence, in M. Perlmutter (ed.) *Minnesota Symposia in Child Psychology* 17: 41–83, Hillsdale, N.J.: Erlbaum.

Sroufe, L.A. (1989) Relationships, self, and individual adaptation, in A.J. Sameroff and R.N. Emde (eds) *Relationship Disturbances in Early Childhood: a Developmental Approach*, New York: Basic Books.

Sroufe, L.A. (1990) An organizational perspective on the self, in D. Cicchetti and M. Beeghly (eds) *The Self in Transition: Infancy to Childhood*, Chicago: University of Chicago Press.

Sroufe, L.A. (in press) *Emotional Development*, New York: Cambridge University Press.

Sroufe, L.A. and Waters, E. (1977) Attachment as an organizational construct, *Child Development* 48: 1184–1199.

Sroufe, L.A., Egeland, B. and Kruetzer, T. (1990) The fate of early experience following developmental change: longitudinal approaches to individual adaptation in childhood, *Child Development* 61: 1363–1373.

Sroufe, L.A., Carlson, E. and Shulman, S. (1993) The development of individuals in relationships: from infancy through adolescence, in D.C. Funder, R. Parke, C. Tomlinson-Keesey and K. Widaman (eds) *Studying Lives through Time: Approaches to Personality and Development*, Washington, D.C.: American Psychological Association.

Steele, H., Holder, J. and Fonagy, P. (1995) Quality of Attachment to Mother at one Year predicts Belief–desire Reasoning at Five years, paper presented at biennial meeting of the Society for Research in Child Development, Indianapolis.

Steele, M., Steele, H. and Fonagy, P. (in press) Associations among attachment classifications of mothers, fathers, and their infants: evidence for a relationship-specific perspective, *Child Development*.

Stern, D.N. (1994) One way to build a clinically relevant baby, *Infant Mental Health Journal* 15: 36–54.

Stern, D.N. (1985) *The Interpersonal World of the Infant*, New York: Basic Books.

Swanson, G.E. (1961) Determinants of the individual's defense against inner conflict: review and reformation, in J.C. Glidwell (ed.) *Parental Attitudes and Child Behavior*, Springfield, Ill.: Thomas.

Thompson, R.A., Lamb, M.E. and Estes, D. (1982) Stability of infant–mother attachment and its relationship to changing life circumstances in an unselected middle-class sample, *Child Development* 53: 144–148.

Treboux, D., Crowell, J. and Cohn-Downs, C. (1992) Self-concept and Identity in late Adolescence: Relation to Working Models of Attachment, paper presented at the biennial meeting of the Society for Research in Adolescence, Washington, D.C.

Treboux, D., Crowell, J., Owens, G. and Pan, H. (1994) Attachment Behaviors and Working Models: Relations to Best Friendships and Romantic Relationships, paper presented at the biennial meeting of the Society for Research in Adolescence, San Diego, Cal.

Urban, J., Carlson, E., Egeland, B. and Sroufe, L.A. (1991) Patterns of individual adaptation across childhood, *Development and Psychopathology* 3: 445–460.

van den Boom, D. (1990) Preventive intervention and the quality of mother–infant interaction and infant exploration in irritable infants, in W. Koops *et al.* (eds) *Developmental Psychology behind the Dikes*, Amsterdam: Eburon.

van den Boom, D. (1994) The influence of temperament and mothering on attachment: an exploration of manipulation with sensitive responsiveness among lower class mothers with irritable infants, *Child Development* 65: 1457–1477.

van IJzendoorn, M. (1992) Intergenerational transmission of parenting: a review of studies in non-clinical populations, *Developmental Review* 12: 76–99.

van IJzendoorn, M. (1995) Adult attachment representations, parental responsiveness, and infant attachment: a meta-analysis on the predictive validity of the Adult Attachment Interview, *Psychological Bulletin* 117: 387–403.

van IJzendoorn, M. and Kroonenberg, P.M. (1988) Cross-cultural patterns of attachment: a meta-analysis of the strange situation, *Child Development* 59: 147–156.

Ward, M.J. and Carlson, E.A. (in press) Associations among adult attachment representations, maternal sensitivity, and infant–mother attachment in a sample of adolescent mothers, *Child Development*.

Waters, E. (1978) The reliability and stability of individual differences in infant–mother attachment, *Child Development* 49: 483–494.

Waters, E., Wippman, J. and Sroufe, L.A. (1979) Attachment, positive affect, and competence in the peer group: two studies in construct validation, *Child Development* 50: 821–829.

Waters, E., Merrick, S., Albersheim, L., Treboux, D. and Crowell, J. (1995) From the Strange Situation to the Adult Attachment Interview: a 20-year Longitudinal Study of Attachment Security in Infancy and early Adulthood, paper presented at meeting of the Society for Research in Child Development, Indianapolis.

Weiss, R. (1982) Attachment in adult life, in C.M. Parkes and J. Stevenson-Hinde (eds) *The Place of Attachment in Human Behavior*, New York: Basic Books.

West, M. and Sheldon-Keller, A. (1992) The assessment of dimensions relevant to adult reciprocal attachment, *Canadian Journal of Psychiatry* 37: 1–7.

Whitebrook, M., Phillips, D. and Howes, C. (1989) *Who Cares? Child Care Teachers and the Quality of Care in America: National Child Care Staffing Study*. Oakland, Cal.: Child Care Employee Project.

Zeanah, C.H., Benoit, D., Barton, M., Regan, C., Hirshberg, L.M. and Lipsitt, L. (1993) Representations of attachment in mothers and their one-year-old-infants, *Journal of the American Academy of Child and Adolescent Psychiatry* 32: 278–286.

Zuravin, S.J. (1987) Unplanned pregnancies, family planning problems and child maltreatment, *Family Relations* 36: 136–139.

Chapter 9

Family and education as determinants of health

Michael Wadsworth

There is increasing evidence for the proposition that in childhood the family and its social circumstances provide the basis for health in later life. It is proposed in this chapter that a fund of what will be referred to as physical health capital is developed in early life, with legacies from the mother in the form of prenatal development, from both parents in the form of genetic endowment and postnatal care, and from the social and physical environment in all its aspects in the early years of life. In this chapter it is suggested that the processes through which the biological endowment may have long-term effects are quite different from the ways in which the family and social influences have their impact. Comparison of the presumptive processes suggests that the determinism that may be inferred from the proposed term 'health capital', or from the processes of what Barker (1994) describes as biological programming, is unlikely to be absolute, and that there are likely to exist opportunities throughout life to augment, as well as to deplete, many aspects of health capital.

THE DEVELOPMENT OF HEALTH CAPITAL

Evidence for a strong early life component in the composition of risk of adult illness has been found in studies of causes of death and of physical and mental function.

In a remarkable series of epidemiological historical studies Barker and his colleagues found that raised risk of death from coronary heart disease, and from all types of cardiovascular illness, was associated with reduced birth weight (Barker 1991). Other, prospective studies showed a similar pattern of relationships of low birth weight with blood pressure and with lower respiratory function in middle life (Wadsworth *et al.* 1985; Mann *et al.* 1992). Barker concluded that growth and development of the cardio-vascular and the respiratory systems take place in a window of biological opportunity before birth and in early life. Babies who do not develop fully during that time are not able to change their biological circumstances later and are, it is argued, in effect programmed for life. Barker concludes that

undernutrition and other adverse influences arising in fetal life or immediately after birth have a permanent effect on the body's structure,
physiology, and metabolism. The specific effects of undernutrition
depend on the time in development at which occurs. In early gestation
undernutrition reduces body size permanently, whereas in late gestation it has profound effects on body form without necessarily reducing
body size.

(Barker 1994)

In studies of respiratory health retarded potential development of
biological capital occurs both through damage experienced *in utero* and
during the early life period of completion of respiratory system development. Babies who had experienced the effects of maternal smoking before
birth had significantly reduced respiratory function in the first months
of life, hypothesized to be caused by the action of maternal smoking on
airway size and on the developing lung's elastic properties (Hanrahan *et
al.* 1992). Lower respiratory illness in early life is also associated with
reduced respiratory function later in childhood (Holland *et al.* 1969; Mok
and Simpson 1984; Strope *et al.* 1991) and in adult life (Strachan *et al.*
1988; Mann *et al.* 1992), and is thought to be the result of damage caused
by the illness to the developing airway system.

Further evidence for the long-term continuation of early life levels of
biological functioning comes from follow-up studies which show that poor
childhood function, in terms of respiratory ability and blood pressure,
predicts continuing poor function. Hibbert *et al.* (1990) showed that
'growth of the respiratory system is occurring in an ordered manner relative to the first time point', and de Swiet *et al.* (1992) showed a comparable
pattern of tracking of blood pressure measurements with increasing age
during childhood. In other words the place of the individual's measured
function, relative to others, tends to stay the same throughout life. Those
with poor measured functional attainment in the early years tend to stay
in that section of the curve at later ages. Thus it is argued that those least
well biologically developed are at most risk of subsequent damage from
illness or other forms of biological stress.

Evidence is beginning to accumulate of similar associations between
early life development and other aspects of later life health, including
mental health. The use of prospective data to compare the early life
circumstances of those known to be schizophrenic with others has shown
that those with schizophrenia were slower in first beginning to speak and
walk (Jones *et al.* 1994). Others have found birth-weight and gestational
age to be associated with psychomotor development (Rantakallio 1988).
Jones *et al.* (1994) speculate that an initiating event early in life may have
been responsible for these observed signs. It was concluded that the initial
events from early life may be part of a dynamic process, in which a range

of factors may 'initiate a self-perpetuating cascade of progressively more abnormal function, culminating in the emergence of psychosis' (Jones *et al.* 1994).

A principal way in which poor or damaged early biological programming may affect a particular organ or system in the long term is to increase vulnerability to stressors or damaging agents encountered later in childhood or adult life. Vulnerability established in early life may be increased by the childhood experience of atmospheric pollution, and the adverse effects of smoking in adult life, which have been shown to have an additional deleterious effect on adult respiratory function, independently of the damaging effects both of poor growth before and after birth, and of lower respiratory illness in the first two years of life (Barker 1991, 1994; Mann *et al.* 1992). Reduced numbers of kidney cells may be a problem if 'the system is stressed, for example, by high salt intake and thereby becomes unable to maintain the volume and composition of bodily fluids' (Barker 1994). Barker and colleagues have also argued that

> diabetes is a consequence of poor nutrition during critical periods of fetal life and infancy with consequent impaired development of beta cell function. If poor nutrition continues the reduced ability to produce insulin is not a disadvantage. It becomes so only if nutrition becomes abundant, when increased demand for insulin outstrips the capacity for production.
>
> (Hales *et al.* 1991)

So far most of the work on early life development of health capital has been concerned with damage to the developing foetus and to the still developing organs of the infant in very early life. But evidence is also being found of a process which may enhance health capital. A number of studies show that premature babies exclusively breast fed for six or eight months or longer tend to score significantly higher on cognitive tests taken later in childhood, in comparison with premature babies exclusively bottle fed for that period (Lucas *et al.* 1992). These findings have been reported even after analysis which takes account of the social and economic circumstances of the family, of parental interest in the child's education, and of parental education (Rodgers 1978). Lucas and colleagues are undertaking a longitudinal study of babies weighing < 1,850 g at birth. When the children were aged $7\frac{1}{2}$–8 years Lucas *et al.* (1992) compared scores on the Weschler Intelligence Scale for Children of those who received mother's milk with those who did not. Babies who received breast milk had a substantial and significant advantage in IQ score over those who had not, after adjustment for mother's age, social class and education, and the child's sex, birth weight, gestational age, birth rank, and the extent of respiratory assistance required immediately after birth. Significantly higher scores were maintained even among babies who received mother's milk by nasogastric tube while they were in hospital, showing that the observed effect was independent of the maternal holding, at least at that time. It was concluded that

> human milk contained various factors that might affect nervous system development ... human milk also contains numerous hormones and trophic factors that might influence brain growth and maturation. Work is needed to explore further whether the advantage in intelligence seen with human milk feeding is due to coincidental parenting or genetic factors or, rather, to factors in human milk itself.
>
> (Lucas *et al.* 1992).

Opportunities for the development of health capital are thus hypothesized to be affected by human behaviour and by social circumstances. If for instance good nutrition is abundantly available then it will be of prenatal value to babies of mothers who choose and are able to afford a good diet; but, for adults who have a legacy of impaired beta cell function from their developmental phase in early life, abundant nutrition in adulthood may present a risk to health. Incomplete or damaged biological programming may be associated with personal and social circumstances which not only help to precipitate a poor biological beginning to life, but are involved also in the development of later risk. Poverty, for example, may be associated with maternal poor nutrition and smoking, which may result in prenatal damage, for example to the developing foetal cardiovascular system, and postnatal damage to the developing respiratory system, and may be associated also with an increased propensity for the child to become, in later life, a smoker (Chollet-Traquet 1992).

Contemporary and historical social and cultural factors in such ways affect health capital, and its maintenance in later life. Maternal smoking and nutrition, for example, have varied over time and with social circumstances, and so too has breast feeding. There has been similar variation in the risks to health encountered in later life. Evidence for social effects on the development of health capital is now reviewed.

THE INFLUENCE OF SOCIAL EFFECTS ON THE DEVELOPMENT OF HEALTH CAPITAL

Social factors affect the development of health capital through processes which have their influence at the individual and at the public level. The development of biological capital takes place in the context of the family, and is strongly influenced by the family's circumstances. Poverty, poor home circumstances and adverse parental health habits all increase the risk of the child's poor growth and development during the biologically critical periods, already described, that occur before birth and in early life.

Poor nutrition in women is more common in those with low or no educational attainment, and in low social class families (Braddon *et al.* 1988), and poor maternal nutrition is associated with poor prenatal development (Butler and Alberman 1969), which is in turn associated with raised risk of hypertension in adult life (Barker *et al.* 1990). Poor growth during the first year of life, which is more common among children living in poor home circumstances (Douglas and Blomfield 1958), increases known adult life biochemical risks for cardiovascular disease (Barker *et al.* 1992), and the risk of raised adult blood pressure (Barker 1994: table 1).

Children in lower social class families have been consistently shown to be at increased risk of lower respiratory illness and lower respiratory function (Wadsworth 1994), for reasons which include prenatal and postnatal poor development (Barker 1994), and home environment (Wadsworth 1994), and may well include diet (Strachan *et al.* 1991). In low social class families smoking is now more common than in others (Wald *et al.* 1988), and maternal smoking has been shown to have a powerful effect on birth weight, independently of a wide range of socioeconomic and other factors (Brooke *et al.* 1989), and a powerful effect on the development of respiratory function (Tager *et al.* 1983). Alberman *et al.* (1991) found that the rate of foetal growth was significantly associated with adult height. Parental smoking seems also to affect height growth in children, even after allowing for birth weight, smoking in pregnancy, overcrowding, and parents' height (Rona *et al.* 1985). Height of children has been found to be adversely affected by paternal unemployment, an effect that looks as if it occurs during the pre-school years (Rona *et al.* 1985; Rona and Chinn 1991).

In addition to the question of how these social factors have their apparent effects on individuals, there is the question of how such effects are influenced by their wider social context. 'Choice' in diet and smoking is influenced by education, by income, by fashion or by perceived acceptability to the individual's peer groups, as well as by current ideas about the beneficial effects or otherwise of such 'choices'. Breast feeding is affected by all of these things, except possibly income. And all of these factors vary greatly over historical time and with age. Smoking, for example, has varied in popularity or fashion over time, with a rise first among men, and later among women, and now a fall in popularity which is varying in relation to education and to gender (Wald *et al.* 1988; Mason 1994; Social Trends 1995). Opportunities for further and higher education began, in Britain, to increase and broaden in the 1960s after a long period at a low and socially strongly differentiated level (Halsey 1988), but did so then mostly for men, and began to improve for women only fifteen years after that (Universities Funding Council 1990). Breast feeding fell in prevalence from the 1920s until the early 1970s, when a striking increase began (Whitehead and Paul 1987) which lasted until 1980. Whereas in one nationally representative sample, born in 1946, 76 per cent of babies were breast fed at age 2 weeks (Douglas 1950), the comparable figure for England and Wales in 1990 was 50 per cent (White *et al.* 1992). Currently the duration of breast feeding is greatest in women with the most years of education, and in those who are non-smokers (White *et al.* 1992).

Since social factors evidently affect the development of health capital it is important to consider also whether there may be an element of capitalization in the social factors and processes that affect health.

THE DEVELOPMENT OF SOCIAL AND EDUCATIONAL CAPITAL

In infancy social factors that affect the development of health capital are also the beginnings of processes of social and educational opportunity. Unlike the hypotheses about health capital, the acquisition of social and educational assets is well documented to be cumulative. Whereas biological capital has been argued to be acquired in the brief period of prenatal growth and in early infancy, social and educational capital is developed over a much longer time span. But, as with health capital, the initial phase of acquisition of social and educational assets is crucial. The key to this process is education.

Before formal education begins, pre-school experience of kindergarten and day care facilities, and parents' education and their degree of concern for education, all begin to shape the child's chances in later life (Douglas 1964; Douglas *et al.* 1968; Osborn and Milbank 1989). Parental interest in school progress, in particular, continues to have a powerful influence on educational attainment. It is exerted regardless of social class, so that the effect of high parental interest is to increase the educational opportunities for children from any socioeconomic background, and this can be seen in children's attitudes to school work, in test scores during the primary school years and later, and in the chances of acquiring higher education or training (Wadsworth 1991). In fact parental enthusiasm for education was found to be associated many years later, at age 43 years, with raised optimism about current and future work, achievements and opportunities, regardless of current social class in men, but in women comparable levels of optimism were found only among those in non-manual occupations (Wadsworth in press). Conversely, children whose parents expressed little interest in their education, or who had persistent material or family disadvantages, including parental divorce or separation, tended to be at greater risk of attaining low or no qualifications than might be expected from scores on tests taken early in their school career (Douglas 1964; Douglas *et al.* 1968; Essen and Wedge 1982; Wadsworth and Maclean 1986).

Like the social effects on health capital, the processes of social capital development are complex, and subject to pressures from the social context. For example, children from manual social class families are still significantly less likely than others to get into higher education, despite its expansion in the 1960s (Douglas 1964; Douglas *et al.* 1968; Association of University Teachers 1995), and, as described in the previous section, women's opportunities for educational attainment at higher levels were greatly restricted until the 1980s (Universities Funding Council 1990). As a result the beneficial effects for the establishment of children's social capital that flow from having parents with further or higher education have been restricted until recently, with a consequent reduction of that benefit in the population of children born before this social change. Findings from one prospective study showed that the benefits of higher educational attainment included a greater likelihood of higher earnings and greater involvement in arts, politics and sport, greater acceptance of new ideas, and higher enthusiasm for the education of offspring (Wadsworth 1991). The effects of such cohort differentiation in opportunity to establish social capital can be exemplified by findings on attitudes to work among women of an earlier generation, born in 1946, and living their childhood at a time when women were not expected to have careers, and were greatly underrepresented in higher education. By mid-life (43 years), in comparison with men, employed women of this generation reported much less ambition in work, and much less perception of having achieved all they wanted to in their working lives (Wadsworth in press). Pressures for this generation to achieve in a male-dominated world may be reflected also in the finding from the same study that women from manual social class families who had further or higher education qualifications and who were employed at age 36 years in non-manual occupations had significantly greater alcohol consumption than other women, more like that of men in similar occupations (Braddon *et al.* 1988). Although further and higher education was, generally, associated in that study with 'good' health related behaviour, in this instance that effect was overridden by what was taken to be peer group pressure at work.

Thus although studies of individuals show the importance of social factors to health, the interpretation of how these apparent effects operate must be undertaken in the light of such wider social factors as educational and occupational opportunity, social and gender differences in what is perceived to be appropriate behaviour, and peer group pressure. In social capital terms these wider social factors condition what it is possible for the individual to achieve, and so leave their mark on each generation. Those who live their childhood in times of sharply gender differentiated opportunity, as happened to the generation now in their 50s, carry the imprint of that effect in later life, as exemplified above (Wadsworth 1991; Hareven 1978). Similarly, those who were children in times of serious economic depression carry the effects in their thinking and behaviour in later life (Elder *et al.* 1984). The implications of this process of period effect for health planning are discussed in the concluding section.

The way in which these social and educational assets, and the progression of experience in these respects, influence the chances of maintenance or depletion of health capital are now described.

EDUCATIONAL, FAMILY AND OCCUPATIONAL EFFECTS ON THE MAINTENANCE OF HEALTH CAPITAL IN LATER LIFE

How is it that social capital provides the child and the young adult with the means of adding interest to or depleting from biological capital? There are, it is suggested, three main ways, namely through the individual's experience of education, family life and occupation.

Men and women with low educational attainment and in manual social class occupations are the least likely or slowest to respond to the messages of health education: they are, for example, those most likely to smoke (Graham 1984; *Social Trends* 1995), to have a poor diet (Braddon *et al.* 1988; OPCS Social Survey Division 1995), and to be obese (Larsson *et al.* 1992). These associations may have been found for a large number of reasons or combinations of reasons; for instance, they may be because poor educational attainment is associated with lower income in adult life (Kuh and Wadsworth 1991), with consequent reduced access to a 'healthy diet', or because in poor circumstances in adult life the accessible comforts of smoking and sweet and fatty foods become irresistible, or because of lack of knowledge about diet, or because of peer group influences. Conversely, the apparently beneficial effects of higher education on health maintenance may be the consequence of an adequate income, a feeling of security, an investment in the future, and easier access to preventive care and ideas about care.

Occupation has also been shown to be strongly associated with health. Unemployment may be associated with poor self-perception and low psychological well-being (Theorell 1992), and the resulting experience of continuing anxiety may also damage physical health (Kaplan 1991). Is it possible that during unemployment the feeling of lack of control over life, and the absence of psychological support that employment provides in terms of self-image, companionship, and another world of roles outside the home, may all be part of accumulating risks to mental and physical health? Similar factors have been shown to affect the health of the employed population. Those with good social support at work have a lower risk of developing cardiovascular symptoms (Marmot and Theorell 1988), and 'adequate' income is associated both with perceived independence and with raised self-esteem (Pahl 1989). But those who feel that work makes high demands on them, yet offers also little opportunity for carrying through decisions of their own, are at greater cardiovascular risk than others (Theorell 1992). Work environment and working hours have also been shown to be associated with health (Theorell 1992).

Studies of family circumstances in relation to health have found comparable risk and protective factors. Perceived strong social support, and a network of relationships, as opposed to apparent poor support and a very small or non-existent social network, has been found to be supportive of better health, particularly in terms of cardiovascular risk (Orth-Gomer and Unden 1990) and mental health (Brown and Harris 1978; Rodgers in press). It may be that similar processes of perceived support and social networks underlie the finding of greater risks to health associated with divorce and separation (Wyke and Ford 1992), as well as the changes in material and economic circumstances also associated with change in marital status (Maclean and Eekelaar 1983; Wadsworth and Maclean 1986). As in employment, disruption in family life, either permanent as divorce or separation, or through other forms of emotional upheaval caused, for example, by moving house, robbery, or serious illness, has been found also to be a risk to health (Blaxter 1990; Theorell 1992). Conversely, strong social support that occurs in cultures or at times when the roles of family and self are well defined, and when values are homogeneous or largely so, and when there is a strong moral tradition, is associated with chances of good health, at least in cardiovascular terms (Marmot and Syme 1976; Prior *et al.* 1974).

BIOLOGICAL FACTORS WHICH AFFECT THE MAINTENANCE AND DEPLETION OF HEALTH CAPITAL

Time and place of birth affect chances of establishment of health capital and its maintenance, through the action of current social and family factors. To have been born in the Depression years, or to have grown up in times of poor educational opportunity, limits the extent of health capital established, and the opportunities for its optimum maintenance, as already described. There are also comparable historical biological period effects which made their mark on the population.

Women who were adolescents or young adults before smoking was fashionably acceptable now have a much lower risk of lung cancer than others born later, who took up smoking to the same extent as men, whose lung cancer rates have been higher for much longer (Chollet-Traquet 1992). The fact that young women are now the group most prone to begin smoking is bad news for the health capital of their offspring, as well as for the maintenance of the health of the women themselves (Jacobson 1986; Mason 1994). Those now in their fifties and older, who were exposed to much heavier doses of parental smoking than is common today (Wald *et al.* 1988), are consequently not likely to be at much less risk of serious lower respiratory illness in later life than earlier generations.

Similarly, in diet, it might be expected that after the years of wartime food rationing in Britain, the following period of increasingly fatty diet – it has been estimated that the fat content of the national diet rose by 30 per cent from the end of rationing to the late 1950s (Burnett 1989) – and high sugar content would have left its mark, both biologically and in terms of taste.

In addition to these long-term effects of changes in health-related habits, the experience of past epidemics may also be detectable in the population's health potential. Martyn *et al.* (1988) suggested that many of those who were children during the poliomyelitis epidemics of the late 1940s and early 1950s would have experienced a subclinical level of this illness, and consequently an irrecoverable brain cell depletion. In adult life these children will, Martyn hypotheses, be particularly vulnerable to infectious and viral illnesses which can further reduce their neurological capacity. Martyn *et al.* suggest that past childhood experience of subclinical poliomyelitis may account for the current rise in such neurological illnesses as motorneurone disease. Similar arguments have been put forward in relation to foetal brain damage caused by maternal experience of influenza, which, it has been suggested, increased the risk of schizophrenia in later life in members of cohorts exposed to such risk (Mednick *et al.* 1988; Susser and Lin 1992).

CURRENT SOCIAL AND EDUCATIONAL CIRCUMSTANCES IN RELATION TO HEALTH CAPITAL AND ITS MAINTENANCE

It has been argued that social, family and educational circumstances affect the chances of establishing a good biological beginning to life or stock of health capital, and that once health capital has been established these same circumstantial factors affect whether it is depleted or maintained. It is now worth thinking forward, by looking at present trends in social circumstances as they affect families and education, in order to speculate about their impact on developmental opportunities for babies recently born, and on the health of older members of the population.

Home circumstances during the last twenty years have improved in many respects (Table 9.1), but the figures hide a powerful underlying current of rising family difficulties in the form of housing loss, and homelessness (Table 9.1). Homelessness of teenagers is particularly an increasing problem of poverty, and of concomitant risk to current and future health in the form of poor housing, poor nutrition, low self-esteem, unhappiness, and raised risk of suicide. There is a serious and rising problem of relative poverty, which hits young parents and children especially

Table 9.1 Changes in family circumstances in Britain (unless otherwise specified) over twenty-two years, 1971–93

Measure	1971	1972	1979	1982	1986	1988	1991	1992	1993
Increases in material wealth:[a] proportion of English households with:									
Central heating (%)		37						83	
Washing machine (%)		66						88	
More than one car (%)		9						24	
UK mortgage repossessions (000)[b]	2.8				24.1	18.5		68.5	58.5
English households in temporary accomodation (000)[b]				10.5	22.7	32.3		67.6	
Households applying to local authorities as homeless (000)									
Accepted and classed as priority need (GB)[b]					107.2		160.7		
Accepted but not a priority need (GB)[b]				10.2		9.8			
Intentionally homeless (England)[a]					3.0		6.0	6.0	
Proportion of children living with both parents and with income below 40% of average (%)[c]			3			12			
As above, but single parents (%)[c]			5			23			
Proportion of families headed by a lone parent (England, %)[a]	8							21	
Families receiving one-parent benefit (GB, 000)[b]			595				1,265		1,409

Sources: (a) Social Trends (1994), (b) Social Trends (1995), (c) Department of Social Security (1992).

hard (Table 9.1). Rising rates of parental divorce and separation may be associated with the increases in homelessness; they increase also the risk to health in parents and children and decrease children's chances in education, as already described. Poverty is not being contained in Britain (Joseph Rowntree Foundation 1995).

> Before housing costs the real median income of the bottom fifth increased by just 3 per cent between 1979 and 1990–1991, while the corresponding figure for the top fifth is 49 per cent. After housing costs the real median income of the bottom fifth actually fell between 1978 and 1990–1991, but increased for all other groups.
>
> (*Social Trends* 1994)

Equally poverty is not being contained in the United States (Fuchs and Reklis 1992), and in both countries it represents a serious threat to health in childhood, and consequently to health in adult life.

Much has been expected of education, and it is no coincidence that the country's education Acts followed close in time to the end of wars, when great change was hoped for and the mechanisms to achieve it were set in motion. It was also the great hope at the turn of the century, when malnutrition and poor sanitation were widespread (Russell 1926). Education has undoubtedly brought great change, and will bring even more as growing numbers are, at last, brought into post-school education (Table 9.2). Increasing educational opportunities for future mothers is likely to be a strategy beneficial both to the health of their children and to the health of working women, and will benefit the development of social and consequently health capital.

The positive benefits of occupation to psychological well-being and to physical health have been described, but the national trend is to the maintenance of a high level of unemployment (Table 9.3). This surely not only has a damaging effect on the mental and physical health of adults (see Chapter 14), but is highly likely to affect the health and social capital of a new generation of children through the reduction in family income, the hopelessness of parents, and the pressures on children to begin earning early to increase family income or to leave home in order to reduce expenditure, with consequent loss of opportunity for further and higher education. Trends in the nature of work may also be conducive to health risk, now that the time and extent of skilled learning are constantly reduced as computer-driven expert systems replace skills learned on the job. This gradual deskilling of the labour force, without loss of product quality, is a valuable resource in bringing developing countries quickly into competing international positions. In Britain it may well present a threat to health in the form of reduced opportunities for pride in work, not to mention the insecurity of work circumstances that it also inevitably brings. In the longer term this trend to deskilling brings the additional

Table 9.2   Undergraduate students at British universities

Measure	1919–20	1938–9	1953–4	1965–6	1988–9
No. of undergraduate students	33,951	50,002	80,602	169,486	317,572
% women	27	23	25	26	42

Source: Universities Funding Council (1990).

Table 9.3 The rise in unemployment over thirty-one years: unemployed claimants of social security benefits in Great Britain (000)

Sex	1961	1971	1981	1991	1992
Men	283	721	1,994	1,773	2,073
Women	101	138	710	540	614

Source: *Social Trends* (1994).

risk of a future reduction in investment in education, at all levels, if it can be argued that it is no longer necessary, on such a wide scale, for the generation of national wealth.

In home and family life, education and occupation, there are at present in Britain disturbing signs of deterioration rather than improvement in risks to the establishment of health and social capital.

CONCLUSIONS

This chapter has emphasized the importance of health and social capital, particularly the apparent power of pre-and postnatal infant circumstances in shaping parameters for health and social opportunities in later life. A poor start in terms of health or social beginnings is likely to be a long-term problem, because health capital seems increasingly likely to be fixed early in life, and although social capital develops more gradually and over a longer period, it becomes in later life the key to maximizing the benefits of health capital. Understanding how these assets come to be established and maintained, particularly health, is in its early stages, but has already some relevance to health policy.

At the level of individual differences new work on the development of health capital is being undertaken or planned at the cellular (Barker 1994) and at the epidemiological levels (Paneth and Susser 1995). New work on social factors should include multidisciplinary investigations of how poor social and psychological circumstances affect physical health, exploring in particular the biological processes, along the lines of recent work by Siegrist *et al.* (1988) and Kaplan (1991). New work is needed to explore the relationship of education with health, including an experimental and evaluated school-life-long course on basic human biology. The current climate of opinion that favours nursery school experience for all children offers great opportunities for innovative and experimental policies in the health education of infants and their mothers. It is important also to investigate receptivity to health education messages in the light of the high value placed on personal freedom and self-expression. Receptivity depends on at least two important factors, namely fashion and the perceived effects of the habit. In children, adolescents and young adults exercise and diet are now strongly subject to fashion and peer group pressure, as smoking, in particular, was in the past. Both smoking and some aspects of diet also continue to be readily available sources of comfort and relaxation. Such 'feel good' effects and the inescapable need for them in everyday life have been too little considered in health education planning.

Whereas at the individual level the effects on health of lack of social integration, perceived low levels of control at work, and low levels of psychological support and companionship are well described, much less is known about their equivalents at the broader social level. Work in this respect has been thorough in defining and describing the extent of poverty (Joseph Rowntree Foundation 1995) and raising awareness, but there needs now to be greater emphasis on how social and health capital could be maximized and how poverty and its effects could be reduced, not only alleviated. To take these questions further it is necessary to reduce the damaging effects of awareness of relative deprivation, and consequent discontent and anxiety. These are surely the social level equivalents of the powerful individual level effects of perceived lack of control and lack of support, already described. Masterman (1909) observed that social discontent 'propagates and triumphs in times of plenty, withers up and vanishes in times of depression. This is exactly the reverse of the accepted belief, which thought that the poor are stung into Socialism by suffering as poets are stung into poetry by wrong' (quoted in Runciman 1966). Politicians, sociologists and historians have therefore been greatly concerned with the social development of perceived discontent and its effects on individuals and families (Runciman 1966; Goldthorpe et al. 1980; Young and Willmott 1973). Work of this kind should now be expanded, and concerned with health. We need to know how such social groups as industries, offices, and districts can optimize the factors that maintain health capital by increasing perceptions of support and control in many aspects of life, and by raising levels of social support and integration. We need also therefore to experiment, and at the same time to develop new measures of integration and contentment for use at this broader social level, in order to increase awareness, to monitor differences between social groups, and to assess the extent of change brought by innovation.

What is known so far about health and social capital might be misinterpreted as deterministic. It must be emphasized that biological programming does not show that the health life course of the individual is fixed, so that good health practice and care of self are pointless in adult life. Biological programming shows the dimensions of the envelope of possibilities for the individual's health, dimensions which will come to be better defined by genetic knowledge. Anything that is known either to expand the dimensions of health capital or to enhance it in adolescence or adult life is of value for policy application.

The long time periods covered by research concerned with health and social capital show that health policy should have a comparably long-term view, in order to appreciate the long-term impact of the past, and the long forward time scale of likely achievement. Health capital research suggests that the burdens of past poor health capitalization cannot be escaped, but may be diminished. However, the health of future adult populations can be improved, relative to those of today, by paying particular attention to the education and health care of today's children and adolescents, and by improving the education and health care of mothers during pregnancy. We must think broadly and boldly about how best to establish capital in both health and social terms, since there is little doubt that the determinants of good health and the risks 'of disease are mainly economic and social, and therefore its remedies must also be economic and social. Medicine and politics cannot and should not be kept apart' (Rose 1992).

REFERENCES

Alberman, E., Filakti, H., Williams, S., Evans, S.J.W. and Emanuel, I. (1991) Early influences on the secular change in adult height between the parents and children of the 1958 birth cohort, *Annals of Human Biology* 18: 117–136.

Association of University Teachers (1995) *Higher Education: Preparing for the Twenty-first Century*, London: Association of University Teachers.

Barker, D.J.P. (1991) *Fetal and Infant Origins of Adult Disease*, London: British Medical Journal.

Barker, D.J.P. (1994) *Mothers, Babies, and Disease in Later Life*, London: British Medical Journal.

Barker, D.J.P., Bull, A.R., Osmond, C. and Simmonds, S.J. (1990) Fetal and placental size and risk of hypertension in adult life, *British Medical Journal* 301: 259–262.

Barker, D.J.P., Godfrey, K.M., Osmond, C. and Bull, A.R. (1992) The relation of fetal length, ponderal index and head circumference to blood pressure and the risk of hypertension in adult life, *Paediatric and Perinatal Epidemiology* 6: 35–44.

Blaxter, M. (1990) *Health and Lifestyles*, London: Tavistock/Routledge.

Braddon, F.E.M., Wadsworth, M.E.J., Davies, J.M.C. and Cripps, H.A. (1988) Social and regional differences in food and alcohol consumption and their measurement in a national birth cohort, *Journal of Epidemiology and Community Health* 42: 341–349.

Brooke, O.G., Anderson, H.R., Bland, J.M., Peacock, J.L. and Stewart, C.M. (1989) Effects on birth weight of smoking, alcohol, caffeine, socioeconomic factors, and psychosocial stress, *British Medical Journal* 298: 795–801.

Brown, G.W. and Harris, T. (1978) *Social Origins of Depression*, London: Tavistock.

Burnett, J. (1989) *Plenty and Want: a Social History of Food in England from 1815 to the Present Day*, London: Routledge.

Butler, N.R. and Alberman, E.D. (1969) *Second Report of the 1958 British Perinatal Morbidity Survey*, Edinburgh: Churchill Livingstone.

Chollet-Traquet, C. (1992) *Women and Tobacco*, Geneva: World Health Organization.

de Swiet, M., Fayers, P. and Shinebourne, E.A. (1992) Blood pressure in the first ten years of life: the Brompton study', *British Medical Journal* 304: 23–26.

Department of Social Security (1992) *Social Security Statistics*, London: HMSO.

Douglas, J.W.B. (1950) The extent of breast-feeding in Great Britain in 1946 with special reference to the health and survival of children, *Journal of Obstetrics of the British Empire* 57: 336–362.

Douglas, J.W.B. (1964) *The Home and the School*, London: MacGibbon & Kee.

Douglas, J.W.B. and Blomfield, J.M. (1958) *Children under Five*, London: Allen & Unwin.

Douglas, J.W.B., Ross, J.M. and Simpson, H.R. (1968) *All our Future*, London: Peter Davies.

Elder, G.H., Liker, J.K. and Cross, C.E. (1984) Parent–child behavior in the Great Depression, in P.B. Baltes and O.G. Brim (eds) *Life-Span Development and Behavior*, New York: Academic Press.

Essen, J. and Wedge, P. (1982) *Continuities in Childhood Disadvantage*, London: Heinemann.

Fuchs, V.R. and Reklis, D.M. (1992) America's children: economic perspectives and policy options, *Science* 255: 41–46.

Goldthorpe, J.H., Llewellyn, C. and Payne, C. (1980) *Social Mobility and Class Structure in Modern Britain*, Oxford: Clarendon Press.

Graham, H. (1984) *Women, Health and the Family*, Brighton: Wheatsheaf.

Hales, C.N., Barker, D.J.P., Clark, P.M.S., Cox, L.J., Fall, C., Osmond, C. and Winter, P. (1991) Fetal and infant growth and impaired glucose tolerance at age 64, in D.J.P. Barker (ed.) *Fetal and Infant Origins of Adult Disease*, London: British Medical Journal.

Halsey, A.H. (1988) *British Social Trends since 1988*, London: Macmillan.

Hanrahan, J.P., Tager, I.B., Segal, M.R., Tosteson, T.D., Castile, R.G., VanVunakis, H., Weiss, S.T. and Speizer, F.E. (1992) The effect of maternal smoking during pregnancy on early infant lung function, *American Review of Respiratory Disease* 145: 1129–1135.

Hareven, T.K. (1978) *Transitions: the Family and the Life Course in Historical Perspective*, New York: Academic Press.

Hibbert, M.E., Hudson, I.L., Lanigan, A., Landau, L.I. and Phelan, P.D. (1990) Tracking of lung function in healthy children and adolescents, *Pediatric Pulmonology* 8: 172–177.

Holland, W.W., Halil, T., Bennett, A.E. and Elliott, A. (1969) Factors influencing the onset of chronic respiratory disease, *British Medical Journal* ii: 205–208.

Jacobson B. (1986) *Beating the Ladykillers: Women and Smoking*, London: Pluto Press.

Jones, P., Rodgers, B., Murray, R. and Marmot, M. (1994) Child developmental risk factors for adult schizophrenia in the British 1946 birth cohort, *Lancet* 344: 1398–1402.

Joseph Rowntree Foundation (1995) *Inquiry into Income and Wealth*, York: Joseph Rowntree Foundation.

Kaplan, H.B. (1991) Social psychology of the immune system: a conceptual framework and review of the literature', *Social Science and Medicine* 33: 909–923.

Kuh, D. and Wadsworth, M. (1991) Childhood influences on adult male earnings in a longitudinal study, *British Journal of Sociology* 42: 537–555.

Larsson, B., Bengtsson, C., Bjorntorp, P., Lapidus, L., Sjostrom, L., Svardsudd, K., Tibblin, C., Wedel, H., Welin, L. and Wilhelmsen, L. (1992) Is abdominal body fat distribution a major explanation for the sex difference in the incidence of myocardial infarction?' *American Journal of Epidemiology* 135: 266–273.

Lucas, A., Morley, R., Cole, T.J., Lister, G. and Leeson-Payne, C. (1992) Breast milk and subsequent intelligence quotient in children born preterm, *Lancet* 339: 261–264.

Maclean, M. and Eekelaar, J. (1983) *Children and Divorce*, Oxford: Oxford University Press.

Mann, S.L., Wadsworth, M.E.J. and Colley, J.R.T. (1992) Accumulation of factors influencing respiratory illness in members of a national birth cohort and their offspring, *Journal of Epidemiology and Community Health* 46: 286–292.

Marmot, M.G. and Syme, S.L. (1976) Acculturation and coronary heart disease in Japanese and Americans, *American Journal of Epidemiology* 104: 225–247.

Marmot, M.G. and Theorell, T. (1988) Social class and cardiovascular disease: the contribution of work, *International Journal of Health Services* 18: 659–674.

Martyn, C.N., Barker, D.J.P. and Osmond, C. (1988) Motorneurone disease and past poliomyelitis in England and Wales', *Lancet* 1: 1319–1322.

Mason, T.J. (1994) The descriptive epidemiology of lung cancer, in J.M. Samet (ed.) *Epidemiology of Lung Cancer*, New York: Dekker.

Mednick, S.A., Machon, R.A., Hultenen, M.O. and Bonnett, D. (1988) Adult schizophrenia following prenatal exposure to an influenza epidemic, *Archives of General Psychiatry* 45: 188–192.

Mok, J.Y.Q. and Simpson, H. (1984) Outcome for acute bronchitis, bronchiolitis, and pneumonia in infancy, *Archives of Disease in Childhood* 59: 306–309.

OPCS Social Survey Division (1995) *Health Survey for England 1993*, Series HS No. 3, London: HMSO.

Orth-Gomer, K. and Unden, A.-L. (1990) Type of behaviour, social support, and coronary risk: interaction and significance for mortality in coronary patients, *Psychosomatic Medicine* 52: 59–72.

Osborn, A.F. and Milbank, J.E. (1989) *The Effect of Early Education*, Oxford: Clarendon Press.

Osmond, C., Barker, D.J.P. and Slattery, J.M. (1990) Risk of death from cardiovascular disease and chronic bronchitis determined by place of birth in England and Wales, *Journal of Epidemiology and Community Health* 44: 139–141.

Pahl, J. (1989) *Money and Marriage*, London: Macmillan.

Paneth, N. and Susser, M. (1995) Early origins of coronary heart disease (the 'Barker hypothesis'): hypotheses, no matter how intriguing, need rigorous attempts at refutation, *British Medical Journal*, 310: 411–412.

Prior, I.A.M., Stanhope, I.M., Evans, J.G. and Salmoral, C.E. (1974) The Tokelau Island migrant study, *International Journal of Epidemiology* 3: 232–255.

Rantakallio, P. (1988) The longitudinal study of the north Finland birth cohort of 1966, *Paediatric and Perinatal Epidemiology* 2: 59–88.

Rodgers, B. (1978) Feeding in infancy and later ability and attainment, *Developmental Medicine and Child Neurology* 20: 421–426.

Rodgers, B. (1996) Reported parental behaviour and adult affective symptoms, 2: Mediating factors', *Psychological Medicine* 26: 63–77.

Rona, R.J. and Chinn, S. (1991) Father's unemployment and height of primary school children in Britain, *Annals of Human Biology* 18: 441–448.

Rona, R.J., Chinn, S. and Florey, C. du V. (1985) Exposure to cigarette smoking and children's growth, *International Journal of Epidemiology* 14: 402–409.

Rose, G. (1992) *The Strategy of Preventive Medicine*, Oxford: Oxford University Press.

Runciman, W.G. (1966) *Relative Deprivation and Social Justice*, London: Routledge.

Russell, B. (1926) *On Education, Especially in Early Childhood*, London: Allen & Unwin.

Siegrist, J., Matschinger, M., Cremer, P. and Seidel, D. (1988) Artherogenic risk in men suffering from occupational stress, *Artherosclerosis* 69: 211–218.

Social Trends (1994) London: HMSO.

Social Trends (1995) London: HMSO.

Strachan, D.P., Anderson, H.R., Bland, J.M. and Peckham, C. (1988) Asthma as a link between chest illness in childhood and chronic cough and phlegm in young adults, *British Medical Journal* 296: 890–893.

Strachan, D.P., Cox, B.D., Erzinclioglu, S.W., Walters, D.E. and Whichelow, M.J. (1991) Ventilatory function and winter fresh fruit consumption in a random sample of British adults, *Thorax* 46: 624–629.

Strope, G.L., Stewart, P.L., Henderson, F.W., Ivins, S.S., Steadman, H.C. and Henry, M.M. (1991) Lung function in school age children who had mild lower respiratory illness in early childhood, *American Review of Respiratory Disease* 144: 655–662.

Susser, E. and Lin, P. (1992) Schizophrenia after exposure to the Dutch hunger winter of 1944–1945, *Archives of General Psychiatry* 49: 983–988.

Tager, I.B., Weiss, S.T., Munoz, A., Rosner, B. and Speizer, F.E. (1983) Longitudinal study of the effects of maternal smoking on pulmonary function in children, *New England Journal of Medicine* 309: 699–703.

Theorell, T. (1992) The psycho-social environment, stress, and coronary heart disease, in M.G. Marmot and P. Elliott (eds) *Coronary Heart Disease Epidemiology: from Aetiology to Public Health*, Oxford: Oxford University Press.

Universities Funding Council (1990) *University Statistics 1988–1989*, Cheltenham: Universities' Statistical Record.

Wadsworth, M.E.J. (1981) Social class and generation differences in pre-school education, *British Journal of Sociology* 32: 560–582.

Wadsworth, M.E.J. (1991) *The Imprint of Time: Childhood, History and Adult Life*, Oxford: Oxford University Press.

Wadsworth, M.E.J. (1994) Prediction of adult disease, in I.B. Pless (ed.) *The Epidemiology of Childhood Disorders*, Oxford: Oxford University Press.

Wadsworth, M.E.J. (in press) Social and historical influences on parent–child relations in midlife, in C.D. Ryff and M.M. Seltzer (eds) *The Parental Experience in Midlife*, Chicago: University of Chicago Press.

Wadsworth, M.E.J. and Kuh, D. (1993) Are gains in child health being undermined? *Developmental Medicine and Child Neurology* 35: 742–745.

Wadsworth, M.E.J. and Maclean, M. (1986) Parents' divorce and children's life chances, *Children and Youth Services Review* 8: 145–159.

Wadsworth, M.E.J., Cripps, H.A., Midwinter, R.A. and Colley, J.R.T. (1985) Blood pressure at age 36 years and social and familial factors, cigarette smoking and body mass in a national birth cohort, *British Medical Journal* 291: 1534–1538.

Wald, N., Kiryluk, S., Darby, S., Doll, R., Pike, M. and Peto, R. (1988) *UK Smoking Statistics*, Oxford: Oxford University Press.

White, A., Freeth, S. and O'Brien, M. (1992) *Infant Feeding 1990*, London: HMSO.

Whitehead, R. and Paul, A.A. (1987) Changes in infant feeding in Britain during this century, in *Infant Nutrition and Cardiovascular Disease*, Southampton: MRC Environmental Epidemiology Unit.

Wyke, S. and Ford, G. (1992) Competing explanations for the association between marital status and health, *Social Science and Medicine* 34: 523–532.

Young, M. and Willmott, P. (1973) *The Symmetrical Family*, London: Routledge.

Chapter 10

Education, social circumstances and mortality

David Blane, Ian White and Jerry Morris

This chapter examines the relationships between education, deprivation–affluence and health. It reviews the mechanisms by which educational attainment could influence health; describes two measures or indices of deprivation which are widely used in Britain; and briefly reports on a study seeking to identify the relative importance to local mortality of levels of education and deprivation–affluence.

EDUCATION AND HEALTH

In many countries education rather than social class is used as the standard indicator of socioeconomic position. When it is used in this way, education levels produce a gradient in *mortality* similar to that produced by social class. The most advantaged individuals in terms of education have the lowest mortality rates, and mortality rates tend to increase in a stepwise fashion as individuals become more educationally disadvantaged. Table 10.1 illustrates this stepwise gradient with recent data for adults of working age in the United States. In 1989–90 those who had received sixteen years or more of formal education had the lowest mortality rates, while those who had received nine to eleven years had the highest rates (NCHS 1994). Other studies in the United States confirm the inverse relationship between education and mortality and suggest that the disparity in death rates of the well and poorly educated has increased in recent decades (Rogot *et al.* 1992; Pappas *et al.* 1993).

The education–health gradient has also been shown with measures of health other than mortality. In The Netherlands (Mackenbach 1993) *self-rated health* was worst and the prevalence of *chronic conditions* highest among those whose formal education was limited to primary school. These measures of health mostly improved in a stepwise fashion as the level of completed formal education increased (Table 10.2). Similarly in Finland (Lahelma *et al.* 1994) *self-rated health* was worst and the prevalence of *chronic conditions*, *long-term disability* and *long-standing illness* highest among those with no formal education, and all these measures of health

Table 10.1 Standardized death rates 1989–90 in the United States per
100,000 persons aged 25–64 of all races by years of education

Years of education	Male	Female
16 or more	318.9	194.4
13–15	501.5	280.7
12	602.1	292.5
9–11	739.8	318.3
0–8[a]	615.3	312.9

Note[a]: Few of those who grow up in the United States spend such a short time in school. The 'off-gradient' mortality rates of this group are probably due to the 'healthy migrant' effect.

Source: Derived from NCHS (1994: table 40).

Table 10.2 Variations in rates of self-reported ill health among those aged
16 years or more by level of education, The Netherlands 1981–5

Highest level of formal education completed	Chronic conditions	Self-rated health less than 'good'
Primary school	1.12	1.41
Lower secondary school	1.00	0.98
Secondary education	0.95	0.81
Vocational college	0.85	0.62
University	0.71	0.64

Note: The rates have been adjusted so that 1.00 is the mean rate for the total population and other scores represent deviations from this mean.

Source: Derived from Mackenbach (1993: table 1) .

improved in a stepwise gradient among both men and women as the level of formal education increased. In the United States (Winkleby *et al.* 1992) the use of *objective measures* of aspects of health thought relevant to cardiovascular risk revealed the same gradient with education, although the relationship appeared to be stronger among women than among men and generally the differences were smaller than for mortality and self-reported morbidity (Table 10.3). An inverse relationship between education and health has thus been found in a number of countries and by studies which have used a variety of measures of health.

Several mechanisms could be involved in the relationship between education and health. The material and cultural resources of the family of origin have been found to have a major influence on a child's educational attainment (Halsey *et al.* 1980). In Britain (OPCS 1990) more than half of the children of fathers in unskilled manual occupations obtained no formal educational qualifications, compared with a very small

Table 10.3 Age-adjusted mean values for cardiovascular risk factors, by
education, among those aged 25–64, United States 1979–86,
males and females separately

Risk measure			Years of education		
		Less than 12	12	13–15	16 or more
Mean systolic	Male	126	127	126	125
blood pressure	Female	117	118	116	114
(mm Hg)					
Mean diastolic	Male	76	77	77	76
blood pressure	Female	73	74	73	71
(mm Hg)					
Mean total	Male	198	198	203	196
cholesterol	Female	201	194	192	190
(mg/1,000 ml)					
Mean HDL	Male	44	44	44	46
cholesterol	Female	52	55	58	61
(mg/1,000 ml)					

Source: Derived from Winkleby *et al.* (1992: table 3).

Table 10.4 Highest qualification obtained by persons aged 25–49 not in
full-time education, by socioeconomic group of father,
percentage of males and females combined, Britain, 1987–8

Highest qualification level attained	[*Socioeconomic group of father*]	
	Professional	Unskilled manual
Degree or equivalent	36	3
Other qualifications	58	41
No qualifications	5	57

Source: Derived from OPCS (1990: table 7.7).

proportion of the children of fathers in professional occupations (Table
10.4). Education thus acts as a marker of material conditions during
childhood.

Second, after leaving formal education, individuals' educational qualifications are strong predictors of their occupation and, consequently, of
their income. In Britain (OPCS 1994) the gross weekly earnings of those
with no qualifications are approximately half of those with a degree or
equivalent (Table 10.5). Education therefore also acts as a marker of a
range of material and psychosocial conditions during adulthood.

Table 10.5 Usual gross weekly earnings of persons aged 20–69 in full-time
employment by highest qualification obtained, Britain 1992,
(£ sterling)

Highest qualification level obtained	Male	Female
No qualifications	220	146
Degree or equivalent	433	346

Source: Derived from OPCS (1994: table 8.6).

Third, educational level may influence receptivity to health promotion messages. In the United States length of education is a strong
predictor of the prevalence of adults with risk factors for coronary heart
disease (cigarette smoking, physical inactivity during leisure time, over-
weight and high blood pressure and cholesterol levels). Among those
with less than twelve years' education, 10.4 per cent of males and 8.5 per
cent of females had none of these risk factors, compared with respectively
25.4 and 26.9 per cent among those with more than twelve years' education (BRFSS 1994). The prevalence of tobacco smoking in the United
States during the period 1979–85 showed a stepwise gradient from 47 per
cent among males and 41 per cent among females who had completed
less than twelve years' education to, respectively, 18 per cent and 12
per cent among those with sixteen years' or more (Winkleby *et al.* 1992).
In Britain educational attainment has been shown to be related, independently of other socioeconomic factors, to dietary preferences (Braddon
et al. 1988) and leisure-time physical activity (Kuh and Cooper 1992)
during adulthood. Education may also affect health by allowing more
informed use of medical services, although some evidence (Leigh 1983)
suggests this may be of less importance than its effect on life style and
behaviour.

Fourth, the relationship between education and health may be spurious,
in the sense that a third variable determines individuals' capacity to
complete a prolonged period of formal education and influences their
capacity to maintain health and cope with disease (Pincus and Callahan
1994). A number of social-psychological constructs have been suggested
which could act as such a third variable, including 'self-efficacy' (Bandura
1991) and 'time preference' (Fuchs 1982). This line of reasoning has been
challenged by analyses of two large US data sets which strongly suggest
that the relationship between education and health is due primarily to the
direct effect of schooling on health rather than the effect of possible third
variables (Berger and Leigh 1989).

Fifth, the relationship between education and health could be due to
ill health during childhood that both limits educational attainment and
predisposes towards adult morbidity and premature mortality (Wolfe

1985). Although this undoubtedly occurs, it is unlikely to make more than a small contribution to the education gradient in health in Western 'developed' societies, where childhood morbidity sufficiently severe to damage educational prospects is too rare to account for the population-wide relationship between education and health.

In summary, there are several mechanisms by which education could be linked with health. Some of these are probably more important than others. Reverse causation, in the sense of childhood ill health interfering with educational attainment, is unlikely to be a major factor. Similarly, the evidence does not support the idea that a pre-existing genetic or personality factor is producing a spurious relationship. The remaining mechanisms are potentially important. Education may influence health behaviours during adulthood and, to the extent that these behaviours produce the desired effect upon health, they may influence the health of adults and that of their children. Also, education may be indexing material conditions during childhood and adulthood, and either or both of these may be influencing adult health. The study reported below attempted to assess the relative importance of these mechanisms. First, though, it is useful to consider the measures of material circumstances which were used.

DEPRIVATION INDICES

Since the 1970s a number of social indices have been developed in Britain. These use decennial census small area statistics to characterize localities (Holterman 1975; Bartley and Blane 1994). The Department of the Environment's index of local conditions (DoE 1994) has been used primarily for distributing central government funds to local authorities. Jarman Underprivileged Area scores (Jarman 1983, 1984) are designed to predict local variation in demand for general medical practitioner services. The Townsend index (Townsend *et al.* 1988) and the Carstairs index (Carstairs 1981; Carstairs and Morris 1989a, b) have been used mainly in social and medical research. As the latter two indices were used in the analyses to be reported here, they need to be considered in greater detail.

The Townsend Deprivation Index combines four variables. The percentage of private households containing economically active members who are unemployed and the percentage of private households with more than one person per room are included in the index as direct measures of deprivation due to unemployment and overcrowding. The percentage of private households which do not possess a car is included as a surrogate for current income. The percentage of private households not owner occupiers acts as a measure of wealth. To calculate the index score, the skewness of the distributions of the unemployment and overcrowding variables is first removed, using the log. transformation; next, the four variables are standardized to mean 0 and standard deviation 1; and finally they are summed to produce the local index score.

The Townsend index has proved to be a powerful predictor of local variations in health. It was first used, based on 1981 census data, in a study of variations in health between the 678 electoral wards of the Northern Region of England; index scores were found to correlate 0.82 with ward-level variations in health (Townsend *et al.* 1988). Local levels of deprivation statistically accounted for some two-thirds of the local variation in health. Recently these analyses have been repeated and extended to include a longer period of mortality follow-up and 1991 census data (Phillimore *et al.* 1994; Phillimore and Beattie 1994); the associations between deprivation and health remain as strong as previously. Interestingly, car ownership alone, the variable intended as an indicator of current income, is as strongly associated as the overall index with the local variation in health.

The Carstairs Deprivation Index is also constructed from four census variables, but unlike the Townsend index these refer to individuals rather than households. The overcrowding and car ownership variables are in other respects the same as Townsend's, but the Carstairs unemployment variable refers only to the proportion of unemployed *men*. Also, the proportion in the Registrar General's social classes IV and V replaces the housing tenure variable in the Townsend index. Each local variable is standardized to mean 0 and standard deviation 1. The Carstairs score is the summation of the four standardized values.

The Carstairs index has been widely used in studies of health inequalities. In Scotland the Carstairs scores are strongly associated with local variation in mortality (Carstairs and Morris 1991) and they have recently been used to demonstrate that differences in mortality experience linked with relative poverty have increased in the decade between the 1981 and 1991 censuses (McLoone and Boddy 1994).

A final issue concerns the interpretation of the results of studies which use area-based measures of deprivation such as the Townsend and the Carstairs indices. Do associations between these deprivation scores and health reflect characteristics of the areas or the characteristics of the individuals and households residing in those areas? And can area correlations between deprivation and health be discounted on the grounds of the ecological fallacy? OPCS longitudinal study data were recently used to compare the effect on mortality of individual-level deprivation and area-level deprivation (Sloggett and Joshi 1994). The comparison indicated that the excess mortality in deprived areas is wholly explained by the concentration in those areas of individuals with adverse personal or household socioeconomic factors. These results add weight to a substantial body of evidence using individuals as the unit of observation and they indicate that ecological correlation studies in which appropriate indices of deprivation have been used cannot be ignored on the grounds of the ecological fallacy (MacRae 1994).

So far in this chapter we have presented evidence that education level is associated with variation in several measures of health and explored a number of mechanisms which could account for this relationship. We have also considered the main indices of social deprivation–affluence which are currently in use in Britain and presented evidence that they too are powerful predictors of variation in health. Education level and deprivation–affluence are important dimensions of social class, and both could be major explanatory pathways in the well established association between social class and health (Morris *et al.* 1996). As well as its intrinsic interest, an exploration of the relationships between education, deprivation–affluence and health is therefore relevant to an understanding of social class differences in health. It was from this point of view that we undertook the following study.

EDUCATION, SOCIAL CIRCUMSTANCES AND MORTALITY IN THE LOCAL EDUCATION AUTHORITY AREAS OF ENGLAND

Our own analyses explore the nature of the relationships between education, deprivation–affluence and mortality. British studies have already examined this issue. The 1946 (Kuh and Wadsworth 1993) and the 1958 (Power *et al.* 1991) British birth cohort studies found that educational attainment and deprivation–affluence, measured in a variety of ways, were independently related to many aspects of health during early adulthood. The OPCS longitudinal study has shown that male adult mortality varies with both educational attainment and occupational social class (Goldblatt 1990). The present study adds to these results. It is an area-based study; unlike the birth cohort studies, its measure of health is mortality; and its measures of deprivation–affluence are more precisely targeted than the longitudinal study's use of occupational social class.

Method

The local education authority area was chosen as our unit of observation because the Department for Education had published these areas' pass rates in the General Certificate of Secondary Education (GCSE) examination for the year 1991/2 (DfE 1993). As our measure of educational attainment we used the proportion of boys and girls in each local education authority area who achieved grades A, B or C in at least five subjects in the GCSE examination at age 15/16. Generous collaborators at St Mary's Hospital Medical School and the Office of Population Censuses

Table 10.6 Rank correlations between educational attainment[a] and
deprivation index scores and several measures of mortality
in the 107 local education authority areas of England

Deprivation/mortality measure	Correlation with education
Carstairs index	−0.93
Townsend index	−0.89
Male all-cause mortality (all ages)	−0.77
Female all-cause mortality (all ages)	−0.64
Male coronary heart disease mortality (ages 15–64)	−0.68
Female CHD mortality (ages 15–64)	−0.69
Infant mortality (both sexes)	−0.60

Note: (a) Passing five or more GCSEs at grades A–C at age 15/16.

Table 10.7 Rank correlations between deprivation indices and mortality in
the 107 local education authority areas of England

Mortality	Carstairs	Townsend
Male all-cause (all ages)	0.86	0.76
Female all-cause (all ages)	0.73	0.60
Male coronary heart disease (ages 15–64)	0.77	0.67
Female coronary heart disease (ages 15–64)	0.75	0.64
Infant (both sexes)	0.63	0.56

and Surveys calculated, respectively, deprivation index scores and
mortality rates for these local education authority areas. Our measures of
deprivation were the Townsend and the Carstairs indices. These have
already been described in some detail, and in the present study the index
scores have been calculated from 1991 census information. Our measures
of mortality for the years 1990–2 were: (1) age-standardized all-cause
mortality per 1,000 at all ages, for males and females separately, (2) age-
standardized coronary heart disease mortality per 1,000 at ages 15–64,
males and females separately, and (3) infant mortality per 1,000 live births,
males and females combined. Several methods have been used to analyse
these data.

Results

The rank correlations of the 107 individual local education authority areas
have been calculated to examine the strength of the relationship between
the examination results and (1) the two deprivation indices and (2) each
of the measures of mortality (Table 10.6). Most strongly associated

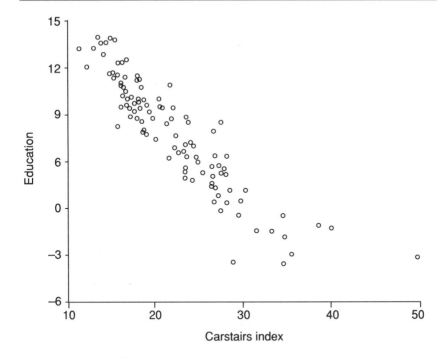

Figure 10.1 Scatter plot of educational attainment (percentage of 15–16 year olds passing five or more GCSEs at grades A–C) against Carstairs index scores in the 107 local education authority areas of England. Negative scores indicate affluence; positive scores, deprivation

were the inverse relationships between the examination results and the deprivation index scores. The rank correlations for the 107 individual LEAs are –0.93 for the Carstairs index (Figure 10.1) and –0.89 for the Townsend index, social deprivation thus statistically 'explaining' more than three-quarters of the variance in educational attainment. The mortality rates showed similar, if weaker, trends, with correlations which range from –0.60 for infant mortality to –0.77 for male all-cause mortality (Figure 10.2). All the rank correlations performed on the 107 individual areas significantly differ from zero at the 0.0001 level.

As well as being strongly associated with educational attainment, the deprivation index scores are also associated with mortality (Table 10.7). The strongest association is between the deprivation indices and male all-cause mortality (Figure 10.3), where deprivation statistically accounts for two-thirds of the variance. The associations with the other measures of adult mortality are somewhat weaker, while those with infant mortality are the weakest of all.

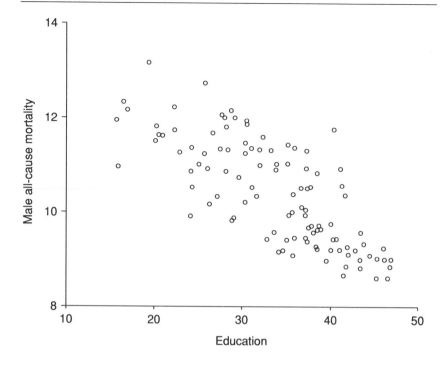

Figure 10.2 Scatter plot of educational attainment (percentage of 15–16 year olds passing five or more GCSEs at grades A–C) against male all-cause mortality (age-standardized, per thousand at all ages) in the 107 local education authority areas of England

Finally, we examined the relative importance of educational attainment and social deprivation–affluence as predictors of mortality. To investigate the hypothesis that local mortality is related to deprivation mainly through local standards of education, a multiple regression of each mortality measure on the GCSE success rate was performed, adjusted for the deprivation index scores (SAS/STAT). These results are presented as the fitted mortality values at the lowest and highest sextiles of deprivation (Table 10.8). To investigate the alternative hypothesis, that local mortality is related to educational attainment mainly through local levels of deprivation, a corresponding analysis was performed on the deprivation index scores, adjusted for GCSE success rate (Table 10.9).

The regression results differ according to whether the Carstairs or the Townsend index is included in the analysis. When the Carstairs index is used, controlling for the deprivation score (Table 10.8) largely abolishes the associations between the measure of educational attainment and local

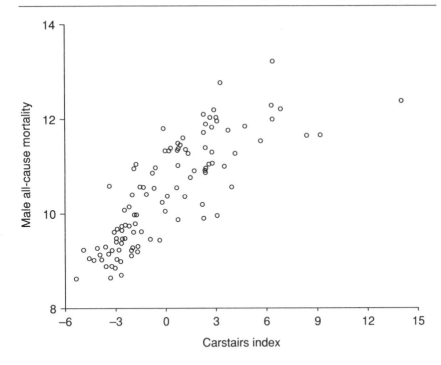

Figure 10.3 Scatter plot of Carstairs index scores against male all-cause mortality (age-standardized, per thousand at all ages) in the 107 local education authority areas of England. Negative scores indicate affluence; positive scores, deprivation

mortality rates. In contrast, the associations between local mortality rates and deprivation scores are largely unaffected by adjustment for the measure of educational attainment (Table 10.9). The Townsend index gives less clear-cut results, which to some extent contradict those obtained when the Carstairs index is used. The associations between education and mortality remain statistically significant after adjusting for the Townsend scores (Table 10.8), while controlling for education (Table 10.9) largely abolishes the associations between the Townsend scores and adult female and infant mortality.

Discussion

Two characteristics of the data analysed in this study should be noted. The data refer to local education authority *areas*, not to individuals. Although the interpretation of such ecological data must be cautious, the strength of the associations revealed by the analyses is striking. More

Table 10.8 Mortality by sextile of education, controlling for deprivation

Mortality index	Mortality (per 1,000), controlling for Carstairs index			Mortality (per 1,000), controlling for Townsend index		
	Least successful	Most successful	p value	Least successful	Most successful	p value
Male all-cause (all ages)	10.40	10.50	0.71	10.80	9.50	0.0030
Female all-cause (all ages)	6.40	6.60	0.40	6.70	5.90	0.0090
Male CHD (ages 15–64)	1.20	1.27	0.50	1.30	1.05	0.0200
Female CHD (ages 15–64)	0.35	0.32	0.55	0.39	0.21	0.0002
Infant (both sexes)	7.60	6.70	0.19	8.00	5.90	0.0020

Table 10.9 Mortality by sextile of deprivation, controlling for education

Mortality index	Sextile of Carstairs index			Sextile of Townsend index		
	Most deprived	Most affluent	p value	Most deprived	Most affluent	p value
Male all-cause (all ages)	12.40	9.50	0.0001	11.30	10.00	0.007
Female all-cause (all ages)	7.50	6.00	0.0001	6.70	6.30	0.230
Male CHD (ages 15–64)	1.69	1.02	0.0001	1.40	1.15	0.030
Female CHD (ages 15–64)	0.49	0.27	0.0001	0.36	0.33	0.600
Infant (both sexes)	8.50	6.80	0.0100	7.60	7.30	0.640

positively, ecological data can suggest area and population level relationships which can be missed by individual level studies. Second, education and mortality in this study refer to different generations. Our measure of local educational attainment is specific to 15/16 year olds, while the mortality measures relate either to infancy or primarily to adulthood.

Educational attainment in our analyses is strongly associated with mortality, 'explaining' between a third and three-fifths of the variance. As the education data refer to 15/16 year olds, and the mortality will have occurred either mostly in their parents' and grandparents' generations or among infants, we must postulate that our education measure is indexing some general characteristic of the community which is important to its members' health. Children's educational attainment is strongly influenced by the material and cultural resources of their parents (Halsey *et al.* 1980). Similar factors determine the conditions under which infants are reared and they also affect adult health. The Black Report (DHSS 1980) instanced smoking behaviour, leisure-time physical activity, dietary preferences and the informed use of health services as behavioural–cultural factors which may have this effect. More than these specific risk factors, however, the educational attainment of a community's children may also act as a summary measure of its general cultural level.

Our regression analyses investigated the relative importance of education and deprivation as predictors of mortality. When the Carstairs index was used as the measure of deprivation, the regression results were clear-cut. Controlling for deprivation largely abolished the associations between education and mortality, while controlling for education had little effect on the deprivation–mortality relationships. These results strongly suggest that deprivation, not education, is the more powerful statistical predictor of mortality. The results of the regression analyses were more complex when the Townsend Deprivation Index was used. The associations between education and mortality largely survived controlling for deprivation, while controlling for education greatly reduced the strength of the associations between deprivation and mortality, particularly female and infant mortality. In contrast to the results obtained by using the Carstairs index, the Townsend results suggest that education remains a significant predictor of mortality.

The interpretation of the results of our regression analyses is thus open to debate. It could be argued that the closer association between the Carstairs index and mortality means it is a better deprivation index than Townsend's. Alternatively, the difference between the regression results may partly reflect differences in the component items of the Carstairs and Townsend indices. The Carstairs index includes social class, more exactly the proportion of the population in social classes IV and V, as one of its components items. The social class component may introduce into the index a range of cultural and educational factors which are less directly associated with material deprivation than the other components of both indices. It is thus possible that, when we controlled for deprivation using the Carstairs index, we to some extent also controlled for education. This possibility raises the question of the independence of our measures of education and deprivation. Since education and deprivation are strongly correlated, our results about their relative importance are highly sensitive to mis-specification of the predictor variables (*Lancet* 1992). Educational attainment, for example, may be a better measure of social deprivation–affluence than the Carstairs and Townsend indices, although if this were so it would cast serious doubt on the current methodology for constructing deprivation indices.

On balance our results suggest that material deprivation is the stronger determinant of mortality in contemporary Britain, but that education retains a residual, independent effect. Since we have postulated that our measure of educational attainment indexes the general cultural and educational level of localities, our results tend to support the point of view that material, rather than behaviour–cultural, factors are the more important determinants of health. Before accepting this conclusion we need to question our methodology and whether we have overinterpreted our results. The many studies which have employed the Carstairs and Townsend indices give confidence in their use as measures of deprivation in an area. The number and grade of GCSE passes are a plausible measure of local educational attainment, which has the advantage of applying to virtually all of the relevant age group. Mortality as a 'hard' outcome measure of health also limits problems of differences in consultation rates, the subjective interpretation of symptoms and provision of medical facilities. Less satisfactorily, our measures of education and mortality refer to different generations and, as noted, our measures of education and deprivation may not be fully independent. Nevertheless, this ecological study has produced results which usefully contribute to current concern about the social determinants of health.

POLICY IMPLICATIONS

Our results have implications for *education* policy. We found that local levels of educational attainment are strongly associated with local levels of social deprivation–affluence, with the deprivation indices explaining some 80 per cent of the variance in GCSE pass rates. A comparable analysis for 1980-3 (DES 1984) found that 66–75 per cent of variation in examination achievement was statistically associated with variation in background social measures. The strength of these associations indicates that school systems at present do not much mitigate the effects of underlying social factors, and the relative stability of the associations during the past decade suggests that in this respect the educational reforms of the 1980s have meanwhile had little effect.

Our results also have implications for the general approach to *health* policy. A concern with health cannot be confined to those with responsibility for medical services. Clearly, material deprivation is still a powerful determinant of mortality risk. The component items of the deprivation indices used in the present analyses refer to income, wealth, housing standards and unemployment levels. Their effect on health indicates that policy in these areas is inescapably also health policy. An appreciation of the social determinants of health would benefit policy-making in many areas of sound governance.

REFERENCES

Bandura, A. (1991) Self-efficacy mechanism in physiological activation and health-promoting behaviour, in: J. Madden (ed.) *Neural Biology of Learning, Emotion and Affect*, New York: Raven Press.

Bartley, M. and Blane, D. (1994) Socioeconomic deprivation in Britain: commentary, *British Medical Journal* 309: 1478.

Behavioural Risk Factors Surveillance System (1994). Prevalence of adults with no known risk factors for coronary heart disease, *Morbidity and Mortality Weekly Report* 43: 61–69.

Berger, M.C. and Leigh, J.P. (1989) Schooling, self-selection and health, *Journal of Human Resources* 24: 433–455.

Braddon, F.E.M., Wadsworth, M.E.J., Davies, J.M.C. and Cripps, H.A. (1988) Social and regional differences in food and alcohol consumption and their measurement in a national birth cohort, *Journal of Epidemiology and Community Health* 42: 341–349.

Carstairs, V. (1981) Multiple deprivation and health state, *Community Medicine* 3: 4–13.

Carstairs, V. and Morris, R. (1989a). Deprivation and mortality: an alternative to social class? *Community Medicine* 11: 210–219.

Carstairs, V. and Morris, R. (1989b). Deprivation: explaining differences in mortality between Scotland and England and Wales, *British Medical Journal* 299: 886–889.

Carstairs, V. and Morris, R. (1991) *Deprivation and Health in Scotland*, Aberdeen: Aberdeen University Press.

Department for Education (1993) *Statistical Bulletin* 15/93.

Department of Education and Science (1984) *Statistical Bulletin* 13/84.

Department of the Environment (1994) *Index of Local Conditions*, London: DoE.

Department of Health and Social Security (1980). *Inequalities in Health: Report of a Research Working Group* ('The Black Report'), London: DHSS.

Fuchs, V.R. (1982) Time preference and health: an exploratory study, in V.R. Fuchs (ed.) *Economic Aspects of Health*, Chicago: University of Chicago Press.

Goldblatt, P. (ed.) (1990) *Mortality and Social Organisation*, LS series No. 6, London: HMSO.

Halsey, A.H., Heath, A.F. and Ridge, J.M. (1980) *Origins and Destinations: Family, Class and Education in Modern Britain*, Oxford: Clarendon Press.

Holterman, S. (1975) Areas of urban deprivation in Great Britain: an analysis of the 1971 census data, *Social Trends* 6: 33–47.

Jarman, B. (1983) Identification of underprivileged areas, *British Medical Journal* 286: 1705–1709.

Jarman, B. (1984) Underprivileged areas: validation and distribution of scores, *British Medical Journal* 289: 1587–1592.

Kuh, D.J.L. and Cooper, C. (1992) Physical activity at 36 years: patterns and childhood predictors in a longitudinal study, *Journal of Epidemiology and Community Health* 46: 114–119.

Kuh D.J.L. and Wadsworth M.E.J. (1993) Physical health status at 36 years in a British national birth cohort, *Social Science and Medicine* 37: 905–916.

Lahelma, E., Huuhka, M., Kunst, A. and Cavelaars, A. *et al.* (1994) Class, Education or Income? Analyzing health inequalities among Finnish men and women, paper presented to European Society of Medical Sociology, Vienna.

Lancet (1992). Measurement imprecision: ignore or investigate? *Lancet* 339: 587–588.

Leigh, J.P. (1983) Direct and indirect effects of education on health, *Social Science and Medicine* 17: 227–234.

Mackenbach, J.P. (1993) Inequalities in health in The Netherlands according to age, gender, marital status, level of education, degree of urbanisation and region, *European Journal of Public Health* 3: 112–118.

McLoone, P. and Boddy F.A. (1994) Deprivation and mortality in Scotland, 1981 and 1991, *British Medical Journal* 309: 1465–1470.

MacRae, K. (1994) Socioeconomic deprivation and health and the ecological fallacy, *British Medical Journal* 309: 1478–1479.

Morris, J.N., Blane, D.B. and White, I.R. (1996) Levels of mortality, education and social conditions in the 107 Local Education Authority areas of England, *Journal of Epidemiology and Community Health* 50: 15–17.

National Centre for Health Statistics (1994). *Health United States 1993*, Hyattsville, Md.: Public Health Service.

Office of Population Censuses and Surveys (1990). *General Household Survey 1988*, London: HMSO.

Office of Population Censuses and Surveys (1994). *General Household Survey 1992*, London: HMSO.

Pappas, G., Queen, S., Hadden, W. and Fisher, G. (1993) The increasing disparity in mortality between socioeconomic groups in the United States, 1960 and 1986, *New England Journal of Medicine* 329: 103–109.

Phillimore, P. and Beattie A. (1994) *Health and Inequality: the Northern Region, 1981–1991*, Department of Social Policy, University of Newcastle upon Tyne.

Phillimore, P., Beattie, A. and Townsend, P. (1994) Widening inequality of health in northern England, 1981–91, *British Medical Journal* 308: 1125–1128.

Pincus, T. and Callahan, L.F. (1994) Associations of low formal education levels and poor health status: behavioural, in addition to demographic and medical, explanations? *Journal of Clinical Epidemiology* 47: 355–361.

Power, C., Manor, O. and Fox, J. (1991) *Health and Class: the early years,* London: Chapman & Hall.

Rogot, E., Sorlie, P.D., Johnson, N.J. and Schmitt, C. (1992) *A Mortality Study of 1.3 million Persons by Demographic, Social and Economic Factors: 1979–1985 follow-up*, NIH Publication No. 92-3297, National Institutes of Health.

SAS/STAT (1987) *Guide for Personal Computers* (Version 6 edition), Cary, N.C.: SAS Institute.

Sloggett, A. and Joshi, H. (1994) Higher mortality in deprived areas: community or personal disadvantage? *British Medical Journal* 309: 1470–1474.

Townsend, P., Phillimore, P. and Beattie, A. (1988) *Health and Deprivation: Inequality and the North*, London: Croom Helm.

Winkleby, M.A., Jatulis, D.E., Frank, E. and Fortmann, S.P. (1992) Socioeconomic status and health: how education, income and occupation contribute to risk factors for cardiovascular disease, *American Journal of Public Health* 82: 816–820.

Wolfe, B.L. (1985) The influence of health on school outcomes: a multivariate approach, *Medical Care* 23: 1127–1138.

ACKNOWLEDGEMENTS

We are grateful to the Analytical Services Branch, Department for Education, the Health Statistics Department, Office of Population Censuses and Surveys, and the Academic Department of General Practice, St Mary's Hospital Medical School, for information and assistance.

Chapter 11

Transmission of social and biological risk across the life course

Chris Power, Mel Bartley, George Davey Smith and David Blane

Some environmental influences are suspected as having particularly long-term effects on health, in that they may be experienced in the early years of life but their major health effects occur several decades later. Both heart and respiratory disease are among the adult diseases for which potential early life influences have been suggested. Evidence relating to heart disease was provided by a Norwegian study by Forsdahl (1977). He reported that deaths from ischaemic heart disease in the 1970s were correlated with infant mortality around the time of birth of those dying in the 1970s. Taking infant mortality as an index of deprivation in childhood, he hypothesized that nutritional deprivation in childhood followed by relative affluence increased the risk of ischaemic heart disease in adult life. Similarly for adult respiratory disease, evidence for a role of childhood influences became available in the 1970s: in a prospective analysis, a higher rate of symptoms was found in adults who had experienced childhood respiratory illness (Colley *et al.* 1973).

Furthermore, long-term effects of environmental influences may extend to the next generation. A study of women who were pregnant during the Dutch Hunger Winter showed that their offspring who had been exposed to famine during the first and second trimester *in utero* later gave birth to lower weight babies when compared with mothers not exposed to famine (Lumey 1992). Thus grandmaternal influences may be relevant to the health of the offspring (Emanuel 1986).

The role of both social and biological mechanisms is raised when considering the transmission of risk across the life course. Since there is now great interest in the early life origins of adult disease, it is especially important to clarify how such mechanisms interrelate. Recent interest in early life has been stimulated by suggestions that events during gestation, as indicated by birth weight and placental weight, and in infancy, as indicated by growth in the first year, are associated with the risk of several important chronic diseases in later life – including cardiovascular disease, obstructive lung disease and diabetes (Barker 1992, 1994). For example, SMRs for cardiovascular disease in men were found to decrease

(a) Programming

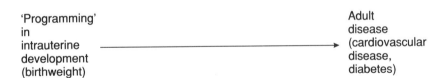

'Programming'
in
intrauterine
development
(birthweight)

Adult
disease
(cardiovascular
disease,
diabetes)

(b) Continuities in lifetime circumstances

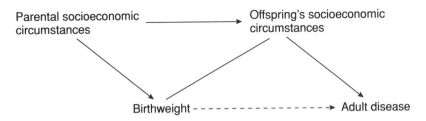

Parental socioeconomic
circumstances

Offspring's socioeconomic
circumstances

Birthweight - - - - - - - - - - - - - - - -→ Adult disease

Figure 11.1 Pathways linking early life with adult disease. (*a*) Programming.
(*b*) Continuities in lifetime circumstances

from 119 for those weighing less than 5.5 lb at birth to 74 for those
weighing more than 8.5 lb (Barker *et al.* 1993). As with other cardiovascular risk factors, the risks associated with birth weight appear to be
continuous and graded.

Two main explanations have been offered, as illustrated in Figure 11.1,
for the link between early life and adult disease. According to the first,
biological explanation (Figure 11.1a), events or circumstances *in utero* or
in infancy 'programme' the individual's risk before other risk factors are
encountered later in life. It is argued that environmental influences at
later ages still play some part in the aetiology of adult diseases, but only
within constraints imposed by early development.

According to the second explanation, birth weight and infant growth
could be acting, at least in part, as markers for other causal factors experienced both in childhood and later on. Given that social and economic
deprivation is known to influence intra-uterine development and early
growth (Butler and Alberman 1969; Wright *et al.* 1994) birth weight may
be a marker of the life chances of the family of origin. In Figure 11.1b
this is shown by the continuous lines linking birth weight and social

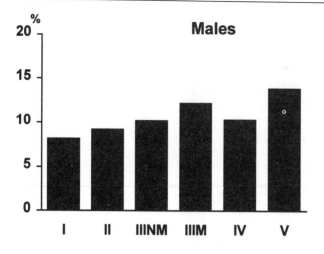

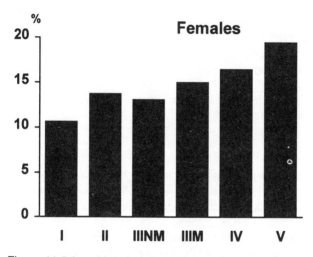

Figure 11.2 Low birth weight (under 6 lb) and social class at birth, 1958 cohort

circumstances and adult disease. Low birth weight babies in particular may be at higher risk of later social disadvantage than others, even within the same broadly defined social group. Paneth (1994) argues that 'a population with lower than average birthweight is a population whose subsequent education, housing and employment will likely differ from that of other populations'.

The two explanations may not be mutually exclusive, and additive or interactive effects may be operating. Thus biological risks established in early life may be exacerbated or attenuated by the consequences of subsequent socioeconomic circumstances. This is represented by the dotted lines linking to the other components in Figure 11.1b. So far, however, lifetime studies from birth to older ages have not been used to investigate early life origins of adult disease.

Although some studies of birth weight and particular risk factors, such as blood pressure, include the intervening period of childhood and young adulthood, only rarely has the relationship between birth weight and subsequent socioeconomic circumstances been examined. An exception is a recent analysis of longitudinal data available from the 1958 birth cohort (National Child Development Study – NCDS) (Bartley *et al.* 1994). This work showed that males born with a lower birth weight were more likely to experience adverse conditions in childhood and adolescence, as indicated by household overcrowding, lacking housing amenities and low social class.

It had already been demonstrated in early reports of the original 1958 birth survey that birth weight was associated with several social indicators, including social class (Butler and Alberman 1969). This is illustrated in Figure 11.2 with low birth weight (defined by a cut-off of under 6 lb) and father's occupation in 1958. As in numerous other studies, including present-day national statistics, there are more low weight babies in the lower social classes, the proportion decreasing with increasing social class.

As noted, Bartley and colleagues (1994) have provided evidence that relationships with birth weight extended beyond the immediate socioeconomic environment in early life to circumstances throughout childhood and adolescence. These analyses were, however, limited to male subjects, and, furthermore, they did not consider socioeconomic circumstances in adulthood in any detail. To illustrate how social and biological risks are linked and can be transmitted across the life course, this chapter extends previous analyses to females and to early adulthood.

A further aim is to investigate whether other factors at birth affect the relationship between birth weight and subsequent socioeconomic circumstances. For the purposes of this preliminary account, mother's parity at birth was selected as one such factor. Associations between parity and birth weight are well documented (Butler and Alberman 1969). Parity is also associated with socioeconomic circumstances, with women of higher parity generally having poorer social conditions. Thus parity may exert an effect on the relationship between early life factors and later adult disease in three ways: through its association with socioeconomic circumstances at birth which continue thereafter; through a biological effect; or through an artefactual association between measures, such as parity and overcrowding. It is possible, therefore, that parity may modify the associations between birth weight and subsequent socioeconomic circumstances. Hence an examination of parity-related effects is included in the

Table 11.1   The 1958 British birth cohort: all living in Great Britain born 3–9
March 1958 (including immigrants 1958–74)

| | PMS 1958 Birth | National Child Development Study | | | | |
		1965 Age 7	1969 Age 11	1974 Age 16	1981 Age 23	1991 Age 33
Target sample	17,773	16,883	16,835	16,915	16,457	16,455
Data sources	Parents	Parents School Tests Medical	Parents School Tests Medical Subject	Parents School Tests Medical Subject Census	Subject Census	Subject Spouse/ partner Children
Achieved sample	17,414	15,458	15,503	14,761	12,537	11,407

present chapter. Analyses are based, as in an earlier report, on longitudinal data available in the 1958 birth cohort study (Ferri 1993).

STUDY SAMPLE

The 1958 British birth cohort (National Child Development Study) is summarized in Table 11.1. Birth weight (in ounces) was recorded for all children in the birth survey (Perinatal Mortality Survey, PMS), which included births to parents resident in Britain in one week in March 1958 (Butler and Bonham 1963). Surviving children were followed up at ages 7, 11, 16, 23 and 33. In general, the sample has remained representative to age 23, although some attrition has occurred. Questions about the social and economic circumstances of cohort members were included in each follow-up. Several indicators of social position were derived from these data (Bartley et al. 1994). Table 11.2 gives details of two such indicators, each of which combines social class with the ownership of assets. As will be shown below, each subgroup contained a sizeable proportion of the population, at least initially at the age 7 follow-up; that is, the indicators were not just reflecting an extreme minority group. Similar measures have not yet been devised to characterize socioeconomic circumstances in adulthood. Hence the preliminary analysis of adulthood circumstances is based on social class. This is derived from the current or most recent occupation reported by the subject at age 33 (in a small number it was obtained

Table 11.2 Socioeconomic measures

Measure	Definition
Social class and overcrowding	I+II IIIN to V and one person per room or less IIIN to V and more than one person per room
Social class and housing amenities[a]	I+II IIIN to V, sole use of household amenities IIIN to V, without sole use of amenities

Note: (a) Inside WC, hot water supply and bathroom.

from the 23-year sweep). Women are classified on the basis of their own occupation.

For birth weight a cut-off of 6 lb (2,721 g) was used for males, identifying approximately 10 per cent of male births as low weight. A similar proportion of females, who tend to be lighter at birth, was obtained with a cut-off of 5 lb 9 oz (2,523 g). Information on parity was also available from the PMS: it was recorded as the number of previous viable pregnancies over twenty-eight weeks.

RESULTS

Table 11.3 shows the relationship between birth weight and socioeconomic circumstances defined by social class and overcrowding in the household for both sexes separately. A greater percentage of children with low weight at birth experienced a combination of lower social class and overcrowding in the household at later ages. For example, at age 7 about 43 per cent of males with low birth weight, compared with 35 per cent not of low birth weight, were in classes III N to V and in overcrowded homes. This association was consistent at each successive age and for both sexes, although for females the trends are slightly weaker.

Table 11.4 shows the relation between birth weight and socioeconomic circumstances as defined by social class and household amenities. A greater percentage of children with low weight at birth subsequently experienced lower social class and lacking or sharing household amenities. The association is consistent at each successive age, and, again, the associations appear to be stronger for males.

These data provide evidence that the relationship between birth weight and social circumstances seen at birth (Figure 11.2) persists throughout childhood. This finding is not surprising, since it reflects continuities in the socioeconomic circumstances of the birth family. However, during early adulthood individuals embark upon their own socioeconomic trajectories, and as a result of intergenerational mobility they may move to

Table 11.3 Birth weight and socioeconomic circumstances in childhood (%), defined according to social class and household overcrowding

			Socioeconomic circumstances (overcrowding)				
Age	Birth weight	Social classes I and II	Social class IIINM to V, no overcrowding	Social class IIINM to V, overcrowded	%	(n)	Overall test of association
Males							
7	Under 6 lb	16.9	40.2	42.9	100	(326)	8.9 (2 df)
	6 lb and over	22.2	42.5	35.3	100	(3,044)	$p = 0.01$
11	Under 6 lb	19.3	41.7	39.0	100	(326)	9.05 (2 df)
	6 lb and over	26.1	41.5	32.4	100	(3,044)	$p = 0.01$
16	Under 6 lb	24.2	54.6	21.2	100	(326)	4.12 (2 df)
	6 lb and over	27.7	55.2	17.1	100	(3,044)	$p = 0.13$
Females							
7	Under 5 lb 9 oz	21.4	39.0	39.6	100	(318)	2.3 (2 df)
	5 lb 9 oz and over	22.4	42.2	35.4	100	(2,879)	$p = 0.32$
11	Under 5 lb 9 oz	23.0	36.5	40.6	100	(318)	10.4 (2 df)
	5lb 9 oz and over	26.5	41.9	31.6	100	(2,879)	$p = 0.006$
16	Under 5lb 9 oz	25.8	54.1	20.1	100	(318)	3.4 (2 df)
	5lb 9 oz and over	28.6	55.2	16.3	100	(2,879)	$p = 0.19$

Table 11.4 Birth weight and socioeconomic circumstances in childhood (%), defined according to social class and household amenities (inside wc, hot water supply and bathroom)

Age	Birth weight	Social classes I and II	Socioeconomic circumstances (household amenities)				Overall test of association
			Social class IIINM to V, sole use of amenities	Social class IIINM to V, lacking/sharing amenities	%	(n)	
Males							
7	Under 6 lb	16.9	63.8	19.3	100	(326)	9.8 (2 df)
	6 lb and over	22.2	63.9	13.9	100	(3,044)	p = 0.008
11	Under 6 lb	19.3	67.8	12.9	100	(326)	12.3 (2 df)
	6 lb and over	26.1	65.6	8.4	100	(3,044)	p = 0.002
16	Under 6 lb	24.2	69.3	6.4	100	(326)	3.41 (2 df)
	6 lb and over	27.7	67.7	4.6	100	(3,044)	p = 0.18
Females							
7	Under 5 lb 9 oz	21.4	61.0	17.6	100	(318)	3.6 (2 df)
	5 lb 9 oz and over	22.4	63.9	13.7	100	(2,879)	p = 0.16
11	Under 5 lb 9 oz	23.0	65.7	11.3	100	(318)	3.9 (2 df)
	5 lb 9 oz and over	26.5	65.0	8.5	100	(2,879)	p = 0.14
16	Under 5 lb 9 oz	25.8	68.6	5.7	100	(318)	2.6 (2 df)
	5 lb 9 oz and over	28.6	67.4	4.1	100	(2,879)	p = 0.28

Table 11.5 Low birth weight and social class at age 33 (%)

	Men		Women	
Social class	Under 6 lb (561)	6 lb and over (5,067)	Under 5 lb 9 oz (608)	5 lb 9 oz and over (5,021)
I	5.9	6.8	1.6	2.2
II	24.1	29.5	23.4	26.8
IIINM	10.7	11.4	40.5	39.9
IIIM	38.0	34.6	8.6	7.9
IV	13.0	13.2	20.1	18.7
V	7.5	4.5	5.9	4.5
χ^2 for trend	11.7 (1 df) $p < 0.001$		5.2 (1 df) $p < 0.05$	

social groups which differ from those of their family of origin. It is therefore also of interest to establish whether the associations shown for childhood extend into adulthood.

Table 11.5 compares adult occupational social class in men and women having had low weight at birth with others who were not low weight. By age 33 there are significant differences in the social class distribution of subjects with low weight at birth and those whose weight was greater, the former being more likely to have a low social class. This is evident for both men and women. Overall, these preliminary analyses of adult social position suggest, therefore, that, in this cohort at least, the relationship between birth weight and social circumstances extends beyond childhood to early adulthood.

Further comparisons of the relationship were made to clarify whether the results were influenced by the well established association between birth weight, social circumstances and parity (Table 11.6). Although the relationship between birth weight and class at age 33 varied slightly according to parity status (with statistically significant trends for some but not all parity groups), in general a smaller proportion of subjects with low weight at birth are classified in social classes I and II at age 33. The association between birth weight and subsequent socioeconomic circumstances did not, therefore, appear to be accounted for by differences in parity status of the low weight births compared with others. Table 11.6 also suggests that mothers' parity at birth is related to the social class of their offspring in early adulthood: a greater percentage with 0 or 1 parity occupy social classes I and II at age 33. Conversely, those with high parity are more likely to occupy unskilled manual positions subsequently at age 33.

Table 11.6 Low birth weight[a] and social class (%) at age 33, according to mother's parity in 1958

Social class	[Parity] [0] Low weight	[0] Not low weight	[1] Low weight	[1] Not low weight	[2] Low weight	[2] Not low weight	[3+] Low weight	[3+] Not low weight
Men	(220)	(1,850)	(160)	(1,663)	(83)	(773)	(98)	(781)
I and II	39.5	40.6	23.8	39.3	24.1	33.2	23.5	22.8
IIIN	12.7	14.1	11.3	11.4	10.8	9.3	5.1	7.6
IIIM	31.8	31.2	48.8	33.1	41.0	40.0	36.7	40.2
IV	11.4	10.6	10.6	11.7	13.3	13.2	20.4	22.5
V	4.5	3.5	5.6	4.6	10.8	4.3	14.3	6.9
χ^2 trend (1 df)		0.55 n.s.		4.6 p = 0.03		4.6 p = 0.03		1.09 n.s.
Women	(265)	(1,812)	(166)	(1,584)	(84)	(817)	(93)	(808)
I and II	27.5	31.7	28.3	30.9	22.6	27.8	14.0	20.3
IIIN	41.1	41.8	36.7	40.5	36.9	40.8	48.4	33.3
IIIM	7.9	7.2	9.6	8.6	7.1	7.6	9.7	8.8
IV	16.2	15.6	21.1	16.5	27.4	18.7	22.6	29.8
V	7.2	3.6	4.2	3.5	6.0	5.1	5.4	7.8
χ^2 trend (1 df)		4.8 p = 0.03		2.5 n.s.		3.8 n.s.		1.07 n.s.

Note: (a) Low birth weight was defined as under 6 lb (males) and under 5 lb 9 oz (females).

DISCUSSION

From the evidence presented here, it appears that birth weight is related to subsequent social circumstances from childhood to early adulthood. It is especially notable that the relationship between birth weight and social circumstances at birth is reproduced thirty-three years later. This has important implications when considering the transmission of biological risks across the life course, and, in particular, in relating early life to adult health outcomes.

Links between early life and adult disease may, as has been proposed, operate through biological 'programming' during the intra-uterine period or during early infancy (Barker 1992, 1994). However, the difficulty of attributing a causal role to developmental factors in the aetiology of later disease has long been recognized. The confounding of development with later socioeconomic and environmental exposure has been seen as particularly problematic in this regard. For example, forty-five years ago when Isabelle Leitch discussed whether optimal growth in early life influenced later health she cautioned that:

> Since all the social circumstances, housing, sanitation, spacing of population and hence exposure to infection, as well as education and, on the whole, facilities for prompt medical attention, improve with, and at about the same rate as growth, it is difficult to judge whether inhibition of growth itself has any effect on morbidity.
>
> (Leitch, 1951)

These comments show how Leitch recognized the need to examine whether aspects of later childhood, adolescence and adulthood could account for the association of early growth with adult disease. Relationships demonstrated here using the 1958 birth cohort support the need for caution.

Continuity in social circumstances has been demonstrated for male cohort members (Bartley *et al.* 1994): the relationship between birth weight and subsequent social circumstances was not limited to a comparison of low weight versus others, but seemed to apply across the birth weight distribution. Using birth weight quintiles, the percentage with poorer socioeconomic circumstances subsequently during their childhood declined with increasing birth weight. This appears to be a fairly evenly graded relationship, mirroring the grading shown in some studies for adult mortality and birth weight. However, repeating the analyses of birth weight quintiles and socioeconomic circumstances for females (unpublished) revealed less consistent relationships.

With the data presented here for females, the relationship between birth weight and social circumstances was consistent but, in general, weaker than that for males. Sex differences are also apparent for some but not all adult disease outcomes, with women having a weaker relationship, for example, between growth in early life and adult chronic bronchitis (Barker, 1992, 1994). The different meaning of birth weight for males and females is raised by the results. Despite their lower birth weights, it is widely accepted that female babies are less susceptible to environmental insult than males. In this cohort, for example, mortality (including stillbirths and neonatal deaths) was higher among males than among females in every 500 g birth weight subdivision, the maximum difference being between 2,501 g and 3,000 g, when male mortality was higher than the female by 60 per cent (Butler and Bonham 1963: 132, table 42). The significantly higher perinatal mortality of males was seen for most causes of death (Butler and Bonham 1963: 268, table 84). In view of these sex differences we used a lower cut-off to define low birth weight for females; none the less the relationships remained, if anything, stronger for males. Extension of analyses initially confined to men to also include women underscores the complexity of relationships between early life and adult diseases. However, further investigation of sex differences may shed light on the relative importance of social and biological pathways.

Birth weight is influenced by many other factors as well as the sex of the infant (Alberman and Evans 1989; Power 1995). Such factors may also affect the association between birth weight and subsequent socioeconomic circumstances. Birth order may be especially important in this regard, given that first and later births tend to be of lower weight: in national statistics for England and Wales 7.3 per cent of births to mothers with no previous live births and 6.2 per cent of births to mothers with three or more previous live births are low weight (less than 2,500 g), compared with 4.7 per cent and 5.0 per cent among those with one or two previous births respectively (Power 1995). Since large family size may indicate poorer social circumstances, disproportionate representation of such families among the low weight group could potentially affect the associations described in this chapter. It was necessary therefore to assess birth order related effects, which was achieved here with information on the mother's parity. From these comparisons it was apparent that continuities in social circumstances had occurred, as indicated by parity at birth and social class at age 33. Associations between birth weight and social class at age 33 varied with mother's parity status, but even so, the general trend of poorer social status among those with low weight at birth emerged within each level of parity status. The association between birth weight and subsequent socioeconomic circumstances is not restricted, therefore, to those in high parity households, where overcrowding and related poor social environment are likely to be more common. It remains to be seen whether other influences on birth weight, such as length of gestation, modify relationships with birth weight, with respect both to subsequent socioeconomic circumstances and to adult disease outcomes.

Indicators of socioeconomic position

In the research into birth weight and adult disease the relationships were found to be independent of social class in subjects for whom an occupation was ascertained (Barker 1992; Barker *et al.*, 1993). This was interpreted as evidence against 'continuity of disadvantage'. However, such conclusions fail to take account of the well documented limitations of social class, especially as a measure of lifetime social conditions. Both here and elsewhere (Bartley *et al.* 1994), analyses of social position are not based solely on occupational class. While social class is a useful measure, it is increasingly recognized that it is only a crude representation of social conditions: income and living standards vary widely within social class groups. Thus socioeconomic indicators were constructed that combined social class and housing conditions. Such measures have been suggested as alternative indicators of socioeconomic position (Goldblatt 1990). Elsewhere we examined additional socioeconomic indicators representing housing adequacy and financial difficulties throughout childhood in order to confirm the relationships with birth weight (Bartley *et al.* 1994).

The preliminary analyses of socioeconomic position at age 33 described here rely on social class. For women in particular own social class at age 33 is a poor indicator of social status and living standards. In future work it will be necessary to develop socioeconomic indicators appropriate to the period in which the adulthood years of this cohort are spent. Indicators that were useful to differentiate socioeconomic circumstances in the 1950s and 1960s, during the cohort members' childhood and adolescence, will be less pertinent to the cohort with increasing age. Even between the ages of 7 and 16 the proportion living in overcrowded conditions and homes lacking or sharing amenities (as defined in Table 11.2) declined substantially. This signifies marked social changes, especially in relation to improved housing standards. Indicators of social circumstances in early adulthood will therefore need to be modified in order to achieve a meaningful social stratification of the population.

Implications

The preliminary analyses of socioeconomic position at age 33 based on social class suggest that the socioeconomic trajectories of individuals will continue to differ systematically according to birth weight into mid- and later life. Thus birth weight appears to be acting as a marker for subsequent socioeconomic circumstances. Confounding may, therefore, be a major problem in studies which have not adequately controlled for socioeconomic circumstances. Another interpretation of the results presented here is that they represent an accumulation of risk, both social and biological. Future work may show this accumulation to be particularly important for later disease. However, the question remains whether these relationships will explain the hypothesized biological 'programming' and consequent adult disease outcome.

Without a clearer understanding of the transmission of biological and social risk across the life course how far should 'programming' hypotheses be considered by those concerned with policies to reduce adult disease risk? Should the emphasis in the prevention of adult disease refocus towards maternal health and environment in infancy? From the perspective of infant and child health the argument is already well established, for example in efforts to reduce infant mortality and disability associated with low birth weight. But, given current uncertainties regarding studies linking early and later life, it can be argued that it is inappropriate to shift efforts to prevent disease in adulthood to maternal nutrition and infant health (Paneth and Susser 1995).

CONCLUSIONS AND FUTURE DIRECTIONS

Work on the effect of early life environment on health in adulthood promises fresh insights into the shaping of adult health and disease, because it may be that later life events do not tell the whole aetiological story. However, it is necessary to take account of intervening factors, since the early life–adult disease relationship could be partly attributable to the later socioeconomic circumstances with which birth weight is associated. Longitudinal data from the 1958 birth cohort provide evidence that a link between birth weight and socioeconomic circumstances exists in childhood and through to age 33. Although birth weight is temporally prior, the associations shown here are not presented as evidence that birth weight 'causes' social deprivation in childhood or subsequently, merely that it is associated with it. In other words, low birth weight may be acting as a marker of a particularly disadvantaged life trajectory.

Differences in socioeconomic circumstances among birth weight groups will also have implications for health-damaging and promoting behaviours to which individuals are exposed. Underpinning this expectation are numerous population studies showing differences in health-related behaviours between social groups. Such differences in life styles have been considered as possible explanations in the Black Report *Inequalities in Health* and in subsequent updates of this topic (Davey Smith *et al.* 1990). Differences in socioeconomic circumstances by age 33 among birth weight groups will similarly have implications for future material circumstances. Those in professional, managerial and technical occupations can look forward to relative job security, incremental pay increases, paid holidays (Reid 1989) and sick leave, and an occupational pension (Reid 1989) in the majority of cases (Giddens 1978). Access to other resources such as privately owned housing and transport will be available (Gallie *et al.* 1994), and, in addition, the risk of work accidents and occupational disease will be low. In contrast, those in skilled manual work will have variable financial security, with poorer provision for holiday and sick pay, and inferior pensions, so that many will be dependent on State benefits in old age. Exposure to hazardous working environments and accidents will also be greater, particularly for those in unskilled manual jobs (Bartley 1991). It is important to extend the study of relationships between birth weight and adult characteristics in further work on the 1958 birth cohort, in order to improve understanding of the transmission of biological and social risks across the life course.

Given the association between birth weight and social class at birth, and between social position at birth and in adult life, it would be surprising if birth weight were unrelated to adult social and economic conditions. Thus, if progress is to be achieved, it will be necessary, in this and other work, to acknowledge the complexity of pathways combining biological, socioeconomic and probably behavioural risk over the life course. For clarification of interrelationships we need to incorporate models of *both* early *and* later life influences. Studies which follow individuals from birth through to adult life will be invaluable in this task.

REFERENCES

Alberman, E. and Evans, S.J.W. (1989) The epidemiology of prematurity: aetiology, prevalence and outcome, *Annales Nestlé* 47: 69–88.

Barker, D.J.P (ed.) (1992) *Fetal and Infant Origins of Adult Disease*, London: British Medical Journal.

Barker, D.J.P. (1994) *Mothers,Babies and Disease in Later Life*, London: British Medical Journal.

Barker, D.J.P., Osmond, O., Simmonds, S.J. and Wield, G.A. (1993) The relation of small head circumference and thinness at birth to death from cardiovascular disease in adult life, *British Medical Journal* 306: 422–426.

Bartley, M. (1991) Health and labour force participation, *Journal of Social Policy* 20: 327–364.

Bartley, M., Power, C., Blane, D. and Davey Smith, G. (1994) Birthweight and later socio-economic disadvantage: Evidence from the 1958 British cohort study, British Medical Journal 309: 1475–1478.

Butler, N.R. and Alberman, E. (1969) *Perinatal Problems*, Edinburgh: Churchill Livingstone.

Butler, N.R. and Bonham, D.G. (1963) *Perinatal Mortality*, Edinburgh: Livingstone.

Colley, J.R.T., Douglas, J.W.B. and Reid, D.D. (1973) Respiratory disease in young adults: influence of early childhood lower respiratory tract illness, social class, air pollution, and smoking, *British Medical Journal* 3: 195–198.

Davey Smith, G., Bartley, M. and Blane, D. (1990) The Black Report on socioeconomic inequalities in health ten years on, *British Medical Journal* 301: 373–377.

Emanuel, I. (1986) Maternal health during childhood and later reproductive performance, in: H.M. Wisnieski and D.A. Snider (eds) *Mental Retardation:*

Research Education Technology Transfer, Annals of the New York Academy of Sciences.

Ferri, E. (1993) *Life at 33: the fifth Follow-up of the National Child Development Study*, London: National Children's Bureau.

Forsdahl, A. (1977) Are poor living conditions in childhood and adolescence an important risk factor for arteriosclerotic heart disease? *British Journal of Preventative and Social Medicine* 31: 91–95.

Gallie, D. and Vogler, C. (1994) Labour market deprivation, welfare and collectivism, in D. Gallie, C. Marsh and C. Vogler (eds) *Social Change and the Experience of Unemployment*, Oxford: Oxford University Press.

Gallie, D., Marsh, C. and Vogler, C. (1994) *Social Change and the Experience of Unemployment*, Oxford: Oxford University Press.

Giddens, A. (1978) *The Class Structure of the Advanced Societies*, London: Heinemann.

Goldblatt, P. (1990) Mortality and alternative social classification, in P. Goldblatt (ed.) *Longitudinal Study: Mortality and Social Organisation 1971–1981*, London: HMSO.

Leitch, I. (1951) Growth and health, *British Journal of Nutrition* 5: 142–151.

Lumey, L.H. (1992) Decreased birthweights in infants after maternal *in utero* exposure to the Dutch famine of 1944–1945, *Paediatric and Perinatal Epidemiology* 6: 240–253.

Paneth, N. (1994) The impressionable fetus – fetal life and adult health, *American Journal of Public Health* 84: 1372–1374.

Paneth, N. and Susser, M. (1995) Early origin of coronary heart disease (the 'Barker hypothesis'), *British Medical Journal* 310: 411–412.

Power, C. (1995) Children's physical development, in B. Botting (ed.) *The Health of our Children: a Review in the Mid 1990s*, London: HMSO.

Reid, I. (1989) *Social Class Differences in Britain*, third edition, London: Fontana.

Wright, C.M., Waterston, A. and Aynsley-Green, A. (1994) Effect of deprivation on weight-gain in infancy, *Acta Paediatrica* 83: 357–359.

ACKNOWLEDGEMENTS

Chris Power is a scholar of the Canadian Institute of Advanced Research and acknowledges its support. We thank Martin Shipley for statistical advice.

Chapter 12

Unpaid work, carers and health

Maria Evandrou

Health and social care provision to people with physical or mental impairments, or to frail elderly people, constitutes a major social policy issue in Britain (Parker and Lawton 1994; Allen and Perkins 1995). With the family providing the bulk of support, informal carers are pivotal in maintaining disabled and frail people in the community. However, only recently have carers been formally placed in the policy arena. It is now the formal responsibility of state service providers to assess carers for community care support. Whilst the government White Paper *Caring for People* (DoH 1989) explicitly located support for carers within state providers' responsibilities, the NHS and Community Care Act 1990 was silent on this. The Carers' (Recognition and Services) Act 1995 redresses this somewhat. Under the 1995 Act, local authorities are formally obliged to carry out a separate assessment of the carer when assessing the cared-for-person for service support. What is critical here is that carers' views, their circumstances and their ability to continue providing care support should be taken into account when the needs of the dependent person are reviewed and a care package developed.

The extent to which the Act's implementation constitutes a real and ongoing 'act of care' is debatable (Clements 1996). Given financing concerns, it remains to be seen whether carers' assessments will contribute to higher levels of support or earlier intervention, and thus help relieve carers' pressures and workload. However, what is clear is that health and social service planners and providers, across statutory and independent sectors, require information about carers: how many carers there are, who they are, what care work they provide and for whom, how such caring impacts on their own lives, and how it affects their own quality of life. There has been a growing number of studies on informal caring; however, little is known about the impact on carers' health, in the short and the longer term, and how this inter-relates to socio-economic position.

The differential impact of caring on carers' lives may further contribute to existing health and income inequalities in society, particularly over the longer term. This chapter discusses the existing research evidence, focusing on the health and socioeconomic position of carers in Britain, and highlights the gaps in our knowledge base, suggesting ways forward for the future. It then goes on to present new evidence regarding the relationship between caring for a dependent person and the carer's health status. Finally some of the policy implications of the research findings are discussed.

WHAT DO WE MEAN BY CARING?

The extent to which caring is a 'natural' part of everyday life, and thus not an issue for public policy, should be debated (Askham *et al.* 1992). Is the provision of care for a sick spouse or infirm elderly relative, every day, over fifty hours per week, for five years or more, part of these 'natural' relations? If not, where should the line be drawn? Should it be according to the relationship with the cared-for person, or to the intensity or duration of care given? Informal caring in the context of this chapter is taken as *additional family responsibilities due to looking after someone who is sick, handicapped or elderly*. It is provided within households and is usually unpaid.

Care can take a variety of forms: physical, practical, personal, social or emotional. It may be light or heavy-duty, intermittent or continuous, short or longer-term. Thus the experience of caring will vary and carers themselves represent a heterogeneous group. There are both positive and negative aspects to caring, and the caring relationship is essentially a dynamic one. Many carers derive gratification and satisfaction at different stages of the caring relationship and for varying lengths of time. The quality of such interaction is infrequently addressed or researched. Studies indicate that many carers are able to adjust successfully to the caring role, taking on new and/or additional demands (Twigg *et al.* 1990; Parker 1990, 1993). Nolan's work shows how high levels of stress among carers can be combined with high levels of satisfaction and demonstrates the reciprocal and dynamic nature of the caring relationship (Nolan and Grant 1992; Grant and Nolan 1993). It is difficult to capture such dynamic aspects of the caring relationship from cross-sectional data. Ideally one requires longitudinal data with representative samples, particularly where the causal nature of any relationship is investigated.

Carers' responses to their caring role have been located within the following three modes: (1) the *engulfed* mode – where carers make their own lives completely secondary to the caring task, and often there is no alternative emotional focus in their lives; (2) the *balancing/boundary* mode – where the carer is able to maintain a distance between her/himself and the caring situation; (3) and the *symbiotic* mode – where caring tasks are integrated with other activities and contribute to a positive self-image, although isolation from the wider society may also be experienced (Twigg *et al.* 1990; Twigg and Atkin 1994). This offers a useful approach to conceptualizing carers' experiences, encompassing both problems and satisfactions.

CARING AND HEALTH

The relationship between caring and health is complex, as caring is carried out within a dynamic process and can have positive and negative experiences, at the same time or sequentially. Caring can have a *direct* effect upon health, such as physical strain, musculoskeletal problems, or emotional strain from the caring experience; or caring may impact upon health *indirectly*, via loss of earnings or reduced family income, and, where the dependent has moved in with the carer, overcrowded housing conditions can adversely affect health status. The indirect link between health and caring may be mediated by the coping strategies and mechanisms adopted by the carer. There may also be positive effects of caring on health, through increased physical activity and/or mental well-being, most notably in the fulfilment of filial or spousal duty. Such emotional and altruistic benefits are less readily quantified than financial costs and opportunities forgone.

The carer 'health effect' may be influenced by a number of factors: (1) the intensity of caring, such as the number of hours of caring carried out per week; (2) the type of care tasks carried out, physical, personal or practical; (3) the nature and extent of the incapacity of the dependant, whether they are physically and/or mentally impaired, or whether their level of independence is related to old age infirmity; (4) the duration of the caring experience, number of months or years; (5) the carer's status or broader level of responsibility towards the dependant, such as whether the caring is done within or outside the carer's own household, whether or not the experience of caring is shared, distinguishing between sole, joint or peripheral caring; (6) the nature of the caring relationship: caring for one's spouse may be very different from the experience of caring for one's elderly parent/parent-in-law, or one's incapacitated child.

Carers' social, psychological and economic positions can be affected whilst caring takes place, and may continue well *after* caring ceases. Some effects may only manifest after caring stops, emphasizing the importance of longitudinal data. Key problems faced by ex-carers include difficulties in re-entering the labour market, a fall in living standards due to the loss of Invalid Care Allowance (ICA) eight weeks after caring stops – ex-ICA recipients become ineligible for unemployment benefit – in addition to deteriorating physical and psychological health (Lewis and Meredith 1988; Glendinning 1992; McLaughlin 1994). The likelihood of re-entry into the labour market diminishes with carers' age, and where they do return to paid work it is usually with lower rates of pay owing to loss of seniority and career opportunities forgone (McLaughlin 1991; Askham et al. 1992). These problematic experiences can have far-reaching effects, impacting upon carers' economic, social and health status, placing them in a disadvantageous position in their own old age, and further contributing to the existing health and income inequalities.

PREVIOUS STUDIES

The number of studies on informal caring in Britain has mushroomed over the last decade, constituting a substantial body of evidence. The majority have been small-scale and qualitative. Research using nationally representative data (Parker and Lawton 1990, 1994; Arber and Ginn 1991, 1995; Evandrou 1992, 1995b) has confirmed many of the findings within the earlier smaller studies, although not all. In particular, it has highlighted the *heterogeneity* among carers in terms of the nature of the caring tasks, the level of support provided, whether the caring role adopted is shared with others, and the relationship to the cared-for person. This heterogeneity has implications for the type and range of services which may be required, and the numbers likely to need them.

Previous research examining the relationship between health and caring has rarely used representative samples. Studies are usually based upon samples of carers who are self-selected out of the carer population, often by having had contact with the community services, hospital or primary health care – either for their dependant or for themselves (Grad and Sainsbury 1968; Gilleard *et al.* 1984).

A wide range of health effects have been reported by carers: physical strain (Cantor 1983); increased levels of emotional strain (Levin *et al.* 1989); stress and social isolation, in particular among mothers caring for mentally impaired children (Quine and Pahl 1985). Two-thirds of members of the National Carers' Association reported that their physical or mental health was adversely affected (Carnegie 1993). Carers often report lack of time or opportunity to consult a GP for themselves, which has the effect of exacerbating their health problems (Wright 1986).

Health effects have been found to vary by the characteristics of the dependant cared for. Baumgarten *et al.* (1992) investigated the physical and psychological health problems of carers of elderly persons. They found a higher likelihood of physical ill health and depression among carers of dementia sufferers than among carers of dependents with no mental impairment. The relationship was found to be stronger among spouse carers than among carers of children. McDowell *et al.* (1994) also found that carers caring for a dementia sufferer were more likely to report chronic health problems and depression than carers supporting dependants without dementia. Nolan and Grant (1992) found that spouse carers experienced greater physical strain than parent carers, and also that spouse carers were more likely to report poor health and consult the GP than other carers (based upon a sample drawn from the National Carers' Association).

None of the above studies was based on a randomly selected national sample. Parker and Lawton (1994) using nationally representative data (1985 General Household Survey) found no health difference between carers and non-carers, standardizing upon age and sex, although they did find some differential between co-resident carers and non-carers: 18 per cent of co-resident carers reported 'not good' general health over the last year, compared with 14 per cent of non-carers. They found the results overall 'puzzling', as no health effect was found among the most heavily involved carers, contrary to prior expectations.

Taylor *et al.* (1995) used the 2007 longitudinal study to examine psychosocial morbidity and malaise among the 55-year-old cohort, first interviewed in 1988 and then once more in 1991 ($n = 858$). Thirty-one per cent were providing regular care. No clear evidence of caring negatively impacting upon health was found; indeed, Taylor *et al.* found a tendency for carers to report better health functioning than their non-carer counterparts, offering support to the findings of Parker and Lawton. A number of reasons are put forward by the authors to account for this 'counter-intuitive finding': the carers in the cohort sample spent few hours per week providing care tasks and support (median of seven hours per week); the carers' population changed significantly between 1988 and 1991, with only 48 per cent of those identified as caring in 1988 continuing to do so by 1991; and 25 per cent of the carers reported either increases or reductions in the number of hours caring in 1991.

Carer selection and self-selection may also help account for this pattern (Taylor *et al.* 1995). Individuals in poorer health may be less likely to take on caring responsibilities, compared with persons whose health is good. Where carers' health deteriorates, they may be more likely to consider options of giving up caring than those carers whose health remains intact. Thus on average the health of the carer population may be more likely to be better than that of a non-carer population.

The American literature on the burden and stress of caring is considerable, focusing on the development of objective measures of stress in order to facilitate evaluations of different interventions. More recently the approach has been subject to criticism (Zarit 1989). As Twigg and Atkin point out, 'stress and burden have been reified, pursued in ways that are detached either from how people cope with their lives or the policy issues posed by caring' (Twigg and Atkin 1994: 5).

However, it is clear that some carers experience extensive satisfaction, gratifications and other benefits from their caring relationship (Motenko 1989; Clifford 1990). Caring can result in an improved caring relationship between carer and dependant, particularly at stages where reciprocity is evident (Townsend and Noelker 1987). The more distant the relationship between carer and cared-for person, the better the carer's mental health (Gilhooly 1984). Nolan and Grant (1992) found in their study that carers combined high stress levels with high levels of satisfaction. The coping strategies which 'protect' and buffer carers and their stresses are not yet fully understood.

THE EXTENT OF INFORMAL CARE IN BRITAIN

Data

It was not until the analysis of the 1985 General Household Survey that nationally representative data shed light on the extent and nature of informal care in Britain. The General Household Survey is an annual cross-sectional survey of individuals (16 years and over) living in households within Great Britain. It offers a rich range of information (demographic, social, economic, behavioural, housing, etc.) on sample sizes of over 26,000 (OPCS 1992a, b).

The screening question used to self-identify respondents as informal carers in the 1985, and repeated in the 1990 General Household Survey, distinguishes between those caring *within* the same households and those caring for dependants *not resident* with them.[1] Informal carers provide care for sick, handicapped or elderly persons.[2] In this chapter, different informal carer types have been distinguished, reflecting the context in which the caring takes place (co-resident with the dependant or not), the intensity of care provided (number of hours per week), whether the caring responsibilities are shared or not (sole, joint or peripheral carer), and the relationship with the cared-for person. Individuals not reporting such regular caring responsibilities are defined as 'non-carers'.[3] The empirical analysis primarily uses the 1990 General Household Survey data, although some 1985 data are also referred to.

Informal care: a national picture

In 1990 one in seven (16 per cent) of the General Household Survey sample were identified as having caring responsibilities for a sick, incapacitated or elderly person, of whom about half provided regular support on their own, i.e. they were *sole carers*. Grossing up these figures nationally, they translate into 3.4 million sole carers in Great Britain, 1.7 million adults caring for someone in their own home, and another 1.7 million people spending at least twenty hours per week providing care and support. Over one in ten of the 1990 General Household Survey sample provided both personal and physical care, approximating to about 500,000 carers, who are involved in substantial levels of caring, for long hours and over lengthy periods of time. Among all carers, carers spent an average of twenty hours per week performing caring tasks.

The proportion of adults reporting such caring responsibilities between 1985 and 1990 rose slightly (Table 12.1). Most of this rise can be attributed to the increase in the proportion caring for dependants *outside* the household. As shown elsewhere, the gender difference in the carers identified in the sample is small, 17 per cent of women, compared with 14 per cent of men (Arber and Ginn 1995). However, women are more likely to

Table 12.1 Percentage of adults (16 years plus) who are carers, by sex, 1985–90

Variable	Men		Women		Total	
	1985	1990	1985	1990	1985	1990
Carers	12	14	15	17	14	16
Not carers	88	86	85	83	86	84
Carers with dependants *inside* household[a]	4	4	4	4	4	4
Carers with dependants *outside* household	8	10	11	14	10	12
Sole carers	6	6	10	10	8	8
Caring for 20 hrs or more per week	3	3	4	4	3	4
Total (*n*)	(8,484)	(8,103)	(9,846)	(9,432)	(18,330)	(17,535)

Note: (a) Includes a small number of carers who have dependants both within and outside their household (sixty-three in 1985; seventy-one in 1990/91).

Source: General Household Survey 1985, 1990/1, author's own analysis.

be caring for someone on their own, that is, as a *sole carer* (i.e. 57 per cent versus 42 per cent), and for longer hours per week. The age group most likely to be caring is those aged 45–59 years (25 per cent), although over a quarter (28 per cent) of all carers are aged 60 or over. The like-lihood of becoming a carer increases for women as they enter stages in their life cycle where their own children are older, in particular 16 plus, and also as they themselves increase in age.

Carers supporting parents and parents-in-law (48 per cent) are most prevalent, with a lower proportion caring for a spouse or child (16 per cent). Nearly three-quarters of carers (71 per cent) care for physically impaired dependants, 5 per cent support dependants with mental impair-ment, 17 per cent have both mental and physical and 5 per cent describe old age or other impairments. One-third of carers provide mainly personal or physical caring tasks.

The 1985 General Household Survey included information on the dura-tion of caring responsibility. It was found that caring tends to be a longer-term experience, with over four out of ten carers (42 per cent) reporting having cared for someone for between one and four years, and a fifth caring for a dependant for at least ten years. Only 12 per cent reported caring for under one year. The length of time spent caring has implications as to the barriers of entering/re-entering the labour market for those carers who wish to return to work and for the impact on health.

Table 12.2 Receipt of social services by dependant, by type of carer (%)

Carers	All 1985	All 1990	Deps in[d]	Deps out[d]	Sole carer[d]	Fifty hours[d]	Twenty hours[d]
					1990		
Doctor[a]	22	17	7	20	13	8	14
Nurse[a]	15	15	13	16	13	14	15
Health visitor[b]	6	4	2	5	3	2	3
Social worker[b]	6	4	2	5	3	4	3
Home Help[b]	24	23	7	28	20	9	13
Meals on Wheels[b]	8	7	1	9	7	1	4
Voluntary worker	4	3	2	4	3	2	3
Other[c]	8	10	6	12	10	11	10
(*n*)	(3,032)	(2,645)	(664)	(1,944)	(1,326)	(289)	(619)

Notes: (a) At least once in the last month.
(b) More than once a month.
(c) Codes changed between 1985 and 1990.
(d) *Deps in*, carer co-resident with dependant. *Deps out*, carer not co-resident with dependant. *Sole carer*, carer providing care on their own. *Fifty hours*, carer providing care fifty or more hours per week. *Twenty hours,* carer providing care for twenty or more hours per week.

Source: General Household Survey 1985 and 1990/1, author's own analysis.

Respite care also is not common; over half of all carers (52 per cent) reported that they had not had a break since caring responsibilities began. Providing consistent care with fewer breaks was found to be more prevalent among co-resident carers than other groups. Given the policy statements above that it is the responsibility of State service providers to support carers, it is instructive to look at what service support is actually provided.

Receipt of health and social service support by the cared-for person is generally limited. Less than half of the people being cared for received any health and social service support. Where they were receiving support, visits from a home help or a doctor were most common, followed by a community or district nurse. With two exceptions, service receipt fell slightly between 1985 and 1990 (Table 12.2). Substantial variation in service receipt across different types of carers was found in the 1990 General Household Survey; those being cared for by relatives in the same household were less likely to receive services (domestic, medical and personal care) than other carers. The likelihood of provision was higher where the carer was a non-relative, irrespective of the dependency of the cared-for person and the caring relationship. Furthermore, home help services were more likely to be provided to women being cared for by men than to men being cared for by women. In short, co-resident carers are more likely to experience a lower level of support than other types of carers, which may in turn have important implications for the levels of stress, general health status and quality of life of these carers in particular.

Charging for home support services is emerging as *the* mechanism by which income is generated and thus the central issue for local authorities faced with implementing community care reforms[4] (Means and Smith 1994). The success of such income generation is unclear, as studies have shown that the amount of revenue generated has in the past tended to be very small; Oldman (1991) reported that the proportion of home help expenditure covered by charges constituted 6 per cent in 1985–6. Price can be a significant barrier: Sinclair *et al.* (1990: 56) conclude that 'the imposition of charges could distort demand, deterring the poor who need home help from applying for it and deflecting services to somewhat richer pensioners who need them less'. Carers' financial position may be affected by charging, especially where they provide support for dependants within the household and the joint financial resources are limited and precarious (Glendinning 1990; Parker 1990), which in turn may impact on health.

YOUNG CARERS

Recent case studies have raised the profile of child carers; describing their experience of providing constant support to incapacitated parents or siblings at home, often with no or little support. Currently there are few targeted community services to assist child carers, and many slip through the social security system owing to the fact that they are minors. Fear of stigma may keep cared-for parents quiet and child carers hidden.

Aldridge and Becker's (1993) in-depth interview study of child carers in Nottingham ($n = 15$) found that the ages they started caring ranged from 8 to 18 years, and the length of time caring ranged from three to seventeen years. There was little support from paid professionals, and many of the families were on low incomes. Many of these child carers adapted to their role as carers, though it raises the question, on humanitarian grounds, whether they should have to. The range of possible effects of such caring includes potential negative psychosocial impact on the child's development; restricted social contacts/friendships, leisure time and hobbies; adverse impact upon education via absenteeism/persistent lateness; as well as disturbed sleep patterns and physical exhaustion. Given the importance of early life experiences (Wadsworth 1991; Power *et al.* 1991), it is likely that the current impact upon the young carers' education, social life and material and psychosocial status will also be carried on into adulthood.

The lack of information concerning the extent and circumstances of child caring represents one of the most significant gaps in current research. Basic facts such as how many child and younger carers there are in Britain, and who they care for, remain unanswered. There has been no nationally representative research into child carers. The exact number of young carers is not known. Small-scale survey estimates conducted in the 1980s suggest there are 10,000 children primary carers under 18 years (O'Neill 1988; Page 1988).

Table 12.3 Percentage of young adults (aged 16–20 years) who are carers, by sex, 1990

Variable	Men	[Women]	Total
Carers	8.0	7.0	7.4
Not carers	92.0	93.0	92.6
Carers with dependants *inside* household	2.5	1.4	2.0
Carers with dependants *outside* household	5.4	5.5	5.5
Sole carers	1.3	1.7	1.5
Caring for twenty hours or more per week	1.3	0.7	1.0
Total (*n*)	(628)	(704)	(1,332)

Source: General Household Survey 1990/1, author's own analysis.

Preliminary analysis of young carers from the 1990 General Household Survey (Evandrou 1995a) indicates that 7.4 per cent of 16–20 year olds are carers, with very little gender difference (Table 12.3). This approximates to over a quarter of a million young carers nationally (i.e. 292,000). This excludes many more who are aged below 16 years. However, many of those identified as carers in the General Household Survey were helpers rather than the main carer, but some did take on greater involvement: an estimated 79,000 16–20 year olds are co-resident carers (2 per cent), whereas 217,000 (5.5 per cent) care for someone outside their home, nearly 40,000 care for at least twenty hours per week (1 per cent). Further research exploring the experience of caring in youth and how it interacts with other spheres of social, familial and economic development is clearly required.

There is a need to develop policies which protect young carers from remaining hidden and neglected in the community. In addition to expanding statutory service support, one approach would be to encourage 'buddying' (a system already gaining success in the support of persons with HIV/AIDS in the community) which would help alleviate stress and anxiety (Haffenden 1991; Cox and Greenwell 1994). Sensitive approaches are called for from the health professionals who are likely to come in contact with child carers.

CONSEQUENCES OF CARING

Health status and health care use

Examining self-reported morbidity over the last year shows that the health of all carers is very similar to that of non-carers (Table 12.4a). Distinguishing between different levels of carer responsibilities and the types of

Table 12.4a Self-reported general health status in last year by carers and
non-carers (16 years plus) (%)

Variable	Good	Fairly good	Not good	(n)
Non-carers	60	28	12	(14,795)
All carers	58	30	12	(2,707)
Sole carer	52	34	14	(1,353)
Joint carer	65	25	10	(379)
Peripheral carer	65	26	9	(932)
Carers with dependant in same household	48	36	17	(668)
Carers with dependant outside household	62	28	10	(2,039)#
Carers of physically impaired dependants	60	30	11	(1,928)
Carers of mentally impaired dependants	57	32	11	(143)
Carers of both physically and mentally impaired dependants	49	34	17	(459)
Carers of frail elderly dependants	69	23	9	(159)
Caring for spouse	40	37	24	(235)
Caring for over twenty hours per week	49	33	18	(621)
Caring for over fifty hours per week	42	39	19	(290)

Source: General Household Survey 1990/1, author's own analysis. $p < 0.001$ except for
where $p < 0.01$.

impairment affecting the dependants changes the health differential. Carers
looking after someone inside their household are more likely to report poor
health over the last year compared with non-carers (17 per cent versus 12
per cent). There is less of difference with sole carers (14 per cent versus
12 per cent). However, this is not the case across all carer types; joint carers,
those caring more peripherally, carers with dependants outside, and carers
of frail elderly dependants report better general health than non-carers. The
highest proportion reporting poor health was among spouse carers (24 per
cent) and those caring for 50 or more hours per week (19 per cent).

As expected, standardizing upon age and sex has the effect of reducing many of these health differences (Table 12.4b). What is clear is that
caring for one's spouse (25 per cent), or caring for a dependant with both
physical and mental impairment (19 per cent), or providing care support
for over fifty hours per week (19 per cent) increases the likelihood
of reporting 'not good' health over the previous year, compared with

Table 12.4b Self-reported general health status in last year by carers and non-carers (16 years plus), age and sex standardized (%)

Variable	Good	Fairly good	Not good
Non-carers	60	28	12
All carers	60	29	11
Sole carer	53	33	14
Joint carer	67	24	9
Peripheral carer	67	25	8
Carers with dependant in same household	50	34	16
Carers with dependant outside household	64	27	9
Carers of physically impaired dependants	62	28	10
Carers of mentally impaired dependants	61	29	9
Carers of both physically and mentally impaired dependants	52	32	19
Carers of frail elderly dependants	71	22	7
Caring for spouse	38	36	25
Caring for over twenty hours per week	51	31	17
Caring for over fifty hours per week	44	36	19

Source: General Household Survey 1990/1, author's own analysis.

non-carers (12 per cent). Co-residence with one's dependant or bearing the main responsibility on one's own is still related to less good health (16 per cent and 14 per cent versus 12 per cent).

Spouse carers where the dependant has both physical and mental impairments report much higher levels of poor health (36 per cent) (Table 12.5). The cumulative effect of caring for a spouse with both types of impairments, bearing the main responsibility as sole carer, and caring for over fifty hours per week becomes clearer when we compare the proportion reporting good health with non-carers, that is, 23 per cent versus 46 per cent – although the cell counts have dropped markedly.

Examining the percentage of carers reporting long-standing illness or disability, a similar pattern emerges (Table 12.6); carers jointly or peripherally involved, or those caring for frail elderly dependants, are less likely to experience such illness or disability compared with their non-carer counterparts. However, being a spouse carer, caring for over twenty or fifty hours per week, living with the person one is caring for, or caring for a dependant with physical and mental impairments raises the proportion

Table 12.5 Self-reported general health status in last year by carers with
specified responsibilities (16 years plus), age and sex
standardized (%)

Variable	Good	Fairly good	Not good	(n)
Non-carers	60	28	12	(14,795)
Caring for *both* physically and mentally impaired dependant *inside* same household	46	36	18	(158)
Sole carer for *both* physically and mentally impaired dependant *inside* same household	40	39	22	(115)
Spouse carer for *both* physically and mentally impaired dependant	28	37	36	(54)
Sole spouse carer for *both* physically and mentally impaired dependant *inside* same household	27	38	35	(52)
Sole spouse carer for *both* physically and mentally impaired dependant *inside* same household for more than fifty hours per week	23	39	38	(31)

Source: General Household Survey 1990/1, author's own analysis.

markedly. The reporting of acute illness or injury (in the last two weeks)
and also consulting one's GP has less marked differences.

The relationship between the number of hours of care provided and self-
reported general health is not straightforward. Carers providing low level
support (under ten hours per week) report better health than non-carers
(65 per cent compared with 60 per cent) (Table 12.7). The heaviest involvement in caring, 100 hours or more per week, reduces the level of reporting
good health to 40 per cent. However, a higher proportion of those caring
for twenty to thirty-four hours reported good health than of those caring
for ten to nineteen hours. Furthermore the level reporting poor health rises
with care hours up to thirty-four hours, then it falls in the next two categories, until the highest category (100 hours plus), where it increases again.
Quite clearly this reflects the possible movement into and out of caring
depending upon the carer's health status. Where health deteriorates from
'good' to 'fairly good' or from 'fairly good' to 'not good', carers may cease
to provide care, thus leaving a higher proportion of healthier carers
continuing to care, up to the most heavily caring category.

Multivariate analysis

The analysis so far has been limited to standardizing for the different
age and sex composition of carers versus non-carers. However, other
characteristics such as marital status, socioeconomic group and education

Table 12.6 Health status and health care use by carers and non-carers (16 years plus), age and sex standardized (%)

Variable	Long-standing illness or disability	Acute illness/ injury in last two weeks	Consulted GP in last two weeks
Non-carers	38	14	18
All carers	40	14	16
Sole carer	45	15	18
Joint carer	36	13	10
Peripheral carer	36	14	16
Carers with dependant in same household	47	15	17
Carers with dependant outside household	38	14	16
Carers of physically impaired dependants	39	13	16
Carers of mentally impaired dependants	45	10	12
Carers of both physically and mentally impaired dependants	47	20	17
Carers of frail elderly dependants	32	6	16
Caring for spouse	60	18	21
Caring for over twenty hours per week	47	18	19
Caring for over fifty hours per week	53	20	19

Source: General Household Survey 1990/1, author's own analysis.

are also known to be associated with health status and as such need to be taken into account when examining the relationship between caring experience and health. Here a logit regression model is employed to allow a greater number of independent variables to be controlled simultaneously. By specifying non-carers as the comparison (or reference) category, the relative probability for subgroups of carers of reporting good health can be calculated, all other things being equal.

Logit models were estimated for two forms of the dependent variable, self-reported health status over the past year. The first form predicted whether an individual reported being in good or fairly good health (as opposed to 'not good' health) over the past year, whilst the second form predicted whether an individual reported being in good health (as opposed to fair or 'not good'). The models were estimated separately for men and for women.

Table 12.7 Self-reported general health status in last year by amount of
time spent caring per week (16 years plus), age and sex
standardized (%)

Variable	Good	Fairly good	Not good	(n)
Not caring	60	28	12	(14,795)
Caring for:				
Less than 5 hours	65	28	8	(937)
5–9 hours	65	25	10	(679)
10–19 hours	57	31	11	(481)
20–34 hours	59	26	16	(245)
35–49 hours	55	30	15	(75)
50–99 hours	51	37	12	(111)
100 hours plus	40	36	24	(178)

Source: General Household Survey 1990/1, author's own analysis.

Table 12.8 Log. likelihood ratios: logistic regression models examining health
and caring amongst men and women (16 years plus)[a]

MODELS change LLR (change df)	[Women]	[Men]
GENH1[b]		
1. NULL MODEL	7,249 (n = 9,176)	5,323 (n = 7,883)
2. MODEL2 (includes AGE, MARITAL, EDLEVEL, CHILDAGE, SEG, OWNEMP, SPOUSEMP)	−707 (21)***	−715 (21)***
3. MODEL 2+CARE	−6.8 (2) *	−4.4 (2)
4. MODEL 2+CARETIME	−10.3 (4) *	−4.9 (4)
5. MODEL 2+IMPAIR	−9.9 (4) *	−13.0 (4) *
GENH2[c]		
1. NULL MODEL	12,632 (n = 9,176)	10,221 (n = 7,883)
2. MODEL 2 (includes AGE, MARITAL, EDLEVEL, CHILDAGE SEG, OWNEMP, SPOUSEMP	−1,034 (21)***	−1,019 (21)***
3. MODEL 2+CARE	−5.9 (2)	−5.2 (2)
4. MODEL 2+CARETIME	−5.4 (4)	−7.0 (4)
5. MODEL 2+IMPAIR	−7.6 (4)	−17.8 (4) **
6. MODEL 2+CARETIME2	−6.2 (6)	−23.3 (6)***

Notes:
(a) Excludes all full-time students.   (b) 1 = good or fairly good health, 0 = poor health.
(c) 1 = good health, 0 = fairly good or poor health.
Changes in models were statistically significant at: ***$p < 0.001$, **$p < 0.01$ and *$p < 0.05$.

Source: General Household Survey 1990/1, author's own analysis.

Table 12.9 Odds ratios of health and the impact of caring for men and women (16 years plus)[a]; baseline model

Variable	Women in good/fair health	Men in good/fair health	Women in good health	Men in good health
AGE				
16–29 years	1.00	1.00	1.00	1.00
30–44 years	0.71*	0.61**	1.07	0.76**
45–59 years	0.58***	0.38***	0.81*	0.55***
60–74 years	1.09	0.44***	0.88	0.51***
75 years plus	0.97	0.32***	0.73*	0.32***
MARITAL				
Single	1.00	1.00	1.00	1.00
Married/cohabiting	0.76*	0.81	0.91	1.07
Divorced/separated	0.60***	0.56**	0.64***	1.00
Widowed	0.85	0.70	0.86	0.81
EDLEVEL				
No qualifications	1.00	1.00	1.00	1.00
O level and other	1.48***	1.30*	1.40***	1.26***
A level	1.19	1.28	1.68***	1.32**
Degree and other	1.73***	1.64**	1.95***	1.91***
Missing information	0.76	1.88***	0.77*	1.52***
CHILDAGE				
No dependent child in family unit	1.00	1.00	1.00	1.00
Youngest child aged under 5 years	1.85***	0.90	1.16	1.12
Youngest child 5–10 years	1.25	1.76**	1.13	1.42***
Youngest child 11–18 years	1.08	1.12	1.00	1.27**
SEG				
I and II	1.00	1.00	1.00	1.00
IIINM	1.08	0.74*	0.96	0.89
IIIM	0.65**	0.64***	0.69***	0.69***
IV	0.71*	0.53***	0.61***	0.65***
V	0.82	0.54**	0.61***	0.60***
Unclassified	0.86	1.44	0.93	1.26
OWNEMP				
Not employed	1.00	1.00	1.00	1.00
Employed	2.89**	4.82***	1.58***	2.43***
SPOUSEMP				
Spouse not employed	1.00	1.00	1.00	1.00
Spouse employed	1.60**	0.84	1.25***	1.01

Notes: (a) Excludes all full-time students. Odds ratios were statistically significant at: ***$p < 0.001$, **$p < 0.01$ and *$p < 0.05$.

Source: General Household Surevey 1990/1, author's own analysis.

Table 12.10 Odds ratios of health and the impact of caring for men and women (16 years plus)[a]

Variable GENH1	Women in good/fair health	Men in good/fair health
CARE		
Not caring	1.00	1.00
Caring for dependant inside own household	0.99	1.18
Caring for dependant outside own household	1.29*	1.29
CARETIME		
Not caring	1.00	1.00
Under 10 hours per week	1.47**	1.37*
10–19 hours per week	0.99	1.09
20–49 hours per week	0.97	1.17
50 or more hours per week	1.04	1.15
IMPAIR		
Not caring	1.00	1.00
Physically impaired	1.33**	1.42**
Mentally impaired	0.99	2.68
Both physically and mentally impaired	0.82	0.73
Frail elderly	1.16	1.32

Notes: (a) Excludes all full-time students.
Odds ratios were statistically significant at: **$p < 0.01$ and *$p < 0.05$.

Source: General Household Survey 1990/1, author's own analysis.

Health was assumed to be influenced by age, marital status, educational qualifications, the age of youngest child, own employment status and whether spouse is in employment. To this base model (Model 2), three different caring variables relating to the intensity of care and type of impairment of the dependant (Models 3–5) were then introduced in turn. Table 12.8 shows how well health status is predicted for both men and women for the two different forms of dependent variable, and the improvement of fit across the models. The parameter estimates for each of the variables in Model 2 are presented in Table 12.9

The changes in the basic health model predicting 'good or fairly good health' with the addition of the caring variables (Models 3–5) were all statistically significant for women. The picture was more mixed for men, with only the addition of IMPAIR (type of impairment affected by dependant) being significant at the 5 per cent level. Under the alternative specification of the dependent variable, the intensity of caring, that is, the number of hours spent caring, distinguishing between dependants inside

Table 12.11 Odds ratios of health and the impact of caring for men and women (16 years plus)[a]

Variable GENH2	Women with good health	Men with good health
CARE		
Not caring	1.00	1.00
Caring for dependant inside own household	0.77*	0.90
Caring for dependant outside own household	1.05	1.19*
CARETIME		
Not caring	1.00	1.00
Under 10 hours per week	1.09	1.06
10–19 hours per week	0.91	1.04
20–49 hours per week	0.91	1.61*
50 or more hours per week	0.76	0.89
IMPAIR		
Not caring	1.00	1.00
Physically impaired	1.05	1.22*
Mentally impaired	0.98	0.87
Both physically and mentally impaired	0.71*	0.64**
Frail elderly	1.11	1.81
CARETIME2		
Not caring		1.00
Care in under 19 hours		0.86
Care in 20–49 hours		1.14
Care in 50+ hours		0.76
Care out under 19 hours		1.10
Care out 20–49 hours		3.22**
Care out 50+ hours		50.11

Notes: (a) Excludes all full-time students.
Odds ratios were statistically significant at: **$p < 0.01$ and *$p < 0.05$.

Source: General Household Survey 1990/1, author's own analysis.

and outside the household (Model 6), was also significant for men. Additional models including other caring variables, such as relationship of carer to dependant, were also estimated but were not found to be significant for either men or women.

The parameter estimates for each of the caring variables are shown as odds ratios in Tables 12.10 and 12.11. Controlling for all other characteristics, there is a negative effect on reporting good health for women caring for a dependant *inside* the same household, whilst caring for someone *outside* appears to have a positive effect on the likelihood of reporting good or good/fair health.

Who you care for also affects the health of the carer. Caring for a dependant who is physically impaired is positively related to health for both men and women, whereas caring for a dependant who has both physical and mental impairments has a strong negative effect. This effect is most clear in the model predicting 'good' health. Caring for longer hours also appears to be negatively associated with health, although here the evidence is more ambiguous. Some of this ambiguity may arise from intensive caring being associated with reporting 'fairly good health' rather than good.

In summary, there may be some health effect, as well as carer selection and self-selection; some carers are able to exercise a real choice as regards taking on caring and when to give it up. Those who experience poor health or long-term illness/disability are less likely to undertake caring initially than those in good health. However, *whilst* caring, carers faced with deteriorating health problems may discuss alternative care arrangements with their dependant and give up caring, compared with carers who continue to enjoy good health. Thus carers on average may report better general health, although *among* carers, and at different intensities of caring, poor health is related to the experience of caring. Ideally these issues require further investigation using longitudinal data, establishing the causal nature of the health patterns observed and exploring how or why people take up caring. The Medical Research Council National Survey of Health and Development has collected data on caring for frail people in the 1946 birth cohort (at 43 years). The data have the potential to shed light on these issues within the context of earlier life experiences.

Social impact

Since time is a limited commodity, it is likely that the greater the time spent undertaking caring responsibilities the less time will be available to spend in alternative ways. In particular with respect to carers who are combining their caring responsibilities with paid employment. Those providing care may face reduced opportunities for pursuing hobbies and generally spend low levels of time engaged in sports, relaxing, going on holiday or going for short breaks, as has been found by a number of studies (Bowling 1984; Wright 1986; George and Gwyther 1986; Clifford 1990; Quereshi and Walker 1989).

The 1990 General Household Survey contains some information on leisure activities and thus allows us to examine the relationship between caring and social activity. Respondents were asked whether they had undertaken a range of outdoor activities within the last year. Standardizing for the different age and sex composition of carers *vis-à-vis* non-carers, co-resident carers were less likely to have participated in either sporting

Table 12.12 Whether participated in physical activity over the past year/
month, by carer's status (16 years plus); age and sex
standardized (%)

Variable	No activity	Walking only	Sport only	Walking and sport	(n)
Participated in activity in last year					
Not caring	18	14	17	50	(14,820)
All carers	14	15	14	57	(2,718)
Carers with dependants					
inside household	28	17	15	40	(688)
Carers with dependants					
outside household	9	14	14	62	(2,030)
Sole carer	20	18	14	48	(1,266)
Caring for spouse	54	18	11	17	(238)
Participated in activity in last month					
Not caring	36	16	25	24	(14,820)
All carers	31	19	21	29	(2,718)
Carers with dependants					
inside household	45	18	18	19	(668)
Carers with dependants					
outside household	26	20	22	32	(2,030)
Sole carer	39	21	16	23	(1,266)
Caring for spouse	71	14	10	6	(238)

Source: General Household Survey 1990/1, author's own analysis.

activities or walking (40 per cent), compared with non-carers (50 per cent)
(Table 12.12). However, joint or peripheral carers were more likely to
take part, 59 per cent and 61 per cent respectively. For sole carers the
proportion fell to 48 per cent.

What is of greater concern is that nearly one in three (28 per cent)
carers who are co-resident with their dependant, and over half of spouse
carers, did not spend time last year doing any sport or any walking as a
leisure activity – this compares with 18 per cent of non-carers. Furthermore, nearly three-quarters of spouse carers had not participated in any
physical leisure activity in the last month (71 per cent) (Table 12.12).
Respondents were also asked whether they had participated in a range
of indoor activity in the last four weeks. Four out of ten non-carers
(39 per cent) had participated in at least one activity, compared with only
29 per cent of sole carers and 35 per cent of joint carers.

Studies have found links between care provision, social isolation and
health (Braithwaite 1990; Parker 1990). Restriction of leisure activities,
hobbies and general social participation is a particularly important issue,
especially as expectations of such activities at the relevant stage of the
carer's life course may be very different. The social stimulation from paid

employment is valued by many carers as much as the income generated (Stevenson 1994). Where carers are not in employment, access to respite and group support has been identified as vital to the well-being of carers, in particular carers from ethnic backgrounds who face language barriers (Baxter 1988; McCalman 1990). Enabling sole carers who are co-resident to participate in some activity outside the home should be a priority for providers of respite care. Yet, as we saw above, it is precisely this group which is least likely to be in receipt of statutory service support.

Economic impact

There are long-term as well as short-term economic effects from caring for someone in terms of the impact on employment status, level of earnings, savings, and additional expenditure incurred from caring. As well as reduced current disposable income, reduced labour force participation and disrupted employment histories among carers, in particular women carers, may affect their economic status in their own old age in terms of income and pension forgone, and lower earnings-related benefits in later life.

Research using the 1985 and 1990 General Household Survey shows that full-time employment rates for both male and female carers are lower than those of their non-carer counterparts (Evandrou and Winter 1992; Evandrou 1995b). Carers are more likely to be employed in part-time jobs than non-carers, standardizing on sex and marital status. However, this tendency is restricted to women, as very few men work part-time, and is less marked for single women. There is significant variation among different types of carer, with the largest differentials in employment when comparing rates for co-resident or sole carers versus non-carers – although this is not consistent across all marital status groups.

Multivariate analysis taking into account age, socioeconomic group, education, spouse's employment, age of the youngest child and morbidity[5] using the 1990 General Household Survey indicated an independent negative effect of caring on employment for both men and women. The odds ratios indicate that a woman caring for an impaired person inside her household is only half as likely to be in full-time employment as her counterpart without such caring responsibilities and is less likely to be in part-time work. Women caring for dependants outside the home are three-quarters as likely to be in full-time employment as female non-carers, but are 30 per cent more likely to be in part-time work. The intensity of caring (i.e. the number of hours of care provided weekly) has the greatest impact upon employment; women caring for over fifty hours per week are five times less likely to be in full-time employment than female non-carers. Caring for a spouse reduces the odds of paid work compared with caring for a parent or parent-in-law.

Carers' average weekly earnings were also found to be below those of non-carers, taking age and sex into account. In short, carers earn less on an hourly rate than non-carers. Co-resident carers and those caring for over twenty hours per week have markedly lower hourly rates of pay compared with non-carers, and also compared with carers caring for a dependant outside their household (Evandrou 1995b). In addition to lower earnings, carers also experience, on average, lower net incomes than non-carers. This is despite the receipt of Invalid Care Allowance[6] (ICA), which is seen by some as an alternative 'wage for caring'. Set at £35.30 per week, ICA is lower than the basic pension (£59.15) and unemployment benefit (£46.45) (April 1995). For many carers it evidently fails to provide any kind of earnings replacement.

In summary, carers' employment, earnings, hourly wage rates and income tend to be lower than their non-carer counterparts' (standardizing on age, sex, and part-time/full-time work). However, the average picture masks enormous variation among different types of carers, reflecting the different demands various caring experiences place on individuals in terms of the labour market. It is questionable whether the existing welfare benefit system, specifically receipt of ICA, compensates carers' financial position sufficiently to place them on a par with their non-carer counterparts.

Do carers recover their economic welfare over the lifetime? Research elsewhere indicates that the lifetime impact upon earnings and other income sources from caring remains (Evandrou and Falkingham 1995). In particular, women with caring responsibilities face lower lifetime earnings and original incomes than women on average. Those women who care for five years or more have on average £13,000 (1985 prices) less lifetime earnings compared with all women. Furthermore, the State benefit system does not redress the position of carers in order to protect their lifetime living standards.

DISCUSSION

Analysis using the General Household Survey has found that there is an economic effect of caring; carers' employment, earnings and family net income have been found to be lower than those of their non-carer counterparts. Multivariate analysis indicated an independent negative effect of caring on employment for both men and women. Analysis of social and physical activity shows that co-resident carers, spouse carers and sole carers are less likely to participate in any sports activities, including going out for a walk.

However, the findings concerning caring and health are somewhat mixed. The self-reported health of carers as a whole is similar to that of non-carers, accounting for age and sex differences. However, distinguishing

Table 12.13 Self-reported general health status in last year by carers, non-
carers and ex-carers[a] (16 years plus) (%)

Variable	Good	Fairly good	Not good
All			
Current carers	60	29	13
Ex-carers	60	30	13
Non-carers	64	24	11
Men			
Current carers	62	27	11
Ex-carers	60	32	9
Non-carers	69	22	10
Women			
Current carers	57	30	14
Ex-carers	57	28	15
Non-carers	60	27	13

Note: (a) Not currently caring but was caring a year ago.

Source: General Household Survey 1985, author's own analysis.

between levels of caring responsibility and intensity of caring does indicate
a significant relationship. Caring for someone co-residentially, bearing the
main responsibility on one's own, caring for someone with both physical
and mental impairments, and caring for over fifty hours per week are associated with less good health. In particular being spouse carer raised the
likelihood of reporting ill health. Multivariate analysis shows that, after
taking into account additional independent factors, these observed patterns
do not all remain. What is clear is that caring for someone who is physically and mentally impaired is negatively associated with carers' health;
male carers are three-quarters as likely to be in good/fair health as men
without such caring responsibilities (0.73 odds ratio). For women the odds
are slightly less, 0.83.

   A number of reasons may contribute to such mixed results. Firstly, the
factors which predispose individuals towards caring may also be important
determining factors for health. Secondly, there is the issue of carer selection and self-selection, discussed above. Thirdly, it has been found by a
number of studies that many carers successfully adjust to their caring
responsibilities, however intensive. More research is called for to gain
greater understanding of the mechanisms involved (Parker 1990; Twigg
1990).

   Fourthly, the non-carer population in the General Household Survey
analysis may include ex-carers. If and where caring does impact upon
some carers' well-being, it is likely that the effects of caring upon health
and socioeconomic activity continue after caring ceases. Thus it is

methodologically important to exclude any ex-carers from the non-carer subsample. Although the 1985 General Household Survey contained information as to whether current non-carers were caring a year ago, unfortunately the 1990 General Household Survey does not distinguish them. Thus the analysis in this chapter could not exclude ex-carers from the non-carers group. It is not certain whether their inclusion does make a difference to the overall findings, although if it does it is likely that it will have the effect of slightly underestimating the proportion of non-carers reporting good health and slightly inflate that of non-carers reporting poor health. Examining self-reported general health among carers, ex-carers and non-carers in the 1985 General Household Survey indicates that ex-carers' health patterns are similar to those of current carers rather than those of non-carers (Table 12.13). This may have the effect of weakening any observed health patterns among the carer and non-carer subgroups.

A key area for future research is the health and socioeconomic position of ex-carers. This needs to be done on a nationally representative basis, possibly using the 1995 General Household Survey, which has ex-carers. Our lack of knowledge of what has been termed 'the legacies of caring' (by McLaughlin 1994) limits our understanding of the causes of health and income inequalities between people approaching pension age and older.

POLICY IMPLICATIONS

Given the emphasis on needs-led service provision, the General Household Survey estimates provide useful information on the caring experience for policy. The results highlight the heterogeneity of this experience, with implications for the range of care packages and policy options developed by care managers. Policies regarding cash and services at national and local level need to reflect the diversity of caring experiences and socioeconomic position of carers and cared-for persons.

We have seen that certain forms of caring are associated with the likelihood of poorer health. This has implications both for the individual and for the State. Individuals may be faced with both a lower income in their own old age (due to interrupted labour market experience) and poorer health, which may in turn result in a higher demand for health and social services. On-going support for carers today may mitigate the cost's of tomorrow's dependants.

Providing community services and respite care to those carers at risk of poorer health should be a priority – that is, carers supporting a dependant with both physical and mental impairments, co-residential carers and spouse carers. At present co-resident carers are least likely to be in receipt of statutory service support. Given financial pressures on the available resources and emphasis on 'ability to pay', this may involve earmarking some funds for such priority targeting.

Community services should be accessible, flexible and responsive to the needs of carers and their dependant (Twigg 1992). Services should include respite options which are offered within or near the carer's home, neighbourhood-based care schemes, as well as information, advice, and carers' network support (Leat 1990; Cox and Greenwell 1994; Stalker 1996). Choice and control should be an explicit element within the care system planned. Carers' organizations emphasize the need to encourage greater involvement of carers and dependants in the planning and also in the evaluation of community care support.

We have seen that carers' needs and rights have begun to be formally recognized within the new care management and assessment procedures, reinforced by the Carers Act 1995. This is vitally important in recognizing the significant contribution made by informal carers in Britain. However, *recognition* of carers' needs does not necessarily translate into *meeting* carers' needs. Given the concern about the extent of community care funding, it remains to be seen whether the policy statements will materialize in any effective support, reducing the work load of carers.

NOTES

1 General Household Survey 1985/90 carers' questions: asked of all aged 16 years or over. '(i) Some people have extra family responsibilities because they look after someone who is sick, handicapped or elderly. May I check, is there anyone living with you who is sick, handicapped or elderly whom you look after or give special help to (for example, a sick or handicapped (or elderly) relative/ husband/wife/child/friend, etc.)? (ii) And how about people not living with you? Do you provide some regular service or help for any sick, handicapped or elderly relative, friend or neighbour not living with you?' These questions identified approximately 2,600 and 2,800 carers in the 1985 and 1990 General Household Survey.
2 Care ranges from personal care, physical help, domestic tasks, keeping an eye on someone, helping with paperwork to giving out medicine.
3 Although they may have other caring responsibilities within their household, such as child care.
4 Local authority charging for domiciliary care is becoming more widespread. However the principle behind it has never had the same level of general acceptance as for charging residential care residents (Glennerster 1992). Lart and Means (1992) usefully distinguish between three policy strategies which local government can adopt regarding domiciliary care service charges; (i) a radical review of charging, (ii) an incremental growth in charges, and (iii) a continued commitment to free services.
5 Self-reported morbidity over the last year and also limited long-standing illness (see Evandrou 1995b).
6 Carers who are earning over £50 per week are not eligible for ICA.

REFERENCES

Aldridge, J. and Becker, S. (1993) *Children who Care – Inside the World of Young Carers*, Loughborough: Department of Social Sciences, Loughborough University.

Allen, I. and Perkins, E. (eds) (1995) *The Future of Family Care for Older People*, London: HMSO.

Arber, S. and Ginn, J. (1991) *Gender and later Life: a Sociological Analysis of Resources and Constraints*, London: Sage.

Arber, S. and Ginn, J. (1995) Gender differences in informal caring, *Health and Social Care in the Community* 3: 19–31.

Askham, J., Grundy, E. and Tinker, A. (1992) *Caring: the Importance of Third Age Carers*, The Carnegie Inquiry into the Third Age, Research Paper No. 6, Dunfermline: Carnegie UK Trust.

Baumgarten, M., Battista, R., Infanterivard, C., Hanley, J., Becker, R. and Gauthier, S. (1992) The psychological and physical health of family members caring for an elderly person with dementia, *Journal of Clinical Epidemiology* 45(1): 61–70.

Baxter, C. (1988) Ethnic minority carers: the invisible carers, *Health and Race* 15: 4–8.

Bowling, A. (1984) Caring for the elderly widowed – the burden on their supporters, *British Journal of Social Work* 14: 435–455.

Braithwaite, V. (1990) *Bound to Care*, London: Allen & Unwin.

Cantor, M. (1983) Strain among caregivers: a study of experience in the United States, *Gerontologist* 23(6): 597–604.

Carnegie UK Trust (1993) *Life, Work and Livelihood in the Third Age*, Final Report of The Carnegie Inquiry into the Third Age, Dunfermline: Carnegie UK Trust.

Clements, L. (1996) A real act of care, *Community Care* 111: 26–27.

Clifford, D. (1990) *The Social Costs and Rewards of Caring*, Aldershot: Avebury.

Cox, L. and Greenwell, S. (1994) *Taking the Pressure off the Carers*, Bristol: University of the West of England.

Department of Health (1989) *Caring for People*, London: HMSO.

Evandrou, M. (1992) Challenging the invisibility of carers: mapping informal care nationally, in F. Laczko and C. Victor (eds) *Social Policy and Older People*, Aldershot: Avebury.

Evandrou, M. (1995a) Child carers – the hidden caregivers: preliminary evidence from the 1990 General Household Survey, mimeo paper, Department of Epidemiology and Public Health, London: University College.

Evandrou, M. (1995b) Paid and unpaid work: the socio-economic position of informal carers in Britain, in J. Phillips (ed.) *Working Carers and Older People*, Aldershot: Avebury.

Evandrou M. and Falkingham J. (1995) Gender, lone-parenthood and lifetime incomes, in J. Falkingham and J. Hills (eds) *The Dynamic of Welfare: the Welfare State and the Life Cycle*, Hemel Hempstead: Harvester–Wheatsheaf.

Evandrou, M. and Winter, D. (1992) Informal Carers and the Labour Market in Britain, Welfare State Programme Discussion paper No. 89, STICERD, London: London School of Economics.

George, L. and Gwyther, L. (1986) Caregiver well-being: a multidimensional examination of family caregivers of demented adults, *Gerontologist* 26(3): 253–259.

Gilhooly, M. (1984) The impact of care-giving on care-givers: factors associated with the psychological well-being of people supporting a dementing relative in the community, *British Journal of Medical Psychology* 59: 165–171.

Gilleard, C., Belford, H., Gilleard, E., Whittick, J. and Gledhill, K. (1984) Emotional distress amongst the supporters of the elderly mentally infirm, *British Journal of Psychiatry* 145: 172–177.

Glendinning, C. (1990) Dependence and interdependency: the incomes of informal carers and the impact of social security, *Journal of Social Policy* 19(4): 469–497.

Glendinning, C. (1992) *The Costs of Informal Care: Looking inside the Household*, London: HMSO.

Glennerster, H. (1992) *Paying for Welfare: the 1990s*, Hemel Hempstead: Harvester–Wheatsheaf.

Grad, J. and Sainsbury, P. (1968) The effect that patients have on their families in a community care and control psychiatric service: a two-year follow up, *British Journal of Psychiatry* 114: 265–278.

Grant, G. and Nolan, M. (1993) Informal carers: sources and concomitants of satisfaction, *Health and Social Care* 1: 147–159.

Haffenden, S. (1991) *Getting it Right for Carers – Setting up Services for Carers: a Guide for Practitioners*, Department of Health and Social Services Inspectorate, London: HMSO.

Jones, D. (1986) *A Survey of Carers of Elderly Dependants Living in the Community*, Research Team for the Care of the Elderly, Cardiff: University of Wales College of Medicine.

Lart, R. and Means, R. (1992) To charge or not to charge? *Community Care*, 17–24 December, p. 21.

Leat, D. (1990) Overwhelming voluntary failure: strategies for change, in I. Sinclair, R. Parker, D. Leat and J. Williams (eds) *The Kaleidoscope of Care*, National Institute of Social Work, London: HMSO.

Levin, E., Sinclair, I. and Gorback, P. (1989) *Families, Services and Confusion in Old Age*, Aldershot: Avebury.

Lewis J. and Meredith B. (1988) *Daughters who Care: Daughters caring for Mothers at Home*. London: Routledge.

McCalman, J. (1990) *The Forgotten People: Carers in the Ethnic Minority Communities in Southwark*, London: King's Fund Centre.

McDowell, I., Hill, G., Lindsay, J. *et al.* (1994) Patterns of caring for people with dementia in Canada, *Canadian Journal on Aging* 13(2): 470–487.

McGlone, F. and Cronin N. (1994) *A Crisis in Care? The Future of Family and State Care for older People in the European Union*, Family Policy Studies Centre Occasional paper No. 19, London: FPSC.

McLaughlin, E. (1991) *Social Security and Community Care: the Case of the Invalid Care Allowance*, DSS Report No. 4, London: HMSO.

McLaughlin, E. (1994) Legacies of caring: the experiences and circumstances of ex-carers, *Health and Social Care* 2: 241–253.

Means, R. and Smith, R. (1994) *Community Care: Policy and Practice*, London: Macmillan.

Motenko, A. (1989) The frustrations, gratifications and well-being of dementia caregivers, *Gerontologist* 29(2): 166–172.

Neal, M.B., Chapman, N.J., Ingersoll-Dayton, B. and Emlen, A. (1993) *Balancing Work and Caregiving for Children, Adults and Elders*, London: Sage.

Nolan, M. and Grant, G. (1992) *Regular Respite: an Evaluation of a Hospital Rota Bed Scheme for Elderly People*, Research Monograph Series, Age Concern Institute of Gerontology, London: ACE Books.

Office of Population Censuses and Surveys (1992a) *General Household Survey: Carers in 1990*, OPCS Monitors, SS 92/2, London: HMSO.

Office of Population Censuses and Surveys (1992b) *General Household Survey 1990 Report*, London: HMSO.

Oldman, C. (1991) *Paying for Care: Personal Sources of Funding Care*, York: Joseph Rowntree Foundation.

O'Neill, A. (1988) *Young Carers: the Tameside Research*, Manchester: Tameside Metropolitan Borough Council.

Page, R. (1988) Report on the initial survey investigating the number of young carers in Sandwell Secondary Schools, Sandwell Metropolitan Borough Council.

Parker, G. (1990) *With Due Care and Attention: a Review of Research on Informal Care*, second edition, London: FPSC.

Parker, G. (1993) *With this Body: Caring and Disability in Marriage*, Milton Keynes: Open University Press.

Parker, G. and Lawton, D. (1990) Further analysis of the 1985 GHS data on informal care, SPRU Working Paper 716, York: University of York.

Parker, G. and Lawton, D. (1994) *Different Types of Care, Different Types of Carer: Evidence from the GHS*, London: SPRU/HMSO.

Power, C., Manor, O. and Fox J. (1991) *Class and Health: the Early Years*, London: Chapman & Hall.

Quereshi, H. and Walker, A. (1989) *The Caring Relationship: Elderly People and their Families*, London: Macmillan.

Quine, L. and Pahl, J. (1985) Examining the causes of stress in families with severely mentally handicapped children, *British Journal of Social Work* 15: 501–517.

Sinclair, I., Parker, R., Leat, D. and Williams, J. (1990) *The Kaleidoscope of Care*, National Institute of Social Work, London: HMSO.

Stalker, K. (1996) Developments in short-term care: breaks and opportunities, *Research Highlights in Social Work* 25, London: Jessica Kingsley Publishers.

Stevenson, O. (1994) Paid and unpaid work: women who care for adult dependants, in J. Evetts (ed.) *Women and Career: Themes and Issues in Advanced Industrial Societies*, Harlow: Longman.

Taylor, R., Ford, G. and Dunbar, M. (1995) The effects of caring on health: a community based longitudinal study, *Social Science and Medicine*, 40(10): 1407–1415.

Townsend, A. and Noelker, L. (1987) The impact of family relationships on perceived caregiving effectiveness, in T. Brubaker (ed.) *Aging, Family and Health: Long-term Care*, Beverly Hills, Cal.: Sage.

Twigg, J. (1990) Carers of elderly people: models for analysis, in A. Jamieson and R. Illsley (eds) *Contrasting European Policies for the Care of Older People*, Aldershot: Gower.

Twigg, J. (1992) (ed.) *Carers: Research and Practice*, London: HMSO.

Twigg, J. and Atkin, K. (1994) *Carers Perceived: Policy and Practice in Informal Care*, Buckingham: Open University Press.

Twigg, J., Atkin, K. with Perring, C. (1990) *Carers and Services: a Review of Research*, London: HMSO.

Wadsworth, M. (1991) *The Imprint of Time: Childhood, History and Adult Life*, Oxford: Clarendon Press.

Wright, F. (1986) *Left Alone to Care*, Aldershot: Gower.

Zarit, S. (1989) Do we need another 'stress and caregiving' study? *Gerontologist*, 29(2): 147–148

Zarit, S., Todd, P. and Zarit, J. (1986) Subjective burden of husbands and wives as caregivers: a longitudinal study, *Gerontologist*, 26(3): 260–266.

ACKNOWLEDGEMENT

I am indebted to OPCS and the ESRC Data Archive, University of Essex, for making the 1985 and 1990/1 General Household Survey data available for analysis.

Part IV

Work and the labour market

Chapter 13

Work and health

Implications for individuals and society

Michael Marmot and Amanda Feeney

Work is crucial in consideration of the social determinants of health for at least three reasons. First, it has central importance in generating prosperity, which in turns allows the development of social conditions conducive to health. Second, it has a direct impact on the individual, the family and the social environment. Third, the production process may have physical and environmental impacts that affect not only the worker, but the general physical environment surrounding the workplace.

It is the third of these that is the traditional focus of occupational and environmental health. Coal miners, cotton workers, agricultural workers, asbestos workers, radiation workers, and numerous others have all been studied to determine whether there are diseases related to chemical and physical exposures. These same exposures have also been studied as possible causes of disease outside the workplace, with much concern directed at the polluting effects of unsafe disposal of toxic waste, as well as the environmental effects of catastrophic accidents in factories and power plants. In addition to chemical and physical exposures, work also involves physical hazards that increase risk of accidents and soft tissue injuries.

Although these occupational exposures continue to arouse much concern, it is arguable that they are not the main causes of ill health related to work. Common diseases such as coronary heart disease, mental illness, and other causes of time lost from work may all be influenced by aspects of work, other than direct physical and chemical exposures. They will be the main focus of this chapter.

The wider social and economic context is important. The state of the economy influences both the quantity and the quality of work available. The productivity of firms, in turn, feeds back into the state of the economy. Hence, work can contribute to the health of the population by its contribution to general prosperity. Prosperity can contribute to health by, among other things, reductions in unemployment and job insecurity and improved working conditions. The general thesis of this chapter is that there may be a virtuous cycle. Wealth creation may improve the prospects for health. Better health may improve the prospects for wealth creation. What is true for the economy as a whole may also be true of the individual workplace. Better working conditions may lead to better health among employees. This may lead to greater productivity and, hence, profitability of the firm.

THE IMPORTANCE OF WORK

Siegrist has suggested four important reasons for the central role of work in industrialized societies (Orth-Gomer and Weiss 1994). First, work is a major determinant of individual income levels, which, of course, have a major impact on living conditions, opportunities, life style, and social and psychological well-being. Second, work may both promote and limit personal growth and development. It shapes life goals and the assessment of self in relation to others. Third, occupation is a measure of social status. Not only is it a criterion of social stratification, but it also relates to esteem and social approval. Fourth, much of social and psychological experience, as well as environmental exposure, takes place in the occupational setting.

For all these reasons work is likely to figure prominently among social determinants of health. For the same set of reasons, it is difficult to separate the effect of work from that of other influences associated with social status. If work defines social status, and if circumstances at work are correlated with other aspects of environment and life style that go along with social status, it will be difficult to isolate the unique contribution of work. The latter part of this chapter will be devoted to analyses from the Whitehall II study that attempt to separate effects of work on health from other influences. We feel that the attempt is justified. In contemplating social gradients in health, such as those described earlier in the book, one response may be that the effects are so pervasive and bound up with the nature of society that there is little that can be done to change them. A major reason for exploring the links between social status and ill health is the search for ways to break the chain linking them. Work is potentially an important link in the chain binding social status to ill health that can potentially be modified without necessarily changing the fundamental nature of social stratification.

THE PSYCHOSOCIAL WORK ENVIRONMENT

Our concern in this chapter is with the effects of the psychosocial work environment on cardiovascular disease and sickness absence. In common parlance, 'psychosocial work environment' is interpreted as 'stress'. Much interest, numerous books (Cooper and Marshall 1976; Cox 1993) and at least one journal are devoted to the issue of work and stress (*Work and Stress* 1994). To the extent possible, we have tried to limit use of the word stress, useful concept though it is. Apart from the old problem of whether stress should be used in the Selye sense of the response of the

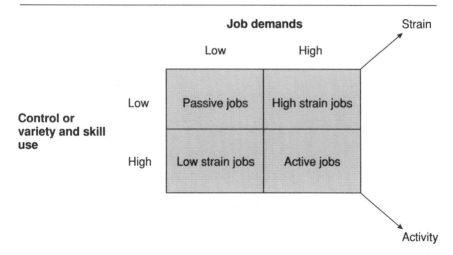

Figure 13.1 The job strain model. (Karasek and Theorell 1990)

organism to outside forces (Selye 1956), or in the engineering sense of outside forces, there is the problem in distinguishing between a subjective response and objective conditions. Both may, of course, be important. One can describe two intellectual positions that are to some extent caricatures. One position would hold that under the same occupational circumstances one individual may be under stress and another not. What is important therefore is to distinguish individual susceptibility to stress. The implication of this line of work would be intervention to change individual susceptibility. The other position would hold that the important sources of stress reside in the social and economic environment, among which the workplace features prominently. The implication of this approach is that attention must be paid not to individual differences in response but to the work environment.

Both positions have validity. Work can only be stressful in so far as it affects the individual in the workplace. Individual responses can never be uniform but will be affected by a variety of factors related to prior experience, other circumstances, and other sources of individual variability.

One particular body of research has used a general stress concept but has proceeded by analysing work conditions rather than subjective reports of stress. This has used the two-factor demand/control model developed by Karasek and Theorell (1990). This two-factor model (Figure 13.1) describes aspects of the work environment along two dimensions that can be described as demand and control, or, more technically, as psychological demands and a combination of skill discretion and decision authority. The hypothesis has been that demands, *per se* may not increase risk. In fact high psychological demands in the presence of high control are

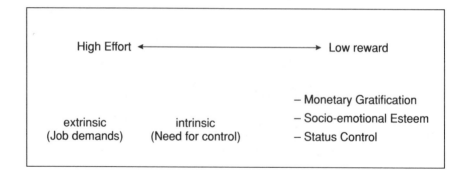

Figure 13.2 The effort–reward imbalance model. (Siegrist and Matschinger 1989)

labelled as the 'active' quadrant in Figure 13.1. The implication is that this may be health-enhancing rather than the reverse. The hypothesis suggests that it is the 'strain' quadrant, high demands and low control, that is associated with increased risk.

This area has been well reviewed by Kristensen (1989). He conducted a review of non-chemical factors in the work environment and cardio-vascular disease. A literature search in the late 1980s yielded 2,000 references, of which 700 were found relevant and evaluated according to precise methodological criteria. He included in his review 'all relevant factors of the work environment' and excluded individual habits or char-acteristics, even though they might be influenced by work conditions. He concluded that physical inactivity in the workplace is associated with increased cardiovascular risk. Turning his attention to stressors related to the organization of work, he observed that they shared one or more common characteristics: (1) lack of control, (2) lack of meaning, (3) lack of predictability, (4) over- or understimulation, and (5) conflict. He found strong and fairly consistent support for a link between the Karasek two-factor model and cardiovascular risk.

Kristensen also found an association between shift work and cardio-vascular disease, although he was concerned at the difficulty in isolating the specific effects of shift work, both from other features of that type of job, and from the characteristics of workers in such occupations.

Siegrist has elaborated a somewhat different two-factor model (Siegrist *et al.* 1990). His model takes into account the role of personal coping and adaptation to work demands. It is illustrated in Figure 13.2. His model stresses effort/reward imbalance. He emphasizes that effort at work is a function of both extrinsic demands and intrinsic motivation. Rather than focus on control, he focuses on rewards of three types: money, esteem and status, and job security. Like the demand/control model, this approach

Table 13.1 Standardized hospitalization ratios (SHR) and 95% confidence
intervals (95% CI) for ischaemic heart disease (ICD-8 = 410–14
in bus and taxi drivers, 1981–4)

Code	Occupation/ Industry	No.	Observed	Expected	SHR	95% CI
Men						
1331	Taxi operator and transport activities n.e.c.[a]	2,829	85	44.94	189	(152.9–233.9)
1339	Forwarding agent n.c.[b]	1,720	55	33.97	162	(124.3–210.9)
4397	Leading position in transport services	505	18	11.78	153	(96.3–242.5)
44342	Salaried employee in bus and carrier service	440	5	2.23	224	(93.3–538.7)
44979	Male urban bus driver	2,664	43	30.14	143	(105.5–192.4)
46974	Male bus driver	4,827	100	73.33	136	(112.1–165.9)
46975	Taxi driver	1,544	25	14.92	168	(113.2–248.0)
46976	Unskilled driver in stevedore and harbour	3,301	60	45.48	132	(102.4–169.9)
46979	Driver, garbage removal and cleaning	38,240	529	450.60	117	(107.8–127.8)
Women						
13310	Taxi operator and transport activities n.e.c.	257	4	0.78	513	(192.5–1,366.4)
4497 +4697	Female transport worker	5,045	18	11.87	152	(95.5–240.7)

Source: Tuchsen *et al.* (1992).

Notes: (a) Not elsewhere classified. (b) Not classified.

posits that high effort and low reward produce sustained distress which
results in increased cardiovascular risk. There is support for this hypothesis in studies of both white-collar and blue-collar occupations (Siegrist
and Matschinger 1989; Siegrist *et al.* 1990, 1991).

APPROACHES TO THE STUDY OF WORK AND HEALTH

Research has addressed the importance of work to health and disease in
at least three different ways. First has been the identification of occupations associated with a high risk of particular diseases. Second, we and
others have raised the question of the contribution of occupational factors
to socioeconomic differences in health. Third has been the study of specific

factors related to occupation that may be related to health risks. This third type of study may involve comparisons across occupations, or within occupational settings.

Table 13.1 shows an example of the first approach from a Danish cohort (Tuchsen *et al.* 1992). It followed a cohort of all people in Denmark aged 20–59 for four years to ascertain death and hospital admission for ischaemic heart disease. The study confirmed the findings of other studies, that people engaged as professional drivers are at increased risk of ischaemic heart disease (Morris *et al.* 1953). It also confirmed other suspected associations, namely increased heart disease risk in bakers, naval officers, fishermen, cooks and waiters, police and salvage corps employees. It also identified a number of other groups at increased risk that had not previously been described.

The problem with this type of study is that it tells us little of the circumstances that may lead to increased risk in those occupations. For example, there are a number of studies of bus drivers pursuing the hypothesis that their increased cardiovascular risk is related to the stressful aspects of the job. It was, however, the observation that drivers of London's double-decker buses had a higher coronary heart disease risk than bus conductors that led Morris to test the hypothesis that lack of physical activity on the job could account for the difference (Morris *et al.* 1953).

Karasek, Theorell and their colleagues have taken this type of study further by classifying occupations according to their mean scores on dimensions of the psychosocial work environment that fit into their two-factor model (Karasek and Theorell 1990). It should be emphasized, that this type of study classifies not individuals but job titles. They have examined coronary heart disease rates for occupations grouped according to their scores on these dimensions and the results of these studies have supported the job strain model.

We tested this approach with data on occupational mortality in England and Wales (Marmot and Theorell 1988). We did not have available a classification of occupations in Britain according to various measures of demand and control, and therefore took the hazardous step of adopting the Swedish system (Alfredsson *et al.* 1982). Table 13.2 shows that people whose jobs were classified as high on monotony and low on the possibility of learning new things had higher mortality ratios from coronary heart disease (Marmot and Theorell 1988). Interestingly, hectic work was not associated with increased risk. The table also illustrates the problem discussed above, i.e. the difficulty in separating the effects of occupation from other phenomena associated with social status. Adjusting for social class reduced the magnitude of the association between work characteristics and coronary heart disease mortality. Two alternative interpretations suggest themselves. First, there is confounding by social class. By this we mean that the apparent association between monotony and cardiovascular

Table 13.2 Mortality from coronary heart disease, expressed as standardized mortality ratios (SMR), in men aged 15–64, by occupation, in England and Wales

Job characteristic	SMR	SMR adjusted for social class
Monotony		
Yes	113	104
No	102	102
Possibility of learning new things		
'Poor'	114	106
'Good'	98	98
Hectic work		
Yes	104	102
No	112	104

Note: Occupations are classified according to the Swedish system of work characteristics. Some occupations were excluded because the Swedish and British occupational codes differed.

Source: Marmot and Theorell (1988).

risk is due not to the work but to the fact that people in such jobs tend to be of lower social status and it is other characteristics associated with such status that are responsible for the increased risk. The other interpretation is that adjusting for social class represents overadjustment. Overadjustment would arise if monotonous work were part of the reason for the association between low social status and increased cardiovascular risk. Adjustment for social class here would actually be adjusting for one of the mechanisms of interest, which would therefore understate the relation between work and cardiovascular disease. We attempt to bypass this problem in our studies of sickness absence, reported below. Similarly, we shall use these studies to illustrate the other two types of investigation, i.e. the contribution of psychosocial work characteristics to generating the social gradient in health; and direct studies of work characteristics and health within one occupation.

WORK AND SICKNESS ABSENCE IN THE WHITEHALL II STUDY

As shown in Chapter 4, the Whitehall studies of British civil servants demonstrate an inverse social gradient in mortality and morbidity: higher rates as one descends the grade hierarchy (Marmot *et al.* 1984; North *et al.* 1993). As social status here is defined on the basis of employment grade, one important question is how much of the differences in health

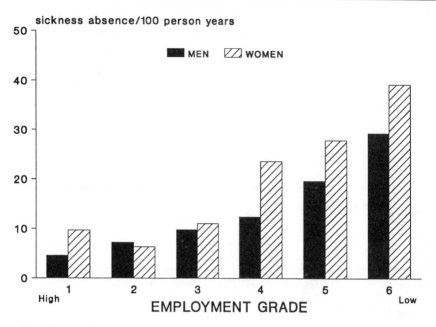

Figure 13.3 Long spells of sickness absence, by employment grade, among British civil servants. (North *et al.* 1993)

can be attributed to circumstances at work. We emphasized at the beginning of this chapter that separating specific effects of work from other social characteristics is far from simple.

In the analyses that follow we present data on the determinants of sickness absence rates, not broken down according to medical diagnosis. This requires some explanation. First, in the original Whitehall study, grade of employment was associated with mortality from a range of specific causes (Marmot *et al.* 1984). This suggested the possibility that, in addition to searching out the determinants of specific medical diagnoses, it was appropriate to search for determinants of general susceptibility to illness. Second, we take the view that ill health is important not only because it may hasten the time of death but because it interferes with social, psychological and physical functioning during life. One way of looking at sickness absence is that it is a measure that integrates decrements in social, psychological and physical functioning. Short spells of absence are more likely to represent decrements in psychological and social functioning; long spells are more likely to represent decrements in physical functioning or 'real illness'. In practice ill health always has physical, social and psychological components. Third, sickness absence is a measure of great economic importance to employers. Studies of the determinants of sickness absence may therefore be of interest not only to those whose primary interest is in the aetiology of illness but to those interested in the health of the economy and of individual firms.

Figure 13.3 shows the clear association between grade of employment and sickness absence rates. Men in the lowest employment grade have six times the absence rate of men in the highest. With the exception of the highest grade, women show a similar gradient. It is of interest that the gradient is similar for short (up to and including seven days) and long spells (over seven days) which require a medical certificate (North *et al.* 1993). Even if it is true that short spells of absence are more likely to represent social and psychological phenomena and long spells 'true illness' it is interesting that short and long spells show an identical social gradient. It suggests that the determinants may be similar and supports the rationale for using sickness absence as an integrated measure of ill health.

Our approach to separating the effects of work from other socioeconomic characteristics is shown in Table 13.3. We look here separately at three dimensions of the psychosocial work environment. 'Work demands' combines five questions on working fast, intensively, with too little time, too many different demands, and a job that is too split up. 'Control' combines eight questions on who decides how and what is done at work, and how much discretion the individual has in deciding on work colleagues, the work environment, and work hours. 'Support at work' combines six questions on help, support, and clarity of information from colleagues and superiors (North *et al.* 1993). The 'age' column of Table 13.3 shows that, adjusting only for age, men and women with high control have lower rates of absence than those with low control. Among men, those with higher support also have lower absence rates. Interestingly, high demands are associated with *lower*, not higher, rates of absence. This is in line with the mortality findings in Table 13.2. Each of these work characteristics varies by grade: high demands, high control and high support are all more common in higher grades. Were we to take the view that grade of employment is a confounder, we would be asking the question of how much of the observed associations between work and sickness absence could be accounted for by the link between these work characteristics and employment grade. An appropriate way to answer this question might be adjustment for grade of employment, as shown in the 'Age, grade' column of Table 13.3. Adjustment for grade appears to account for all of the association between work characteristics and long spells of absence, with the exception of conflicting demands, where women who report high levels have higher rates of long spells of absence.

This may, however, be overadjustment. Grade of employment is not only a social status measure, it gives a fairly precise guide to the type of job pursued. It is the nature of low-grade jobs to have less control and fewer demands. Adjusting for grade is therefore largely to adjust for the variables of interest. Further, grade is measured with greater precision

Table 13.3 Long spells of sickness absence (over seven days), by self-reported work characteristics

Work character-istic	Rate (no. of events)[a]	[Rate ratio (95% confidence interval) adjusted for]		
		Age	Age, grade	Age, other SES indicators[b]
MEN				
Work demands (n = 4,753)				
Low	14.5 (290)	1.00	1.00	1.00
Medium	11.8 (284)	0.82 (0.69–0.96)	1.02 (0.87–1.21)	0.86 (0.73–1.02)
High	9.9 (232)	0.69 (0.58–0.82)	1.03 (0.86–1.24)	0.76 (0.64–0.90)
Control over work (n = 4,760)				
Low	17.0 (275)	1.00	1.00	1.00
Medium	11.2 (271)	0.67 (0.57–0.79)	1.03 (0.86–1.24)	0.74 (0.62–0.88)
High	9.7 (265)	0.57 (0.48–0.67)	1.05 (0.87–1.26)	0.66 (0.55–0.78)
Support at work (n = 4,764)				
Low	12.8 (293)	1.00	1.00	1.00
Medium	12.1 (270)	0.94 (0.79–1.10)	1.02 (0.86–1.20)	0.95 (0.81–1.12)
High	10.9 (247)	0.84 (0.71–1.00)	0.91 (0.77–1.08)	0.87 (0.73–1.03)
WOMEN				
Work demands (n = 2,066)				
Low	31.9 (458)	1.00	1.00	1.00
Medium	29.4 (261)	0.94 (0.81–1.10)	1.10 (0.94–1.29)	1.01 (0.87–1.18)
High	30.6 (190)	1.00 (0.85–1.19)	1.34 (1.12–1.60)	1.08 (0.91–1.29)
Control over work (n = 2,070)				
Low	38.6 (516)	1.00	1.00	1.00
Medium	23.2 (196)	0.62 (0.53–0.73)	0.71 (0.60–0.83)	0.65 (0.55–0.76)
High	24.5 (134)	0.66 (0.55–0.80)	0.91 (0.75–1.10)	0.73 (0.61–0.89)
Support at work (n = 2,085)				
Low	34.5 (391)	1.00	1.00	1.00
Medium	26.3 (237)	0.77 (0.65–0.90)	0.80 (0.68–0.94)	0.78 (0.67–0.92)
High	32.6 (307)	0.95 (0.82–1.10)	0.94 (0.81–1.09)	0.91 (0.79–1.06)

Notes: (a) Rates of sickness absence per 100 person years. (b) Other indicators of socioeconomic status (SES) are: level of education, type of housing, access to a car.

Source: North *et al.* (1996).

than are work characteristics, constructed from a principal component analysis of self-reported items. Therefore, if both grade and, for example, low control are put into the same statistical model, it is more likely that the more precise measure will appear to have the greater independent predictive power. It is not, therefore, necessarily correct to assume that all of the associations between work and sickness absence are due to characteristics associated with differing social status, although these may play a role.

What is the way out of this dilemma? If we adjust for grade there is overadjustment. If we do not adjust for grade there may still be confounding by social status. Our approach was therefore to repeat the analysis (last column of Table 13.3), adjusting not for grade but for other indicators of socioeconomic status, i.e. level of education, housing tenure, and access to a car. As shown, this adjustment makes little difference. It is consistent with the interpretation that the associations between work characteristics and sickness absence are not due to other characteristics associated with social status. The relation, therefore, may be causal.

A different type of issue is not whether employment grade is a confounder, as described above, but whether the association between work and sickness absence is similar in different grades. In Figure 13.4 we have combined the six grades into three broad levels: senior administrators, executives, and clerical and office support. High demands are associated with lower rates of absence in the high grades, but with higher rates in the clerical and office support grades. High control appears to be protective in the high grades but not in low grades. By contrast, high support appears to offer protection in low grades but not in high grades.

Perhaps these contrasting findings are telling us something important about the nature of adverse work characteristics. For a long time we have speculated, consistent with the findings in Table 13.2, that high demands may not be a source of stress, as, in general, high demands are characteristic of high-grade jobs. One might almost speculate that high demands may be a feature of what makes high-grade jobs interesting and challenging and leads to enhanced self-esteem. Given the nature of low-grade jobs, low variety and under-use of skills (North *et al.* 1993), high demands may simply make the job less attractive and contribute to stress-related illness.

Why should high control appear to be protective in high but not in low grades? The answer may relate in part to differential perception of what constitutes 'control' in the workplace. Although high control showed a clear status gradient, higher control in higher grades, some men and women in lower grades did report high control. This is surprising, given the hierarchical nature of large bureaucratic organizations. There may well be a discrepancy between degree of control as perceived by the employee and as assessed objectively.

As an approach to this question, we asked personnel managers to rate jobs according to work demands and control over work. These external assessments were available in eighteen of the twenty civil service departments in the study. These assessments showed marked differences by grade of employment: 7.6 per cent of the combined senior administrative

SHORT SPELLS OF SICKNESS ABSENCE (RATE RATIOS)

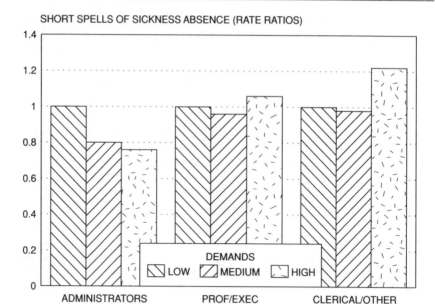

Figure 13.4 Rate ratios for short spells of sickness absence. (a) By work demands (tertiles) within employment grade. (North *et al.* 1996)

SHORT SPELLS OF SICKNESS ABSENCE (RATE RATIOS)

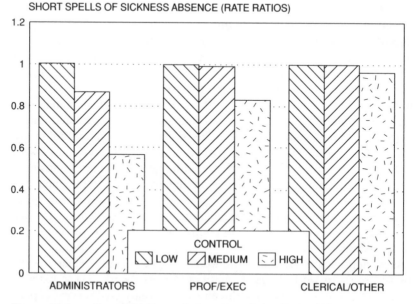

Figure 13.4 continued (b) By control over work (tertiles) within employment grade. (North *et al.* 1996)

SHORT SPELLS OF SICKNESS ABSENCE (RATE RATIOS)

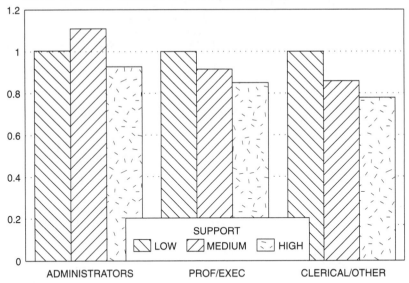

Figure 13.4 continued (c) By support at work (tertiles) within employment grade. (North *et al.* 1996)

group showed low control, compared with 77.5 per cent of the clerical and office support grades. At the individual level, however, the correlation was quite poor between self-reports and external assessments: work demands (0.20 in men and 0.19 in women) and control over work (0.33 in men and 0.32 in women). Within grades the correlations were even lower. Despite these low correlations between external assessments and self-reports, they are both associated with sickness absence rates (North *et al.* 1996) (Table 13.4). In these analyses we have taken account not only of social status (level of education, housing tenure, and access to a car) but also of two other classes of predictors of sickness absence, i.e. health-related behaviours (smoking status, alcohol consumption and physical activity) and social circumstances outside work (difficulty paying bills and negative aspects of social support).

These analyses tie into a long-standing question in stress research: is subjectively perceived, or objectively defined, stress more important in generating adverse health consequences? Given the low order correlation between the two, the data in Table 13.4 suggest that both subjectively perceived and externally assessed characteristics of the work environment play a role in generating sickness absence rates.

In view of the apparent protection associated with high demands in the high grades, we would not have been surprised at the lack of support for

Table 13.4 Long spells of sickness absence (over seven days), by self-reported and externally assessed work demands and control over work, adjusted for confounding factors[a]

	Adjusted rate ratio[a] (95% CI)	
Work characteristic	*Self-reports*	*External assessments*
MEN		
Work demands	(*n* = 4,585)	(*n* = 4,186)
Low	1.00	1.00
Medium	0.84 (0.70–0.99)	0.83 (0.70–1.00)
High	0.73 (0.61–0.87)	0.67 (0.55–0.80)
Control over work	(*n* = 4,593)	(*n* = 4,185)
Low	1.00	1.00
Medium	0.82 (0.68–0.98)	0.80 (0.67–0.95)
High	0.77 (0.64–0.93)	0.61 (0.50–0.76)
WOMEN		
Work demands	(*n* = 1,962)	(*n* = 1,800)
Low	1.00	1.00
Medium	1.03 (0.88–1.21)	0.76 (0.64–0.92)
High	1.20 (1.01–1.44)	0.74 (0.61–0.86)
Control over work	(*n* = 1,962)	(*n* = 1,797)
Low	1.00	1.00
Medium	0.69 (0.58–0.81)	0.92 (0.78–1.09)
High	0.82 (0.67–0.99)	0.86 (0.70–1.10)

Note: (a) Confounding factors: age, socioeconomic status (level of education, type of housing, access to a car), ethnicity, health-related behaviours (smoking status, frequency of alcohol consumption, physical activity), and social circumstances outside work (difficulty paying bills, negative aspects of support).

Source: North *et al.* (1996).

the two-factor demand-control model of Karasek. In fact, when stratifying for grade, there was a clear suggestion of higher absence rates among those with high demands who also had low control over work (North *et al.* 1996).

A different type of question is the contribution of these work characteristics to generating the social gradient in ill health as measured by sickness absence rates. We have, to date, approached this in a rather conventional statistical way, using Poisson regression and a multivariate model. Figure 13.5 shows long spells of absence by grade, adjusted first for age and then for the other predictors of sickness absence, including psychosocial work characteristics. This analysis suggests that about 25 per cent of the social gradient in men and about 35 per cent of the gradient

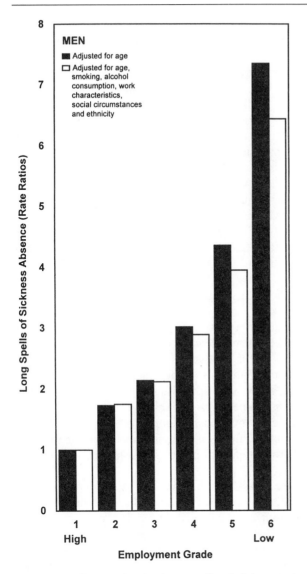

Figure 13.5 Rate ratios for long spells of sickness absence, by grade of employment among male British civil servants. (North *et al.* 1993)

in women is accounted for by these characteristics (North *et al.* 1993). The caveat of measurement precision must, once again, be borne in mind; many of our measures are quite crude. As we have already discussed with work, so also with other social characteristics linked with social status, grade may be a more precise guide than our actual measures of them.

The estimate therefore, of explaining between a quarter and a third of the social gradient on the basis of these characteristics must be a minimum estimate.

Doubtless, better conceptualization and measurement of both the work domain and circumstances outside work would enhance our ability to explain the social gradient in ill health. We must nevertheless consider that there are other factors unmeasured. Quite apart from other circumstances of adult life, there may be important determinants acting earlier in the life course. One implication of the work, reviewed in other chapters, on the British birth cohorts, is that social and family background and early experiences shape ability to cope with adult life experiences. One major feature potentially distinguishing men and women in different jobs is their ability to rise to challenges, perhaps related to the psychological concept of mastery. A review of the evidence on pre-school education for deprived children suggests that such education can teach mastery which has effects lasting into adulthood (Ball 1994).

SICKNESS ABSENCE AND THE VIRTUOUS CYCLE

At the beginning of this chapter we suggested the existence of a virtuous cycle. Better working conditions may lead to better health of employees, which in turn may lead to better productivity of the firm. This may in turn allow for better working conditions. Hence there is a virtuous cycle. The Whitehall II data are consistent with this. It is a reasonable supposition that the differences in sickness absence relate also to differences in productivity. The virtuous cycle may have wider effects. Spread across a whole economy, better output of firms is in the interest of primary wealth creation, which may in turn benefit the health of the population (Frank and Mustard 1994).

It is important therefore to ask whether the findings on civil servants may be generalizable. First, absence rates in the civil service do not differ markedly from those in other employment sectors. The number of days of absence in the Whitehall II study averaged eight per person. In a survey carried out for the Confederation of British Industry (1993), the number of days of absence in 1992 was eight per person in the manufacturing sector and in financial services. It was lower than that in some other sectors, and higher in local government and the National Health Service. Second, the same work factors shown here to predict sickness absence have been shown to be predictive of cardiovascular and other diseases. It is a reasonable working assumption that these findings are generalizable to other large white-collar employment sectors.

In Chapter 4 the favourable life expectancy of the Japanese was discussed, with speculation that it might in part relate to the organization of society. One specific feature of this organization may relate to work.

Table 13.5 Volume car producers, 1989 averages

Characteristic	Japanese in Japan	Japanese in United States	American in United States	All Europe
Productivity (hours/vehicle)	16.8	21.2	25.1	36.2
Quality (defects/100 vehicles)	60.0	65.0	82.3	97.0
% of work force in teams	69.3	71.3	17.3	0.6
Job rotation (0 = none 4 = frequent)	3.0	2.7	0.9	1.9
Suggestions/employee	61.6	1.4	0.4	0.4
Training of new workers (hours)	380.3	370.0	46.4	173.3
Absenteeism	5.0	4.8	11.7	12.1

Source: Womack et al. (1990).

As was pointed out, the relative improvement in Japanese life expectancy occurred at the same time that the country's economic fortunes soared.

An MIT group conducted an international study of the car industry (Womack et al. 1990). Table 13.5 summarizes some results from that study. Among volume car producers, it compares Japanese manufacturers in Japan, Japanese manufacturers in the United States, American manufacturers in the United States and all European manufacturers. The bottom line of the table shows that the level of absenteeism in the Japanese-owned firms is half that in the American and European firms. This lower rate of absence appears to go along with two crucial markers of success: productivity and quality. The number of working hours per vehicle produced was lowest in Japan, next among Japanese-owned firms in the United States, and highest in Europe. The number of defects found per 100 vehicles showed a similar gradient. The MIT study showed that, in general, there is an inverse association between the quality and the productivity of car firms. However, the Japanese-owned firms were the exception to this rule.

How is it possible to have people work harder, to higher standards, and yet apparently have lower absence rates? It cannot simply be the cultural background of the workers in Japan. Japanese-owned firms in the United States, employing American blue-collar workers showed better performance than American-owned firms in the United States. Part of the answer may lie in the management style. The table also shows that a high percentage of the work force in the Japanese-owned firms work in teams. There is a higher frequency of job rotation, and in Japan a higher number of suggestions per employee. It also shows that the Japanese-managed firms have a much greater investment in training new workers. The Americans trail badly in this respect.

These data from the car industry are consistent with other reports from Japan suggesting a higher degree of participation in decision-making, a more highly trained work force, and in addition greater job stability

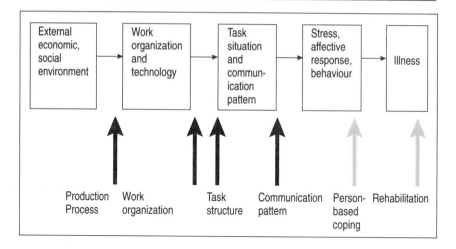

Figure 13.6 A model of the work stress development process. (Karasek 1992)

(Tasker 1987). It has also been suggested that work offers a high degree of social supports in Japan (Matsumoto 1970).

IMPLICATIONS

We should start with a limitation. In this chapter we have focused only on work and in particular on findings from office-based workers in Whitehall II. We have said nothing about the health impact either of unemployment or of job insecurity. One major way in which the broader economy affects the world at work is through its effects on both unemployment and job insecurity, which in turn have health impacts discussed elsewhere in this book.

If the virtuous circle hypothesis is correct and there is no trade-off between the health of employees and the health of firms, it is in the firms' interest to examine management styles that may lead to improved health and wealth. One question arises: is it possible to make changes in the workplace to improve health? This is an important question. However, it is beyond our competence to discuss the vast literature on management styles, productivity and stress in the workplace.

The International Labour Organization commissioned nineteen case studies of stress prevention programmes at the workplace in industrialized and developing countries (International Labour Office 1992). In a review of these interventions, Karasek (1992) produced a schematic model of the work–stress development process (Figure 13.6). He reviewed interventions at each of the points represented by the arrows and found some evidence of effectiveness. Person-based interventions commonly involve individual strategies to relax and/or cope with challenge. He cites examples from Sweden at the other end of the scale, where there have been interventions on work organization and the production process. His general conclusion is that the success of anti-stress programmes is related to workers' participation. This requires institutional support. Karasek suggests that workers' participation involves three stages: awareness of the problem and its links with task organization and work systems; evolving explanations that lead to action plans; and evolving system solutions that extend to change at the work organization level.

One step forward would be to develop models of good practice, based on international experience, to show that the problem of 'stress' in the workplace can be tackled, to improve health, with possible benefit to the organization as well as its employees.

REFERENCES

Alfredsson, L., Karasek, R. and Theorell, T. (1982) Myocardial infarction risk and psychosocial work environment: an analysis of the male Swedish working force, *Social Science and Medicine*, 16: 463–467.

Ball, C. (1994) *Start Right: The Importance of early Learning*, London: Royal Society for the Encouragement of Arts, Manufactures and Commerce.

Confederation of British Industry (1993) *Too much time out?*, CBI/Percom survey on absence from work, London: CBI Percom.

Cooper, C.L. and Marshall J. (1976) Occupational sources of stress: a review of the literature relating to coronary heart disease and mental ill health, *Journal of Occupational Psychology* 49: 11–28.

Cox T. (1993) *Stress*, London: Macmillan.

Frank, J.W. and Mustard, J.F. (1994) The determinants of health from a historical perspective, *Daedalus* 123: 1–21.

International Labour Office (1992) Preventing stress at work, *Conditions of Work Digest*, 11: 1–275.

Karasek, R. (1992) Stress prevention through work organization, *Conditions of Work Digest* 11: 23–40.

Karasek, R. and Theorell, T. (1990) *Healthy Work: Stress, Productivity, and the Reconstruction of Working Life*, New York: Basic Books.

Kristensen, T.S. (1989) Cardiovascular diseases and the work environment: a critical review of the epidemiologic literature on nonchemical factors, *Scandinavian Journal of Work, Environment and Health* 15: 165–179.

Marmot, M.G. and Theorell, T. (1988) Social class and cardiovascular disease: the contribution of work, *International Journal of Health Services* 18: 659–674.

Marmot, M.G., Shipley, M.J. and Rose, G. (1984) Inequalities in death – specific explanations of a general pattern, *Lancet* 1: 1003–1006.

Matsumoto, Y.S. (1970) Social stress and coronary heart disease in Japan, *Millbank Memorial Fund Quarterly* 48: 9–36.

Morris, J.N., Heady, J.A., Raffle, P.A.B., Roberts, C.G. and Parks, J.W. (1953) Coronary heart disease and physical activity of work, *Lancet* 2: 1053–1057.

North, F., Syme, S.L., Feeney, A., Head, J., Shipley, M.J. and Marmot, M.G. (1993) Explaining socioeconomic differences in sickness absence: the Whitehall II study, *British Medical Journal* 306: 361–366.

North, F.M., Syme, S.L., Shipley, M., Feeney, A. and Marmot, M. (1996) Psycho-social work environment and sickness absence: the Whitehall II study *American Journal of Public Health* 86: 332–40.

Orth-Gomer, K. and Weiss, S. (1994) *Behavioural and psychosocial aspects of prevention: First International Teaching Seminar in Behavioural Medicine, Stockholm*, Stress Research Reports 245, Stockholm: Karolinska Institute.

Selye, H. (1956) *Stress of Life*, New York: McGraw-Hill.

Siegrist, J. and Matschinger, H. (1989) Restricted status control and cardiovas-cular risk, in A. Steptoe and A. Appels (eds) *Stress, Personal Control and Health*, Chichester: Wiley.

Siegrist, J., Peter, R., Junge, A., Cremer, P. and Seidel, D. (1990) Low status control, high effort at work and ischaemic heart disease: prospective evidence from blue-collar men, *Social Science and Medicine* 31: 1127–1134.

Siegrist, J., Peter, R. and Georg, W. *et al.* (1991) Psychosocial and biobehavioral characteristics of hypertensive men with elevated atherogenic lipids, *Atherosclerosis* 86: 211–218.

Tasker, P. (1987) *Inside Japan: Wealth, Work and Power in the new Japanese Empire*, London: Penguin.

Tuchsen, F., Bach, E. and Marmot, M.G. (1992) Occupation and hospitalization with ischaemic heart diseases: a new nationwide surveillance system based on hospital admissions, *International Journal of Epidemiology* 21: 450–459.

Womack, J.P., Jones, D.T. and Roos, D. (1990) *The Machine that changed the World*, Don Mills: Collier Macmillan.

Work and Stress (1994) 8(2): 77–204.

ACKNOWLEDGEMENTS

The Whitehall II study is supported by the Medical Research Council, the Health and Safety Executive, the British Heart Foundation, the National Heart Lung and Blood Institute, the Agency for Health Care Policy Research, the New England Medical Centre Division of Health Improvement, the Institute for Work and Health, Toronto, the Volvo Foundation and the John D. and Catherine T. MacArthur Foundation Research Network on Successful Midlife Development.

Chapter 14

Health and work insecurity in young men

Mel Bartley, Scott Montgomery, Derek Cook and Michael Wadsworth

All studies show higher rates of ill health, however measured, both psychological (Warr 1984, 1985; Heady and Smyth 1989) and physical (Moylan *et al.* 1984; Cook *et al.* 1982; Bartley 1988; White 1991) in women and men who are unemployed. However, there is continuing debate about the meaning of this association (Gravelle 1985; Cook and Shaper 1984; Bartley 1994). Ill health may predispose men to lose their jobs (Stern 1983); it would be economically rational for managers to select those with poor health records when reducing the size of their work force. During a time of recession, health is obviously a lesser consideration in job loss – the vast majority of lay-offs and redundancies take place because of a general decline in the demand for labour. Health may still play a role, however, in the likelihood of re-employment (Morris and Cook 1991).

There is abundant evidence that men who experience unemployment are also at higher risk of additional forms of labour market disadvantage (Ferman and Gardner 1979; Daniel 1983, 1990). After a period of unemployment, however it is caused, the risk of downward social mobility from higher to lower status occupations appears to be increased. The next job will often be in a smaller firm with less security and training or fewer promotion opportunities. In men the first spell of unemployment seems greatly to increase the risk of further unemployment, so that a large proportion of all days of unemployment is experienced by a small proportion of working age men (Stern 1979; White 1983). Those who are unemployed may also therefore be experiencing a complex of interrelated disadvantages of which unemployment is only one aspect (Harris 1987; White 1983; Westergaard *et al.* 1989). When studies observe a high rate of ill health among the unemployed it may at least in part be due to a more general experience of work insecurity.

The most recent research on this question in Britain is that carried out as part of the ESRC's Social Change and Economic Life Initiative (SCELI), which examined work histories in six discrete geographical areas chosen to represent different economic patterns during the 1980s recession. Findings from this study describe a group of men employed in low paid and low status jobs to which they had moved by a process of downward mobility who were no better off in terms of psychological well-being than those who were actually unemployed at the time of the survey (Gallie *et al.* 1994). In SCELI, men with insecure work who had been obliged to take lower-status jobs in the recent past had a score on the General Health Questionnaire not significantly different from the unemployed (Burchell 1994). Insecure jobs also tend to involve high exposure to work hazards of various kinds which may affect physical health (Robinson 1986).

During the 1980s the labour market in Britain underwent major changes and job insecurity was greatly increased (Hamnett *et al.* 1989). Secure unskilled or semi-skilled work in the old style smokestack industries became much harder to find. The proportion of all jobs which required education and training rose sharply. Demand for traditional manual skills, which had depended upon the older heavy industries, declined. The manual work career involving either apprenticeship or on-the-job training followed by many years of relative security became less and less available. It is within this context that the relationship between work insecurity and health needs to be addressed.

THEORETICAL MODELS

There are four ways in which work histories could be related to health: two of these may be regarded as 'causal models' in which some characteristics of the unemployment situation increase the risk of poor health; the other two may be regarded as 'selective models' in which some characteristic of the individual, in terms of health or of 'human capital', is causally related both to the type of work history and to the risk of ill health.

1 *Unemployment as a direct cause of ill health.* In this model, the experience of unemployment causes stress, material hardship and behavioural changes, in some combination, which lead to an increased risk of ill health and even mortality.
2 *Unemployment as an indicator of more general insecurity and work hazard.* In the second causal model, those who are found to be unemployed at the time of a census or survey are regarded as at higher health risk because a single spell of unemployment is more often than not experienced as part of an insecure work history with, in many cases, relatively poor working conditions and low pay.
3 *'Direct selection': ill health as a cause of unemployment.* It may be, alternatively, that ill health and higher mortality in the unemployed are a result of the higher levels of disease in those who lose, and find difficulty in regaining, employment.
4 *'Indirect selection'.* This model once again takes a longer view and considers the possibility that those at high risk of unemployment may

also have social and individual characteristics such as lower levels of educational attainment which are independently associated with health risk.

In both the causal and the selective models we may distinguish three possible types of hazard to which the unemployed are exposed: it may be that the experience of unemployment itself is harmful to health, it may be that the degree of insecurity even when employed constitutes a risk factor, or health may be impaired more directly by hazardous working conditions characteristic of insecure occupations (Olsen and Lajer 1979). This chapter compares the physical and mental health of young men aged 23–33 with more and less secure employment histories in the period 1981–91.

MEASURES AND METHODS

Sample

Information for this investigation comes from the National Child Development Study (NCDS), a national longitudinal study of all those born in the week 3–9 March 1958 and living in Great Britain (Butler and Bonham 1963). The original cohort included 17,414 births, and there have been five subsequent sweeps: at ages 7, 11, 16, 23 and 33. The target sample for the most recent data collection was 16,455, which included all members of the cohort who had ever taken part in any previous survey; 86 per cent of the target sample were traced and 11,407 interviewed in 1991, 69 per cent of the target sample. Despite this attrition, it has been shown that the sample remains satisfactorily representative, despite some underrepresentation of the most disadvantaged groups (Ferri 1993). In this chapter only men have been included, owing to the difficulty of classifying women's economic position accurately; data are presented on approximately 4,400 men, with complete information on the variables studied.

Work insecurity

Data collected at ages 23 and 33 include information on all occupations and all spells of unemployment experienced between labour market entry and age 33. Work insecurity is defined here in two different ways. At age 23 work insecurity is defined as the number of spells of unemployment experienced between labour market entry and age 22. At this young age, men will have been in the labour market, and therefore at risk of unemployment, for different periods of time depending upon when they left full-time education. Therefore, previous unemployment is measured in terms of the number of spells experienced rather than the amount of time unemployed. At age 33 the great majority of male cohort members will have been economically active for the past ten years. Work insecurity at this age is therefore defined as the total number of months of unemployment experienced between ages 23 and 33. In the process of checking the consistency of data collected at ages 23 and 33 it was found that spells of unemployment of less than three months' duration were less likely to be reported accurately by members of the manual social groups than by members of the non-manual, introducing a danger of bias. Because of this, only spells of three months or more have been included in the analysis reported here.

Economic position

Only those men who were either unemployed and seeking work or in full-time employment have been included in the analysis. Those who were not in employment owing to long-term ill health are excluded, as are part-time workers and those whose work consisted of full-time home and family care.

Occupation

The social class of the cohort members' fathers at the time of their birth was classified by means of the Registrar General's classification of occupations. Social mobility of cohort members was defined as mobility between the Registrar General's social classes between ages 23 and 33. The Registrar-General's classification is conventionally regarded as a measure of status or 'general standing in the community'. It has six categories: class I consists of professionals and senior managers; II consists of other managers; IIIN are clerical and sales workers; IIIM are skilled manual workers; IV are semi-skilled and V are non-skilled manual workers. 'Upward' mobility is defined as movement from any lower status to any higher status class, for example, V to IV, IIIM to IIIN; 'downward' mobility includes movement from any higher status to any lower status class; the 'stable' are those who have remained in the same class throughout the period of observation.

Health

Men were also asked questions about their health at the time of the interview, and were administered a validated measure of psychological well-being, the Malaise Inventory (Rutter *et al.* 1970). In this chapter, self-reported general health and Malaise Inventory score are used. A score of 8 or more on the Malaise Inventory is regarded as indicative of a risk of depression.

Table 14.1 Work insecurity and self-reported general health at age 23

Previous spells of unemployment up to age 22	[Self-reported general health at age 23 (%)]		
	Excellent/good	Fair/poor	n = 100%
0	94	6	3,140
1	92	8	860
2+	84	16	426
n	4,090	336	4,426

Note: $\chi^2 = 48.6$, 2 df, $p < 0.001$.

We are therefore able to make some assessment of how current economic position, previous unemployment patterns and the status of previous and present occupations related to self-reported general health and to psychological health at the time of two data collections when the men were aged 23 and 33.

RESULTS

Work insecurity and health at age 23

Table 14.1 shows the risk of reporting fair or poor self-rated health at age 23 in relation to the number of previous spells of unemployment. Men of this age are, on the whole, healthy, as can be seen from the small proportion who report themselves in other than excellent or good health. However, the proportion reporting fair or poor health rises from 6 per cent in those who have experienced no spells of unemployment up to the age of 22 to 16 per cent in those who have experienced two or more.

Table 14.2 shows the relationship of the Malaise inventory score to previous work insecurity: once again, most cohort members score within the normal range. However, the proportion scoring within the range indicative of a risk of depression rises from 3 per cent of those with no previous unemployment to 6 per cent of those with two or more spells. When looking at these two tables it has to be remembered that they include both the employed and the unemployed at the time of the survey: the number of spells of unemployment could be associated with health just because those with more spells were more likely to be unemployed when interviewed.

A 'selective' theoretical model would propose that the observed relationship between work insecurity and health could be due to some prior variable which explains both the risk of work insecurity and that of poorer health. For example, it is known that frequent job changing, and the resulting risk of having many spells of unemployment, is related to the social class of the family of origin (Cherry 1976).

Table 14.2 Work insecurity and Malaise Inventory score at age 23

Previous spells of unemployment up to age 22	[Malaise Inventory score at age 23 (%)]		
	Normal 0–7	Depressed 8–24	n = 100%
0	97	3	3,135
1	95	5	860
2+	94	6	427
n	4,268	154	4,422

Note: χ^2 = 23.6, 2 df, p < 0.001.

In order to test these two possibilities – that the relationship between work insecurity and health could be due to unemployment at the time of the survey or to prior circumstances increasing both the risk of unemployment and of poor health – logistic modelling was used. The relation between work insecurity and present health state was adjusted for whether or not the person was unemployed at the time their health was measured and the social class of their father, as a measure of prior social circumstances.

Table 14.3 shows the model of self-reported general health. In the first column the relationship between each variable on its own and the risk of fair or poor self-reported health at age 23 is shown. Work insecurity and unemployment and the time of the interview are statistically significant. The unemployed had a 70 per cent higher risk of 'fair or poor' health than the employed, and in those with two or more previous spells of unemployment the risk was almost threefold. In the second column the relative odds of fair or poor health associated with each variable are shown after the effect of the others has been taken into account. In this adjusted model, father's social class remained significant when treated as a continuous variable: the differences between class I and classes II to IV could have arisen by chance, but those whose fathers were in social class V were considerably more likely to report fair or poor health, producing a significant trend. Work insecurity also remained significant. The extent to which it increased the risk of fair or poor health was somewhat reduced by introducing employment status at the time of interview and family background variables; however, the excess risk associated with being unemployed at the time of the interview was no longer significant once the effects of the other two variables had been taken into account.

In Table 14.4 logistic modelling has been used in order to see whether the relationship between work insecurity and psychological health varied according to economic position at the time of interview and social background. In the first column the relationship of each variable on its own to the risk of scoring in the depressed range of the Malaise Inventory is shown. Those who were unemployed had almost double the risk of those in full-time employment. Those with two or more spells of unemployment

Table 14.3 Relationships between work history variables, social background
and self-reported general health at age 23

	Relative odds of reporting poor or fair general health at age 23			
Variable	Unadjusted odds (95% CI)	Significance	Adjusted odds	Significance
Spells of unemployment up to age 22		0.0000		0.0000
0	1 (ref.)		1	
1	1.21		1.14	
	(0.91–1.61)		(0.83–1.56)	
2+	2.76		2.41	
	(2.05–3.71)		(1.07–3.42)	
Economic position at age 23		0.0049		0.7996
Employed	1		1	
Unemployed	1.60		1.05	
	(1.15–2.21)		(0.72–1.54)	
Father's social class				
Overall trend		0.0044		0.0168
I	1		1	
II	1.43		1.51	
	(0.67–3.01)		(0.71–3.20)	
IIIN	1.65		1.74	
	(0.77–3.54)		(0.81–3.75)	
IIIM	1.70		1.72	
	(0.85–3.38)		(0.86–3.42)	
IV	2.06		2.05	
	(0.98–4.31)		(0.98–4.31)	
V	2.49		2.31	
	(1.16–5.34)		(1.07–4.97)	

since leaving full-time education had two and a half times the risk. Taken
on its own, father's social class was also significantly related to psychological health at age 23. In the second column the risks of each single variable
have been adjusted for each other. Once again, the relationship between
being unemployed at the time of the survey and the risk of poor health
was no longer significant. In contrast, whereas the relative risk associated
with job insecurity was somewhat reduced, it remained highly significant.

Work history and health at age 33

We also investigated the relation between work insecurity and health at
age 33. Because between the ages of 23 and 33 the amount of unemployment was not affected by age at leaving school the measure of work

Table 14.4 Relationship between work history variables, social background and Malaise Inventory score at age 23

	[Relative odds of scoring 8+ on Malaise Inventory]			
Variable	⎡Unadjusted⎤ odds ⎣95% CI ⎦	Significance	⎡Adjusted⎤ odds ⎦	Significance
Spells of unemployment up to age 22		0.0000		0.0044
0	1(ref.)		1	
1	1.98		1.68	
	(1.36–2.88)		(1.11–2.53)	
2+	2.48		2.11	
	(1.59–3.88)		(1.26–3.52)	
Economic position at age 23		0.0022		0.5702
Employed	1		1	
Unemployed	1.97		1.16	
	(1.28–3.04)		(0.69–1.96)	
Father's social class				
Overall trend		0.0001		0.0008
I	1		1	
II	1.40		1.45	
	(0.39–5.02)		(0.41–5.20)	
IIIN	1.94		1.97	
	(0.54–6.94)		(0.55–7.07)	
IIIM	2.22		2.20	
	(0.70–7.12)		(0.69–7.04)	
IV	4.28		4.12	
	(1.29–14.2)		(1.24–13.70)	
V	3.65		3.20	
	(1.05–12.60)		(0.92–11.10)	

history used here is the total number of months' unemployment experienced (in spells of over three months) rather than the number of spells.

Tables 14.5–6 show the relationship of work insecurity to self-reported general health and to score on the Malaise Inventory. Table 14.5 shows that there are slightly more cohort members reporting fair or poor general health at age 23 than at age 33. Among those with no spell of unemployment longer than three months in the intervening period, 10 per cent report fair or poor health, in contrast to 16 per cent of those who have experienced over twelve months' total time unemployed. Table 14.6 shows that 4 per cent of those in the lowest unemployment category scored as at risk of depression on the Malaise Inventory, in contrast to 10 per cent of those with over twelve months out of work.

Table 14.5 Work insecurity and self-reported general health at age 33

Months of unemployment between ages 23 and 33	[Self-reported general health at age 33 (%)]		
	Excellent/good	Fair/poor	n = 100%
0	90	10	2,929
≤12	86	14	622
13+	84	16	421
n	3,530	442	3,972

Note: χ^2 = 21.6, 2 df, p < 0.0001.

Table 14.6 Work insecurity and Malaise Inventory score at age 33

Months of unemployment between ages 23 and 33	[Malaise Inventory score at age 33 (%)]		
	Normal 0–7	Depressed 8–24	n = 100%
0	96	4	2,946
≤12	93	7	623
13+	90	10	424
n	3,780	213	3,993

Note: χ^2 = 26.3, 2 df, p < 0.00001.

Social mobility, economic position and existing health

At age 33 we were also interested in any effect on health of the direction of social mobility, and in the effect of 'selection' whereby an apparent relationship between work history and health may be due to those with health problems at the beginning of the period being more vulnerable to insecurity. Social mobility is a routine occurrence between labour market entry and age 23, while young people are finding their feet in the world of work. Between 23 and 33, however, such changes are less common and can be a more threatening experience: it is known that after a spell of unemployment men are more likely to experienced 'job demotion' (Daniel 1983; Westergaard et al. 1989).

Over 40 per cent of economically active cohort members experienced some social mobility as they moved from their 20s into their early 30s during the 1980s: 30 per cent moved upwards and 13 per cent downwards. Tables 14.3–4 indicate that the degree of previous work insecurity largely accounted for the health differences between the employed and the unemployed at age 23. At age 33 we ask first whether work insecurity has the same relationship to health. Next, in order to see whether this could in turn be partly due to job status changes associated with such insecurity, social mobility is introduced into a logistic model including work insecurity and

Table 14.7 Relationships between work insecurity, economic position, social mobility and self-reported general health at age 33

	Relative odds of reporting poor or fair general health at 33			
Variable	Unadjusted odds (1)	Adjusted for social mobility (2)	Adjusted for mobility and economic position (3)	Adjusted for mobility, economic position and health at age 23 (4)
Months of unemployment between ages 23 and 33				
0	1 (ref.)	1	1	1
≤12	1.48	1.47	1.40	1.32
	(1.14–1.92)	(1.14–1.91)	(1.08–1.82)	(1.00–1.74)
13+	1.80	1.79	1.53	1.25
	(1.35–2.39)	(1.34–2.39)	(1.12–2.11)	(0.90–1.74)
Social mobility between ages 23 and 33				
Upward	1	1	1	1
Stable	1.01	1.06	1.05	0.99
	(0.81–1.27)	(0.84–1.32)	(0.84–1.32)	(0.78–1.26)
Downward	1.25	1.22	1.21	0.99
	(0.91–1.72)	(0.89–1.68)	(0.89–1.68)	(0.71–1.39)
Economic position at age 33				
Employed	1		1	1
Unemployed	2.17		1.68	1.44
	(1.53–3.08)		(1.14–2.47)	(0.96–1.51)
General health at age 23				
Excellent	1			1
Good	2.57			2.53
	(2.02–3.28)			(1.80–3.55)
Fair/poor	12.2			11.47
	(8.94–16.50)			(10.22–12.87)

economic position at the time of the interview. In order to test the 'selection' model, a variable measuring self-reported general health at age 23 is also included in the model, to see how strongly health at the earlier age may be related to work insecurity between 23 and 33.

Table 14.7 shows the results of taking each variable into account jointly. Column 1 shows the simple univariate relationships between each variable and the risk of reporting fair or poor health at age 33. As at age 23, work insecurity and unemployment at the time of the interview are both statistically significant, and remain so when adjusted for each other. Adjusting for social mobility does not affect the relationship between insecurity and health: this relationship is therefore unlikely to have been

Table 14.8 Relationship between work insecurity, economic position, social mobility and Malaise Inventory score at age 33

| | *Relative odds of scoring 8+ on Malaise Inventory* | | | |
Variable	Unadjusted odds	Adjusted for social mobility	Adjusted for social mobility and economic position	Adjusted for health at age 23 mobility, economic position and malaise
Months of unemployment between ages 23 and 33				
0	1 (ref.)	1	1	1
≤12	1.63	1.65	1.58	1.60
	(1.14–2.33)	(1.15–2.36)	(1.10–2.27)	(1.09–2.34)
13+ months	2.42	2.45	2.17	1.76
	(1.68–3.48)	(1.70–3.54)	(1.45–3.25)	(1.14–2.72)
Social mobility between ages 23 and 33				
Upward	1	1	1	1
Stable	1.25	1.33	1.33	1.25
	(0.81–1.93)	(0.96–1.85)	(0.96–1.85)	(0.89–1.76)
Downward	1.50	1.43	1.42	1.34
	(0.96–2.34)	(0.92–2.24)	(0.91–2.22)	(0.83–2.15)
Economic position at age 33				
Employed	1		1	1
Unemployed	2.31		1.50	1.32
	(1.45–3.65)		(0.90–2.47)	(0.76–2.30)
Malaise at age 23				
Normal	1			1
Depressed	17.74			16.29
	(11.92–25.50)			(11.10–23.90)

produced by insecure workers moving down the social scale. However, by far the most important precursor of health at age 33, not surprisingly, is health at age 23. Perhaps rather more surprisingly, once this is introduced into the multivariate model, neither work insecurity between 23 and 33 nor unemployment at the time of the survey remains significantly related to self-reported health at 33.

Table 14.8 shows the same logistic model for the Malaise Inventory. Considering the variables singly, both the unemployed and those who, regardless of their present economic position, had over twelve months of unemployment since age 23 are at more than double the risk of a high Malaise score. When account is taken of previous work insecurity and social mobility the risk associated with current unemployment is greatly reduced and becomes statistically non-significant. Adjustment for current unemployment and social mobility does not, however, account for the excess risk associated with over twelve months' previous unemployment: it is still more than double. Once again the variable most strongly related to malaise at 33 is malaise at 23. However, in this case there does seem to be an effect of work insecurity over and above predisposing ill health: though reduced, the relationship remains statistically significant.

DISCUSSION

At age 23 it is previous work insecurity rather than economic position itself which is associated with poor self-reported health, and this association is independent of the relationship of class background with the risk of unemployment in the early years of working life. Work insecurity also appears to be an important factor in psychological health at age 23, accounting for most of the association between Malaise Inventory score and current economic position and acting independently of class of origin.

Social mobility between ages 23 and 33 did not seem to play a very great role in the link between labour market experience and health at age 33. This may seem to contradict the evidence that loss of employment acts on health via an increased risk of poor working conditions. Evidence relating economic status to mortality in Scandinavian countries and in Italy has found morbidity to be considerably higher among the unemployed than in any category of employed men (Isaksson 1989; Lahelma 1992a, b; Rudas et al. 1991). This implies that unemployment is less 'healthy' than any type of employment, although the studies did not record social mobility or patterns of previous unemployment.

Work insecurity had a significant independent relationship with psychological health at age 33. Although reduced by the introduction of current economic position and social mobility, the relationship remained significant. In contrast, the relationship between psychological health and unemployment at the time of interview was no longer significant once adjustment was made for work insecurity and social mobility. When Malaise Inventory score at age 23 was introduced, it further reduced the strength of the relationship between work insecurity and the risk of depression at the time of the interview, but a significant effect remained. The finding that work insecurity as well as unemployment *per se* may have implications for psychological health is consistent with previous evidence that health begins to be affected at the time when people are still at work but begin to feel their jobs are at risk (Cobb and Kasl 1977; Beale and Nethercott 1985; Iversen and Klausen 1981).

In the case of self-reported general health the results are somewhat different. We have taken this to be a measure of physical health, and studies have shown answers to this type of question to be predictive of mortality (Wannamethee and Shaper 1990). Unlike the Malaise Inventory, however, self-reported health is not a clinically validated indicator. We do not know whether those who report 'good' rather than 'excellent' health at an interview are objectively more likely to be suffering from clinically definable disease. Once the effect of the equivalent variable measured at age 23 is taken into account, there is no remaining significant relationship between either unemployment at the time of interview or the amount previously experienced and self-reported general health at age 33. This result needs to be interpreted cautiously: even those who report 'good' as opposed to 'excellent' health at 23 have over double the risk of later 'fair or poor' health at 33. Self-reported general health may in part reflect conditions of life themselves: a mismatch between the demands of life and normal variations in physical energy, which could only crudely be interpreted as 'selection' (Stern 1983; Wagstaff 1986; Valkonen and Martikainen 1992). And this result also needs to be seen in the context of findings from much larger studies which show that the association between unemployment and mortality, a far clearer end-point, is unlikely to be due to selection of those with clinically life-threatening disease into unemployment (Morris *et al.* 1994; Moser *et al.* 1984, 1990).

CONCLUSION AND POLICY IMPLICATIONS

In this chapter we have asked whether the poor health observed in studies of the unemployed could be in part a consequence of more general work insecurity, or of a deterioration in work conditions and occupational status in men who experience unemployment. We have shown that the association between unemployment at the time of interview and psychological ill health can to a large extent be explained in terms of the extent of unemployment in the previous seven to ten year period. Mobility from a more to a less favourable type of work (as indicated by changes in social class) was not seen to play a significant role, either in itself, or as a moderator of the relationship between health and labour market experience. In contrast, unemployment at age 33 is related to self-reported general health independently of previous work insecurity. However, neither unemployment nor work insecurity is associated with general health at 33 independently of reported health status at age 23.

The strength of pre-existing health as a predictor of health at age 33, and the extent to which it reduces the excess risk of ill health in those with greater job insecurity, indicate some support for the role of health selection (Gravelle 1985; Stern 1983; Wagstaff 1986). However, further research is needed into the determinants of health in young people. By their early 20s few women or men have yet developed significant clinically definable disease. In other related work we have shown that such disease, as measured by a medical examination at age 16, is not an important cause of future unemployment. More important are unfavourable early family circumstances and the associated deficits in physical growth, psychological development and educational attainment (Montgomery *et al.* 1995). These in turn increase the risk of unemployment between labour market entry and age 23. Cohort members who felt that their health was generally less than 'excellent' at age 23 may have been those who had already experienced various forms of disadvantage which affected both their health and their occupational histories; this chapter has shown a significant relationship between fathers' social class at the time of cohort members' birth and health at age 23. This possibility needs further examination. The relationship of health at 23 to health at 33 and labour market experience may itself be a long-term outcome of earlier unfavourable circumstances.

The likelihood that 'indirect selection' plays a role in the relationship between work insecurity and health makes it more rather than less important to consider labour market policies which promote training and employment, especially of those who have experienced less favourable conditions in earlier life. It is widely considered inequitable that the costs of social change fall most heavily on those in the heaviest and least well paid jobs. Particularly in the 1980s recession, those in professional and administrative jobs were more or less untouched, while skilled manual jobs declined sharply. The analysis presented here suggests that those with some degree of vulnerability in terms of social background and health were also at higher risk of job insecurity over long periods of time. Nearly thirty years ago Sinfield (1970) pointed out that the insecurity and arduous conditions of the work often obtained by those at high risk of unemployment should be as great a policy concern as unemployment itself. This, of course, is even more true if we believe that those in poorer health are at higher risk of unemployment.

Much has been made of the virtues of a more 'flexible' labour market – one in which a higher proportion of all jobs are temporary, and a higher proportion of all workers are on short-term contracts, or are formally self-employed freelance workers (Hutton 1995). In the 1980s, the period dealt with here, many of the newly flexible work force were ex-steelworkers, shipbuilders, hospital and factory cleaners whose jobs had been contracted out (Dale 1986; Harris 1987; Westergaard *et al.* 1989; Fevre 1991). Under these conditions the same jobs were in some cases being done by the same workers for less pay, and with none of the forms of protection that go along with permanent regulated employment. The 1980s shake-out affected mostly people in jobs which would always have entailed a fair degree of hazard and were often not well paid. The 1990s recession may be different: flexible working is now increasingly seen as a virtue by employers of professional, technical and managerial staff. The fact that, in this cohort, job insecurity was associated with poorer health regardless of social mobility implies that extending work casualization to the middle classes may have a similar effect on their health to that which has been shown for the 1980s. Firstly, job insecurity may fall most heavily on those with some, even minor, degree of health impairment; second, it may equally increase the risk of depression and become, literally, a 'feel bad factor' for those who previously have held more protected positions.

REFERENCES

Ashton, D.N. (1986) *Unemployment under Capitalism: the sociology of British and American labour markets*, Brighton: Wheatsheaf.

Bartley, M. (1988) Unemployment and health, selection or causation: a false antithesis?, *Sociology of Health and Illness* 10: 41–67.

Bartley, M. (1994) Unemployment and health: understanding the relationship, *Journal of Epidemiology and Community Health* 48: 333–337.

Beale, N. and Nethercott, S. (1985) Job-loss and family morbidity: a study of a factory closure, *Journal of the Royal College of General Practitioners* 35: 510–514.

Burchell, B. (1992) Towards a social psychology of the labour market: or why we need to understand the labour market before we can understand unemployment, *Journal of Occupational Psychology* 65: 345–354.

Burchell, B. (1994) The effects of labour market position, job insecurity, and unemployment on psychological health, in D. Gallie, S. Marsh and C. Vogler (eds) *Social Change and the Experience of Unemployment*, Oxford: Oxford Univerity Press.

Butler, N.R. and Bonham, D.G. (1963) *Perinatal Mortality: the first report of the 1958 British Perinatal Mortality Survey*, Edinburgh: Livingstone.

Cherry, N. (1976) Persistent job changing: is it a problem?, *Journal of Occupational Psychology* 49: 203–221.

Cobb, S. and Kasl, S.C. (1977) *Termination: the Consequences of Job Loss*, US National Institutes for Occupational Safety and Health, Publication No. 77–224, Cincinnati: DHEW–NIOSH.

Cook, D.G. and Shaper, E.G. (1984) Unemployment and health, in J.M. Harrington (ed.) *Recent Advances in Occupational Health* II, Edinburgh: Churchill Livingstone.

Cook, D.G., Cummins, R.O., Bartley, M.J. and Shaper, A.G. (1982) The health of unemployed middle aged men in Britain, *Lancet* 1: 1290–1294.

Dale, A. (1986) Social class and the self-employed, *Sociology* 20: 430–434.

Daniel, W.W. (1983) How the unemployed fare after they find new jobs, *Policy Studies* 3: 246–260.

Daniel, W.W. (1990) *The Unemployed Flow*, London: Policy Studies Institute.

Fallon, P. and Verry, D. (1988) *The Economics of Labour Markets*, Oxford: Philip Allan.

Ferman, L. and Gardner, J. (1979) Economic deprivation, social mobility and mental health, in L. Ferman and J. Gordus (eds) *Mental Health and the Economy*, Kalamazoo, Mich.: W.E. Upjohn Institute for Employment Research.

Ferri, E. (ed.) (1993) *Life at 33: the Fifth Follow-up of the National Child Development Study*, London: National Children's Bureau.

Fevre, R. (1991) Emerging 'alternatives' to full time and permanent employment, in P. Brown and R. Scase (eds) *Poor Work: Disadvantage and the Division of Labour*, Milton Keynes: Open University Press.

Gallie, D., Marsh, S. and Vogler, C. (1994) *Social Change and the Experience of Unemployment*, Oxford: Oxford Univerity Press.

Gravelle, H.S.E. (1985) Does unemployment kill?, Nuffield/York Portfolio No. 9, Leeds: Nuffield Provincial Hospitals Trust.

Hamnett, C., McDowell, L. and Sarre, P. (eds) (1989) *The Changing Social Structure*, London: Sage/Open University.

Harris, C.C. (1987) *Redundancy and Recession*, Oxford: Blackwell.

Heady, P. and Smyth, M. (1989) *Living Standards during Unemployment*, London: HMSO.

Hutton, W. (1995) *The State We're In*, London: Jonathan Cape.

Isaksson, K. (1989) Unemployment and mental health and the psychological functions of work in male welfare clients in Stockholm, *Scandinavian Journal of Social Medicine* 17: 165–169.

Iversen, L. and Klausen H. (1981) *The closure of the Nordhavn shipyard*, Kobenhauns Universitat Publikation 13, Copenhagen: Institute of Social Medicine

Lahelma, E. (1992a) Unemployment and mental well-being: elaboration of the relationship, *International Journal of Health Services* 22: 261–274.

Lahelma, E. (1992b) Paid employment, unemployment and mental well-being, *Psychiatrica Fennica* 23: 131–144.

Montgomery, S., Bartley, M., Cook, D. and Wadsworth, M. (1995) Are young unemployed men at greater risk of future illness, even before they experience any unemployment?, *Journal of Epidemiology and Community Health* 49: 552.

Morris, J.K. and Cook, D.G. (1991) A critical review of the effect of factory closures on health, *British Journal of Industrial Medicine* 48: 1–8.

Morris, J.K., Cook, D.G. and Shaper, A.G. (1994) Loss of employment and mortality, *British Medical Journal* 308: 1135–1139.

Moser, K.A., Fox, A.J. and Jones, D.R. (1984) Unemployment and mortality in the OPCS longitudinal study, *Lancet* ii: 1324–1328.

Moser, K., Goldblatt, P., Fox, J. and Jones, D. (1990) Unemployment and mortality, in P.O. Goldblatt (ed.) *Longitudinal Study: Mortality and Social Organisation*, London: HMSO.

Moylan, S., Millar, J. and Davis, R. (1984) *For Richer, for Poorer – the DHSS Cohort Stody*, London: HMSO.

Olsen, J. and Lajer, M. (1979) Violent death in two trade unions in Denmark, *Social Psychiatry* 14: 139–145.

Robinson, J.C. (1986) Job hazards and job security, *Journal of Health Politics, Policy and Law* 11: 1–18.

Rudas, N., Tondo, L., Musio, A. and Mosia, M. (1991) Unemployment and depression. Results of a psychometric evaluation, *Minerva Psichiatrica* 32: 205–209.

Rutter, M., Tizard, J. and Graham, P. (1970) *Education, Health and Behaviour*, London: Longman.

Sinfield, R.A. (1970) *Poor and Out of Work in South Shields,* in P. Townsend (ed.) *The Concept of Poverty*, London: Heinemann.

Sinfield, R.A. (1981) *What Unemployment Means*, Oxford: Martin Robertson.

Stern, J. (1979) Who bears the burden of unemployment?, in W. Beckermann (ed.) *Slow Growth in Britain*, Oxford: Clarendon.

Stern, J. (1983) The relationship between unemployment, morbidity and mortality in Britain, *Population Studies* 37: 61–74.

Valkonen, T. and Martikainen, P. (1992) The association between unemployment and mortality: causation or selection?, Paper to IUSSP Seminar *Premature Adult Mortality in Developed Countries*, Taormina, Italy, 1–5 June.

Wagstaff, A. (1986) Unemployment and health: some pitfalls for the unwary, *Health Trends* 18: 79–81.

Wannamethee, G. and Shaper, A.G. (1990) Weight change, perceived health status and mortality in middle-aged British men, *Postgraduate Medical Journal* 66: 910–913.

Warr, P.B. (1984) Job loss, unemployment and psychological well-being, in V. Allen and E. van de Vliert (eds) *Role Transitions*, New York: Plenum.

Warr, P. (1985) Twelve questions about unemployment and health, in B. Roberts, R. Finnegan, D. Gallie (eds) *New Approaches to Economic Life*, Manchester: Manchester University Press.

Westergaard, J., Noble, I. and Walker, A. (1989) *After Redundancy: the Experience of Economic Insecurity*, Cambridge: Polity Press.

White, M. (1983) *Long Term Unemployment and Labour Markets*, London: Policy Studies Institute.

White, M. (1991) *Against Unemployment*, London: Policy Studies Institute.

ACKNOWLEDGEMENT

This research was supported by ESRC Grant no. R000234697.

Chapter 15

The social and biological basis of cardiovascular disease in office workers

Eric Brunner

Men and women working in higher employment grades in the British civil service live longer and report better health than those in lower employment grades. An important component of these differences in health is the large occupational gradient in the risk of circulatory disease which has existed on both sides of the Atlantic for the past thirty years (Hinkle *et al.* 1968; Marmot *et al.* 1978). During this period rates of coronary heart disease mortality have fallen, but the decline in coronary heart disease (Marmot and McDowall 1986; McLoone and Boddy 1994) as well as in all-cause mortality (Phillimore *et al.* 1994) has been greater among the more affluent, and socioeconomic inequalities in coronary heart disease have grown larger. For this reason the importance of work-related differences in cardiovascular disease is today perhaps greater than at the height of the epidemic.

The focus of this book is on the links between social structure and health. Measures of social and economic status, including occupation, are extremely powerful discriminators of health expectations. They are more powerful than, for example, the combination of smoking, serum cholesterol and blood pressure in predicting premature heart disease (Marmot *et al.* 1978). To state the obvious: social phenomena require social explanations. Yet health research remains dominated by a biomedical model which looks for the molecular mechanisms responsible for disease. Political and economic interests, such as those of the pharmaceutical industry, are paramount in shaping this unbalanced allocation of research funding (Judge 1994). There is, however, a further reason to give attention to biology. The case for remedial action to reduce the burden of preventable ill health can be strengthened if the biological pathways connecting low social status with specific diseases are understood. As Kaplan and Keil (1993) have suggested, socioeconomic status is found to be an 'independent' risk factor in prospective studies only because our knowledge of causation is inadequate. As we learn more about the social, environmental, psychological, behavioural and biological pathways by which socioeconomic status affects cardiovascular disease its independent predictive power will tend to diminish. Recent research, for example, on the fetal and infant origins of the disease (Barker 1992) has highlighted the effects of intrauterine growth. When lifelong follow-up studies have been carried out it seems likely that low birth weight and slow growth in early life will emerge as some of the consequences of socioeconomic disadvantage (Bartley *et al.* 1994). This would add to our understanding of the relevant pathways, and reduce the 'independent' effect of socioeconomic status measures in a multivariate statistical model, but it would not detract from the importance of socioeconomic factors such as occupation as primary determinants of cardiovascular risk.

The approach in this chapter is to look at some of the existing evidence for the biological pathways which connect lower socioeconomic status with increased risk of cardiovascular disease and non-insulin-dependent diabetes, and to consider in particular whether the data support a psychosocial stress mechanism.

PATHWAYS

There is strong evidence of social gradients in the functioning of lipid metabolism and components of the blood clotting system (Kaplan and Keil 1993; Brunner *et al.* 1993). The evidence is based on coronary heart disease risk factor measurements, which may be seen not only as predictors of future disease but also as markers of the atherosclerotic and thrombotic processes leading to disease. The gradients are inverse, with the least favourable levels in the lowest social strata and, in general, stepwise improvements as the strata are ascended. Surveys of adults drawn from population and occupational groups show trends with several measures of social position, including Registrar General's social class, civil service employment grade, education level and material circumstances. The pattern of risk factor trends is not uniform. Serum total cholesterol, for instance, appears weakly or not at all associated with social position.

Novel evidence presented here suggests that differences in carbohydrate metabolism may be involved in the inverse social gradient of cardiovascular risk. Hyperinsulinaemia is linked with the male-type pattern of obesity – apple rather than pear shape – and both of these are linked with elevated risk of coronary disease. Though comparatively little research has been carried out in this area, both central obesity and high blood levels of insulin have been more frequently observed in adults of lower occupational status. Taken together, the findings based on studies of lipids, clotting factors and carbohydrate metabolism are consistent with an increased prevalence in individuals of lower socioeconomic status of the clustering of coronary risk factors known as *insulin resistance* or *metabolic* syndrome. This syndrome (more fully described below) is linked with an increased likelihood of diabetes as well as heart disease.

If this pattern of metabolic disturbances emerges as a coherent and widely applicable description of the physiological and health consequences of lower social and occupational status in affluent societies two key questions need to be considered. Can we explain the processes leading to this pattern of metabolic disturbances? Can this explanation provide a useful approach to policies for the reduction of health inequalities?

EVIDENCE FROM THE WHITEHALL STUDIES

The first Whitehall study

The British civil service provides a highly valuable population for studying the determinants of health. Within one institution, where broad similarities in the environment may be expected to minimize differences in health, quite the reverse is found to be true. The first Whitehall study was set up in 1967 to examine the role of conventional risk factors, i.e. smoking, blood pressure and serum cholesterol. It found the relative risk of coronary heart disease among male office support staff was 4 compared with top level administrators after seven and a half years of follow-up (Marmot *et al.* 1978). Intermediate grades had intermediate rates of coronary heart disease incidence. The difference between the top and bottom of the employment grade hierarchy is an order of magnitude larger than the Registrar General social class V/social class I difference of 26 per cent in 1971 (Rose and Marmot 1981). Finer subdivision of socioeconomic position often shows additional grading of risk differentials, and in Whitehall (Davey Smith *et al.* 1990) car ownership predicted lower coronary heart disease risk within employment grade.

The three classic risk factors accounted for only a quarter of the differences in premature coronary heart disease between civil service employment grades. This surprising finding is partly explained by problems of measurement. The proportion accounted for would be larger if repeated rather than single measurements had been taken, in view of the biological variability of blood pressure and the difficulty of accurately determining smoking histories. Despite this caveat, the conventional risk factor model was seen to be inadequate: quantitatively because it could not explain variations in risk well enough, and qualitatively because it did not tackle the upstream structural and psychological aspects of health differences. In response, a younger cohort of civil servants is now being followed in which repeated measurements are being taken of a much expanded set of biomedical measures and an array of psychosocial variables.

The Whitehall II study

The Whitehall II study of 10,308 civil servants in London began in 1985–8. The questionnaire and medical examination were repeated, in modified

Table 15.1 Basic salary levels at 1 August 1992, by civil service employment grade (£)

Civil service employment grade	Minimum	Maximum
Unified Grade 1 Permanent secretary	–	87,620
Unified Grade 2 Deputy secretary	62,504	73,216
Unified Grade 3 Under-secretary	51,272	59,280
Unified Grade 4 Deputy under-secretary	46,121	51,732
Unified Grade 5 Assistant secretary	37,589	49,790
Unified Grade 6 Senior principal	28,904	44,390
Unified Grade 7 Principal	25,330	36,019
Senior Executive Officer	18,082	25,554
Higher Executive Officer	14,456	20,850
Executive Officer	8,517	16,668
Administrative Officer (Clerical officer)	9,729	11,917
Administrative Assistant (Clerical assistant)	6,483	9,620
Other, e.g. messengers, porters, telephonists, typists	7,387	9,054

form, at the second follow-up in 1991–3, and results from the two surveys are presented in this chapter. Participants were aged 35–55 at the baseline, and so the emphasis is on processes taking place in adult life. The importance of earlier influences in the life course to health is also relevant. Anthropometric and biochemical data were collected at both phases of the study. Self-report questionnaires provide data on social, economic, psychological and behavioural factors.

Salary levels in 1992 (Table 15.1) show the differentials in income across employment grades. The grade classification identifies a clear hierarchy in the material circumstances of the men and women in the civil service. More than 97 per cent of those in the higher administrative grades owned their own home in 1987, compared with some 60 per cent in clerical and office support jobs. Likewise, a car was available to some 90 per cent of senior staff but to only 60 per cent in the lowest employment grade. Notably, none of the study participants was in absolute poverty, and at the time of the baseline survey none was unemployed. Whitehall study and other data (Wilkinson 1986) show that health and well-being are related to income and other measures of material wealth at all levels. It is, however, not clear which of the many features of social stratification most profoundly influence health. Those with higher disposable incomes may be able to buy health in the form of better housing conditions, private medicine and expensive holidays. The phenomenon can be interpreted in other ways. Income in affluent societies, as international ecological data suggest (Wilkinson 1992), may be not the key to longevity but a marker for the cultural and psychological differences which are its underlying determinants.

Table 15.2 Employment grade and risk factor status at the Whitehall II baseline (1985–8): serum cholesterol, apolipoproteins, and clotting factors by employment grade (age-adjusted means)

Factor	Sex	[Employment grade[a]]						Total sample	Test for trend P
		1 highest	2	3	4	5	6 lowest		
Serum cholesterol (mmol/l)	Men	5.89	5.87	5.84	5.97	5.89	5.87	6,860	n.s.
	Women	5.70	5.73	5.64	5.67	5.82	5.80	3,374	n.s.
Apo-AI (mg/dl)	Men	150.8	148.4	146.4	147.1	143.3	142.4	5,176	0.0001
	Women	171.1	170.1	167.6	169.1	163.0	159.3	2,634	0.0001
Apo-B (mg/dl)	Men	103.2	103.9	101.0	105.1	102.5	103.7	5,176	n.s.
	Women	88.5	90.3	90.2	91.1	93.9	95.2	2,634	0.0010
Apo-B/apo-AI ratio	Men	0.69	0.70	0.69	0.71	0.72	0.73	5,176	0.0001
	Women	0.52	0.53	0.54	0.54	0.58	0.60	2,634	0.0001
Plasma fibrinogen (g/l)	Men	2.59	2.60	2.60	2.68	2.69	2.80	2,095	0.0001
	Women	2.52	2.54	2.69	2.82	2.87	2.89	1,190	0.0001
Factor VII activity (% standard)	Men	83.9	87.1	84.3	85.4	87.6	87.0	1,525	n.s.
	Women	81.6	87.9	86.3	88.2	91.8	89.4	847	n.s.

Note: (a) Grade 1, unified grades 1–6; 2, unified grade 7; 3, senior executive officer; 4, higher executive officer; 5, executive officer (and professional equivalents in employment grades 3–5); 6, clerical officer/office support. n.s. $p > 0.05$.

Indirect evidence suggests that genetic explanations for health inequalities are not important. The apparent inversion of the social class distribution of coronary heart disease among men in mid-century, and the increased inequalities observed in the Britain in the past twenty years, make the eugenic argument seem weak. Studies of ABO blood group prevalence provide additional evidence of genetic homogeneity across social classes in England (Mascie-Taylor 1990: 128). Evidence of gene–environment interaction is likely to be sought increasingly in the near future as research into the human genome continues to expand. Health-related social selection has been shown to account for only a small part of health inequality in recent British studies (Fox *et al.* 1985; Power *et al.* 1986).

Blood lipids

In the first Whitehall study with the baseline in the late 1960s and the British Regional Heart study in the late 1970s, mean serum cholesterol levels were paradoxically higher in those with higher socioeconomic status. Among individuals and between populations the data show that coronary heart disease risk is partly accounted for by serum cholesterol levels. The same explanation does not appear to extend to differences in risk according to socioeconomic status. In Whitehall II mean cholesterol levels by employment grade in both men and women varied by no more than 0.1 mmol/l at baseline and in follow-up screening examinations (Table 15.2). Among women, whose socioeconomic status may be less well measured by employment grade because of the husband's or partner's occupation, small social differences were seen. Women who had been in higher education and those who were owner-occupiers had cholesterol levels 0.1 mmol/l below those of their less advantaged female colleagues.

At the baseline of Whitehall II more detailed lipid profiles were obtained (Brunner *et al.* 1993), including measurements of apolipoprotein-A-I (apo-AI) and apolipoprotein-B (apo-B). Apo-AI is a key protein component of high density lipoproteins (HDL) and high levels appear to protect against atherosclerosis by promoting 'reverse transport' of cholesterol away from peripheral tissues. Apo-B, the apoprotein of low density lipoproteins (LDL), delivers cholesterol to the arterial wall. Prospective studies in numerous Western populations (Manolio *et al.* 1992) show that LDL cholesterol and apo-B levels predict new cases of coronary heart disease, while HDL cholesterol and apo-AI levels are inversely related to it, both in men and in women.

In contrast to the null findings with total cholesterol, there are considerable gradients across civil service grades in apo-AI in both sexes (Table 15.2). Apo-B is higher in lower grade women, but not in lower-grade men. The findings for apo-AI are consistent with other studies of HDL

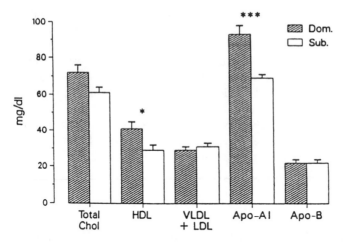

Figure 15.1 Lipids and social hierarchy in baboons. Total cholesterol, lipoprotein cholesterol and apolipoprotein levels according to social rank among male Serengeti baboons. A similar pattern is observed in male civil servants, classified by occupational status. *Dom.* dominant males. *Sub.* subordinate males. $*p < 0.05$, $***p < 0.001$. (Sapolsky and Mott 1987) Reproduced with permission.

cholesterol levels according to education level (Heiss *et al.* 1980) and social class (Gregory *et al.* 1990), and suggest that determinants of the protective lipoprotein fraction may be important in understanding socio-economic differences in coronary heart disease risk. Remarkably, the same lipid and lipoprotein pattern has been found in the dominance hierarchy of male baboons. Sapolsky and Mott (1987), studying wild baboon communities in the Serengeti, split a troop into dominant and subordinate groups. Total cholesterol and apo-B were similar (Figure 15.1), just as in Whitehall II men, but there were higher HDL cholesterol and apo-A1 levels in the dominant as compared with the subordinate males, again mirroring findings in civil servants. Speculatively, these parallels may reflect the psychosocial effects of position within the two primate hierarchies. Production of the more favourable lipid levels in dominant baboons may be the direct consequences of their assertion of supremacy and consequent feelings of well-being, or alternatively perhaps the result of easier access to the best available food. It would, however, be treading dangerously to take the analogy too far into the realms of health research. Subordinate (non-smoking) baboons, according to Sapolsky, have poorer health than their superiors, again in parallel with the effects of socioeconomic status in human societies. The violence involved in the production and maintenance of the baboon hierarchy suggests that the human primate would be well advised to take this animal model, if anything, as a cautionary tale.

Clotting factors

Soluble fibrinogen circulates in the blood to provide the material from which insoluble fibrin is formed during the process of clotting. Raised plasma levels of fibrinogen and factor VII, one of the proteins of the extrinsic clotting cascade, have been shown to predict coronary disease in prospective studies (Meade *et al.* 1986; Wilhelmsen *et al.* 1984; Kannel *et al.* 1987; Yarnell *et al.* 1991; Heinrich *et al.* 1994). These two clotting factors were measured in Whitehall II as potential explanatory variables for employment grade differences in incident coronary heart disease, and in order to study their respective determinants (Brunner *et al.* 1993). Coronary risk indexed by fibrinogen is substantially higher in lower grades in men and women, but though factor VIIc predicted coronary heart disease in the Northwick Park study (Meade *et al.* 1986) there is no gradient across Whitehall grades (Table 15.2).

There is not consensus on the role of fibrinogen. It is usually present in plasma at high levels of around 3 g/l, even in populations at low coronary risk. As an acute phase reactant, fibrinogen levels increase in response to infection and other stresses. Fibrinogen may therefore predict overt coronary disease not because it is a causal factor, but because levels start to rise during the early stages of vessel wall damage many years before symptoms develop. A third explanation for the association with coronary disease is also possible. If recent work (Mendall *et al.* 1994) is confirmed showing the links between past or present infection with the gut bacterium *Helicobacter pylori*, fibrinogen levels and heart attack, we would have evidence of an infectious mechanism for coronary heart disease. The finding of antibodies to *H. pylori* is not unusual in British adults, suggesting there are high rates of undetected infection. Infection is associated with poor childhood living conditions and in particular with overcrowded housing (Patel *et al.* 1994).

Importance of the metabolic gradients

Estimates have previously been made of differences in the incidence of coronary heart disease according to plasma levels of HDL cholesterol and fibrinogen. These effect estimates, derived from the Framingham study (Gordon *et al.* 1981; Kannel *et al.* 1987), suggest that grade differences in apo-AI and fibrinogen may account for about one-third of the excess coronary deaths predicted in the lower grades, if it is assumed that the excess is similar to that seen in the ten-year follow-up of the first Whitehall study (Brunner *et al.* 1993). This is doing quite well. The British Regional Heart Study took account of smoking, systolic blood pressure and serum cholesterol differences between white and blue collar men (Pocock *et al.* 1987). Only 45 per cent of the 1.44 heart attack rate ratio of manual versus

Table 15.3 Height and coronary risk

Risk factor	Men	Women
Cholesterol (mmol/l)		
Height Q4–Q1	0.23	0.20
Adjusted for civil service grade	0.23	0.20
Fibrogen (g/l)		
Height Q4–Q1	0.12	0.16
Adjusted for civil service grade	0.09	0.11

Notes: Whitehall II baseline (phase S1). Q4–Q1 interquartile difference. Data adjusted for age.

non-manual workers was explained using this relatively insensitive social stratification.

Early influences

Adult height is a reflection of early growth and development and in cross-sectional analyses of Whitehall II data shows some specific associations with coronary risk factors (Table 15.3). The relationships of serum cholesterol and plasma fibrinogen with height are consistent with Barker's view (1992) that early influences are important to individual risk in adulthood. Serum cholesterol is substantially lower in the taller men and women. Mean cholesterol is not associated with civil service grade, and adjustment for grade does not alter this height effect. Fibrinogen is also lower in taller subjects, but in that case factors associated with employment grade, such as smoking and drinking rates, seem to account for around 30 per cent of the effect.

Blood pressure

Blood pressure tends to be lower among individuals of higher socioeconomic status (Kaplan and Keil 1993; Pocock *et al.* 1987) but this relation appears to be weak. For example, blood pressure was inversely associated with education level in the Intersalt study (Stamler *et al.* 1992) in men (–1.3 mm Hg per ten additional years of education) and women (–4.5 mm Hg per ten additional years of education). In the first Whitehall study of men screened in 1967–8 mean age-adjusted systolic blood pressure (BP) was 4.2 mm Hg higher in unskilled office staff compared with senior administrators (Marmot *et al.* 1978). The proportion of hypertensives (systolic BP > 160 mm Hg) fell stepwise from 17 per cent to 11 per cent from lower to higher employment status. Perhaps because of better detection and treatment, blood pressure gradients were diminished among civil

Table 15.4(a) Mean body mass index in the Whitehall studies (kg/m²⁾

Sex	Administrative		Professional/ executive		Clerical/ support		Trend p
	Mean	SE	Mean	SE	Mean	SE	
	Whitehall						
Men	24.5	0.09	24.7	0.03	24.7	0.06	0.15
	889		11,081		3,232		
	Whitehall II (S3)						
Men	25.0	0.06	25.2	0.07	25.5	0.22	< 0.005
	2,404		2,300		334		
Women	24.5	0.24	25.4	0.14	26.5	0.19	0.0001
	352		1,006		821		

Note: Age-adjusted (40–59 years).

Table 15.4(b) Prevalence of obesity in the Whitehall studies (body mass index greater than 30 kg/m²)

Sex	Administrative		Professional/ executive		Clerical/ support		Trend p
	%	SE	%	SE	%	SE	
	Whitehall						
Men	1.7	0.33	1.9	0.09	3.1	0.23	< 0.001
	889		11,081		3,232		
	Whitehall II (S3)						
Men	6.6	0.51	7.6	0.56	10.1	1.65	< 0.05
	2,404	2,300	334				
Women	11.3	1.78	14.6	1.11	18.8	1.48	< 0.005
	352		1,006		821		

Note: Age-adjusted (40–59 years).

servants screened some 20 years later. Resting blood pressure differences were absent in women and small in men: 1–2 mm Hg across grades. Stroke mortality rates do increase as the social classes are descended, and it may be that larger blood pressure differences would have been obtained at work rather than in the clinic, under stress rather than basal conditions.

Cigarette smoking

Although it has not always been the case, the prevalence of cigarette smoking is now inversely related to socioeconomic status in most industrialized countries, including Britain (Gregory *et al.* 1990) and the United States (Kaplan and Keil 1993). Prevalence rates of smoking are inversely

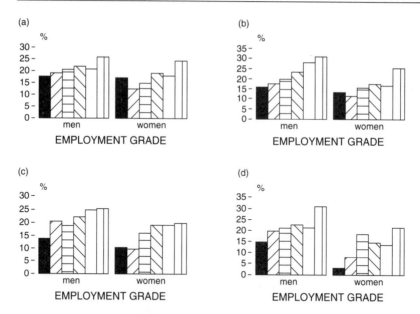

Figure 15.2 Body mass index, waist–hip ratio, high-density lipoprotein choles-terol and serum triglycerides, by employment grade, at phase 3 (1991–3) of the Whitehall II study (available data), age-adjusted. (a) Body mass index in upper quintile; men $p < 0.05$, women $p < 0.01$. (b) Waist–hip ratio in upper quintile; men $p < 0.0001$, women $p < 0.0001$. (c) HDL-C in lower quintile; men $p < 0.0001$, women $p < 0.0001$. (d) 2H triglyceride in upper quintile; men $p < 0.01$, women $p < 0.05$. Employment grades range from high at the left (solid black: senior administrative civil servants) to low on the right (vertical hatching: clerical/office support staff)

related to occupation in the Whitehall studies (Marmot *et al.* 1978) as well as to other indicators of social position, including income (Kaplan and Keil 1993) and social class (Baker *et al.* 1988). The inverse relation appears to have become stronger in recent years, as those in higher social strata appear to have higher quitting rates (Kaplan and Keil 1993). Rates at the Whitehall II baseline fell steadily with higher employment grade from 34 per cent to 8 per cent among men, and from 28 per cent to 18 per cent among women. Women in Whitehall II are more likely to be smokers than men in all except the lowest employment grades (Marmot *et al.* 1991).

Obesity and body fat pattern

In Whitehall II obesity, defined as a body mass index greater than 30 kg/m^2, is inversely related to employment status (Table 15.4). Comparison of the first and second Whitehall cohorts shows the considerable increase in obe-sity between the late 1960s and late 1980s, which is mirrored in nationally

Table 15.5 Waist–hip ratio and socioeconomic status in population surveys

Men	Women
Inverse association	*Inverse association*
Brent	Brent
Caerphilly	Heartbeat Wales
Heartbeat Wales	Health Survey, England
Health Survey, England	Health and lifestyle
Whitehall II	Hertfordshire
EFDS (six cities)	Whitehall II
Finland	Finland
Gothenburg	Gothenburg
Cardia	Cardia
	Iowa
No association	
Health and lifestyle	*No association*
Hertfordshire	Preston
Preston	Sheffield
Sheffield	

representative data comparing 1980 with 1987 (Gregory *et al.* 1990). Differences in average body mass index across grades are small in both sexes.

There is considerable evidence of differences in body fat pattern according to occupational status. Abdominal fatness, as opposed to fatness on the thighs, is linked strongly with civil service grade. Figure 15.2 shows that the probability of being in the top fifth of waist–hip ratio in the clerical/support grades is twice that in the top administrative grade. Adjustment for overall degree of obesity reduces this little.

Published and unpublished data from Britain, Europe and the United States show that the linkage between central adiposity and socioeconomic status is a common finding in surveys conducted in the last two decades (Table 15.5). The significance of this little recognized link is twofold. First, it ties in with the key features of the metabolic syndrome, and, second, it is consistent with a psychogenic explanation of health inequalities.

Metabolic syndrome

In the first Whitehall study the pre-diabetic state of *impaired glucose tolerance*, and non-insulin-dependent diabetes, both of which are common features of ageing in Western countries, increased in prevalence down the employment grades (Fuller *et al.* 1983). Both impaired glucose tolerance and non-insulin-dependent diabetes are linked with an increased risk of cardiovascular disease. Other prospective studies have shown that a high plasma insulin level, an imperfect marker of insulin resistance, predicts coronary disease (Eschwege *et al.* 1985; Pyorala *et al.* 1985).

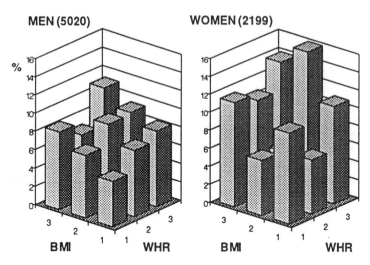

Figure 15.3 Prevalence of impaired glucose tolerance by tertiles of body mass index (BMI) and waist–hip ratio (WHR) at phase 3 (1991–3) of the Whitehall II study (available data), age-adjusted

Data from Whitehall II show that impaired glucose tolerance, defined according to the WHO criterion by serum glucose two hours after 75 g of glucose, rises both with overall fatness and with abdominal fatness (Figure 15.3). In women the U-shaped relationship suggests that extreme thinness in middle age may not be ideal. Impaired glucose tolerance shows a clear stepwise and inverse trend with employment grade in men, and a less clear but similar trend in women. Impaired glucose tolerance is related to the degree of central obesity and, over and above that, to occupational status. At any given level of waist–hip ratio, impaired glucose tolerance tends to be more common in lower grades (Figure 15.4), indicating that other factors, in addition to obesity, appear to be operating.

As might be expected, the regulation of lipid and carbohydrate metabolism is not independent. South Asians in Britain are at increased risk of both non-insulin-dependent diabetes and coronary disease compared with the native UK population. Relative to Europeans, many healthy South Asian adults in the United Kingdom exhibit the characteristic pattern of disturbances which involves both carbohydrate and lipid metabolism (McKeigue *et al.* 1991). These are central adiposity, impaired glucose tolerance, raised serum insulin and triglycerides, and low HDL cholesterol, known variously as Reaven's syndrome X, the metabolic syndrome or the insulin resistance syndrome (Reaven 1988).

Results from Whitehall II suggest there may be an analogy between ethnicity and socioeconomic status. Each of the components of the insulin resistance syndrome shows less favourable levels in lower employment

(a)

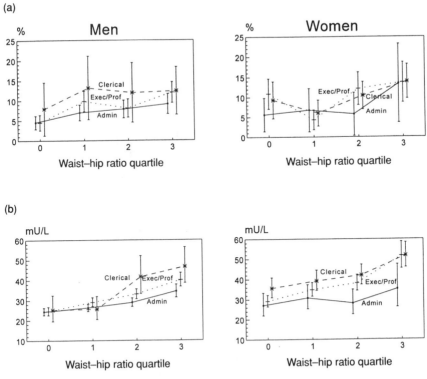

Figure 15.4 Prevalence of impaired glucose tolerance and mean post-glucose load serum insulin in civil service employment grades at phase 3 (1991–3) of the Whitehall II study by quartiles of waist–hip ratio. (a) Prevalence of impaired glucose tolerance, adjusted for age. (b) Two-hour insulin (normoglycaemics only), adjusted for age, menopause and body mass index

grades (Figure 15.2) and in those who have more abdominal fat. Serum insulin levels two hours after a glucose load are a good proxy for insulin resistance in those with glucose tolerance in the normal range. The grade effect is particularly clear in women (Figure 15.4), suggesting that additional grade-related factors must be operating. Triglyceride levels also rise markedly with degree of central obesity, but in this case grade effects are absent or weak. The data for HDL cholesterol – more rather than less is better – replicate the findings for apo-A1, the HDL apoprotein, which were obtained at the Whitehall II baseline.

A BEHAVIOURAL EXPLANATION?

The stepwise inverse social gradients in lipid and clotting factors do not appear to be entirely accounted for by health-related behaviours (Brunner

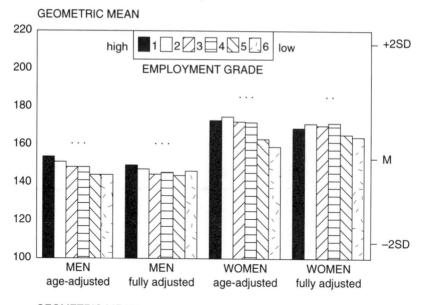

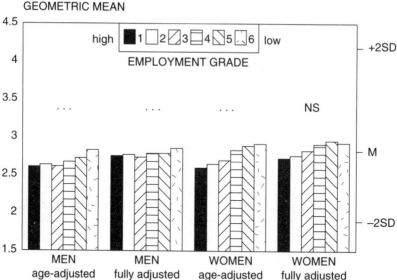

Figure 15.5 Relation between employment grade and (a) Serum apolipoprotein Al. (b) Plasma fibrinogen, showing the effects of adjusting for degree of obesity, reported smoking, alcohol intake, exercise and dietary pattern. The histograms show age-adjusted grade mean values (labelled 'age-adjusted') and grade mean values after controlling for ethnicity, adiposity and health-related behaviours as well as age (labelled 'fully adjusted'). The population geometric means (M) and standard deviations (SD) are marked on the right-hand vertical axes. $*p < 0.05$, $**p < 0.02$, $***p < 0.0001$. (Brunner *et al.* 1993: 203)

et al. 1993). Using linear modelling, adjustment for smoking rates, alcohol consumption, exercise and dietary pattern, as well as age, ethnicity, body mass index, report of symptoms, and menopausal status in women (Figure 15.5, the fully adjusted means) reduced the strength of association for apo-AI with employment grade by 43 per cent in men and 70 per cent in women. The corresponding reductions for fibrinogen were 47 per cent and 35 per cent. The residual social gradients may be due to measurement imprecision in the adjustment variables, unmeasured behavioural factors, or effects unrelated to behavioural factors.

Smoking rates in Whitehall II are strongly and inversely related to employment grade, consistent with an important contribution to the excess cancer and cardiovascular risks among those of lower social status. It should be noted, however, that comparable coronary mortality gradients have been observed in never smoking men in the first Whitehall study and in a Copenhagen-based cohort (Hein *et al.* 1992).

MATERIAL AND PSYCHOSOCIAL FACTORS

In the baseline data of the Whitehall II study several occupational, social and psychosocial factors and material circumstances are associated with fibrinogen, apo-AI and the apo-B/apo-AI ratio (Brunner 1994), which is an index of atherogenicity equivalent to the LDL/HDL cholesterol ratio. We obtained self-reports of pace, control, variety and skill use, conflicting demands, and social support at work. Subjects give a scaled response – often/sometimes/seldom/never – for example, to the variety and skill use item 'Do you have the possibility of learning new things through your work?', and the discretion item 'I have a great deal of say in planning my work environment'. Greater variety in tasks and levels of skill use at work is associated with more favourable levels of apolipoproteins and fibrinogen in both sexes. Work pace and demands of the job show less consistent relationships with risk factors. In both sexes financial difficulties are associated with less favourable levels of apolipoproteins.

Cross-sectional analyses suggest, bearing in mind their limitations, that fatalism, or external locus of health control, may influence blood lipids and haemostasis. Measurement problems and multiple collinearity make the interpretation of grade-related effects difficult. Grade adjustment, for example, will tend to eclipse the effects of less precisely measured psychosocial factors such as fatalism.

Type A behaviour illustrates the grade issue (Figure 15.6a). Men and women in the top tertile of Framingham type A score tend, if anything, to have lower coronary risk, indexed by fibrinogen and apo-AI. This is, of course, not surprising, since many of the type A components – need for control, ambition and competitiveness – are linked with occupational

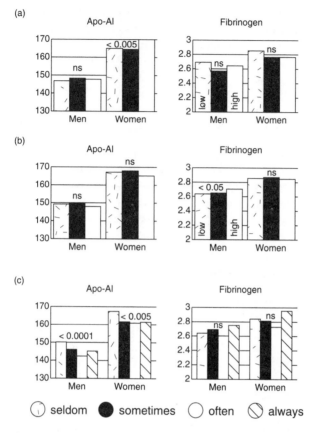

Figure 15.6 Coronary risk factors. (a) Framingham type A score (need for control/ambitious/impatient/competitive/hostile), grouped into tertiles, low on the left, high on the right. (b) Cook–Medley hostility score (thirty-eight-item questionnaire: suspicion/paranoia/need for revenge/sense of isolation), grouped into tertiles, low on the left, high on the right. (c) Reported financial problems (difficulty paying for food and clothing) at phase 1 (1985–8) of the Whitehall II study. Data adjusted for age. Apo-AI serum apolipoprotein AI

success, and therefore with lower fibrinogen and higher apo-AI. Upper tertile type A scores are some four times more common in the top, compared with the bottom, grade. On the other hand, self-rated hostility, which is more commonly reported by lower grade staff, shows the expected pattern (Figure 15.6b). Some researchers (Matthews *et al.* 1977; Siegler *et al.* 1992) have found hostility to be the crucial component of type A with respect to coronary risk. Whitehall II data, in parallel with this, show a tendency to higher risk with higher hostility. Multivariate

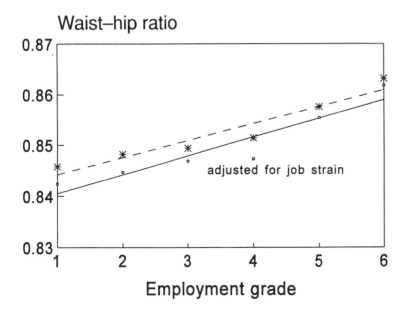

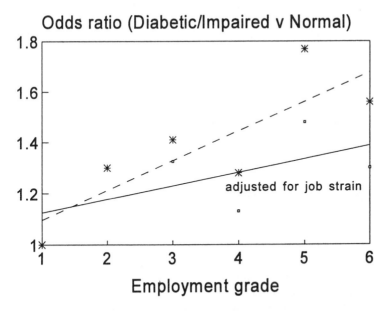

Figure 15.7 Relation between civil service employment grade and (a) Waist –hip ratio. (b) Likelihood of being diagnosed diabetic/glucose intolerant, according to interim results from phase 3 (1991–3) of the Whitehall II study. Data adjusted for age, sex, menopausal status and body mass index. The solid lines are adjusted for work characteristics

analyses suggest that the associations between hostility and apo-AI/ fibrinogen are mediated by health-related behaviours.

A clearer psychosocial effect is obtained with self-report of financial problems (Figure 15.6c), which is strongly related to lower grade. Increasing reported frequency of financial problems is associated with declining apo-AI, and, by implication, HDL cholesterol. A residual effect with apo-AI is seen in men after controlling for health-related behaviours and grade.

Other cross-sectional analyses give some support to the psychosocial hypothesis. Lower apo-AI levels are seen with poorer quality of social networks, assessed with Stansfeld and Marmot's (1992) close persons questionnaire, and with the impact of bereavement in the past year reported in Ruberman's (1984) life events questionnaire.

Job strain

An analysis (Nanchahal 1994) using impaired glucose tolerance (IGT) or new diabetes as the disease outcome gives evidence that job strain may be important in explaining the poorer health status of individuals in lower civil service grades (Figure 15.7). When grade differences in work pace, discretion, variety and conflicting demands were controlled for in a logistic model, the IGT/diabetes gradient across grades was no longer statistically significant. The association of grade with waist–hip ratio remained unchanged. In other words, work-related stress appears to mediate the link between grade and impaired glucose tolerance, but not the link between grade and central obesity. Further work will clarify these observations.

A PSYCHOENDOCRINE PATHWAY?

Lower grade office staff tend to experience their work as monotonous and lacking in opportunities to control how and what they do. A relatively low income will often accompany these characteristics of work. The long-term psychological demands imposed by such life circumstances, compared with those of higher status workers, may produce an excess of psychiatric illness such as depression (Dohrenwend 1990), but is it plausible that an adverse psychosocial environment could produce an excess of coronary disease?

If the biologically important gradients shown in Whitehall II and other data are put together, i.e. those relating to impaired glucose tolerance, insulin resistance, fibrinogen, HDL cholesterol, triglycerides, and central obesity, a coherent explanation can be proposed to account for these specific effects. This pathway links the chronic stress response of the hypothalamic pituitary adrenal system (Figure 15.8) with resulting elevated levels of corticosteroids, to central obesity, insulin resistance, poor lipid

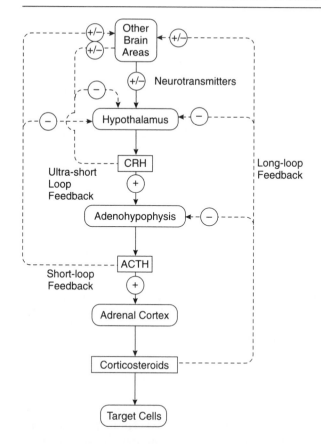

Figure 15.8 The hypothalamic–pituitary–adrenal system. Feedback regulation is complex: it depends on the levels of intermediate hormones as well as on the response of the adrenal gland. *CRH* corticotrophin releasing hormone, *ACTH* adrenocorticotrophic hormone. Reproduced by permission Cambridge University Press

profile and an increased tendency for the blood to clot (Bjorntorp 1991). The importance of this mechanism in the context of health inequalities is as yet unknown, but several lines of evidence suggest its plausibility.

This pathway implies a *direct* psychoendocrine mechanism which disturbs normal physiological functioning. *Indirect* mechanisms which place health-related behaviours, such as increased rates of smoking, on the causal pathway are also relevant and have been referred to above.

Cushing's syndrome, due to excessive secretion of cortisol, is characterized by central obesity, diabetes, high triglyceride levels and insulin resistance, and sometimes depression. Also linking depression with cortisol levels, depressed patients have been successfully treated with

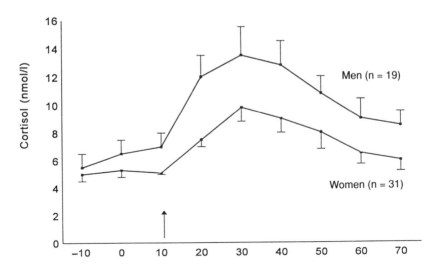

Figure 15.9 Salivary cortisol response to experimental stress in volunteers. At time 0 the subjects were told they would have to take on the role of a job applicant making a five-minute introductory speech to a selection panel. The arrow marks the start of the speech. (Kirschbaum *et al.* 1992)

metyrapone, a drug which inhibits the final step in cortisol biosynthesis (Checkley 1992). At the population level, depression has been shown to predict the incidence of coronary heart disease in a follow-up study of an American national survey sample (Anda *et al.* 1993). Though by no means conclusive, the findings suggest there may be a common pathway to coronary heart disease and depression in some populations.

Sapolsky and Mott in their study of male baboons (1987) have shown an inverse association between early morning cortisol and HDL cholesterol. The reason for this association is not understood. It is consistent with the proposal that in primates the stress response of the hypothalamic pituitary adrenal axis may be linked with cardiovascular risk status. Experimental findings with cortisol are consistent with another aspect of the epidemiology of coronary disease. There is a well known excess risk among men compared with women, and a sex difference has been shown in the cortisol response to psychological stress (Figure 15.9). Men seem to be more responsive to conflict, anticipatory and performance anxiety but not to cycle ergometry (Kirschbaum *et al.* 1992). One explanation for the null finding with the exercise stress test is that the phenomenon is a psychological rather than a physiological difference.

Another experimental study, in which women with and without central obesity (Moyer *et al.* 1994) were required to perform stressful tasks, including public speaking, supports a direct association between waist–

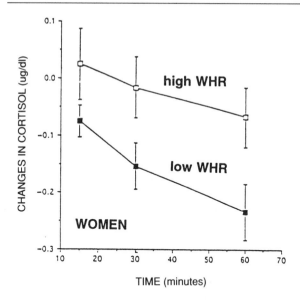

Figure 15.10 Salivary cortisol response to stressful tasks in centrally obese women and controls. *WHR* waist–hip ratio. (Moyer *et al.* 1994). Reproduced with permission.

hip ratio and the cortisol response (Figure 15.10). Salivary cortisol levels at baseline and during stress were higher in the centrally obese group. The observed overall decline in cortisol is due to the diurnal rhythm in secretion. Cortisol levels are at their highest in the early hours and fall during the day.

Moving attention to the controls on cortisol secretion, there is evidence for the involvement of the autonomic nervous system together with neuroendocrine pathways in patterning the response to stress. For example, in a study (Delitala *et al.* 1991) where the acute stress reponse was obtained by the administration of methoxamine, a drug which mimics the action of adrenalin, rising levels of cortisol were provoked over a two-hour period. The rise could be blocked by giving subjects a synthetic opiate, which emulates the effect of endogenous opioid peptides (Figure 15.11). These findings are consistent with a protective effect of well-being, induced for example by exercise, which limits the adverse effects of stress.

A variety of environmental stimuli may influence the endocrine and immune systems simultaneously. Figure 15.12 shows schematically the hypothalamic pituitary adrenal axis down the right-hand side. On activation, cells of the immune system release cytokines and peptide hormones which act on the brain, neuroendocrine system and other immune cells.

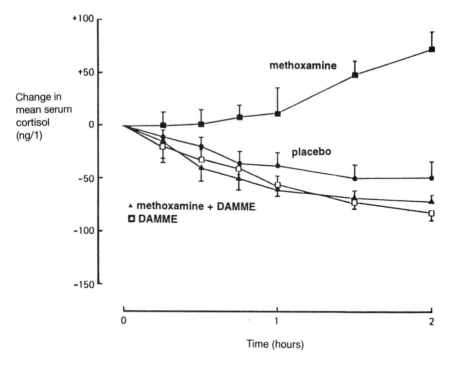

Figure 15.11 Abolition of the cortisol response by the administration of a synthetic opiate peptide. DAMME (D-alanine-methylphenylalanine-met-enkephalin) has pharmacological properties similar to those of met-enkephalin, an endogenous opioid peptide. (Delitda *et al.* 1991) Reproduced with permission.

The brain is able to influence immune function via the autonomic nervous system, which innervates all tissues of the immune system, i.e. bone marrow, thymus, spleen and lymph nodes. Several pituitary and gonadal hormones have effects on the immune system.

A non-cognitive stimulus such as recurrent infection (which is more common in groups with low socioeconomic status) may not be perceived by the central nervous system, but will induce an immune response. As part of this acute phase response, white blood cells known as macrophages will secrete the cytokine hormone interleukin-1, which in turn stimulates the increased secretion of fibrinogen by the liver. Fibrinogen, as discussed above, is a risk factor for coronary heart disease.

As a note of caution, it should be remembered that the mechanisms summarized in this last section have been demonstrated only in the laboratory. Their importance in determining the pattern of degenerative disease in the population at large has yet to be established even in an illustrative way.

Neural, endocrine and immune systems intercommunication

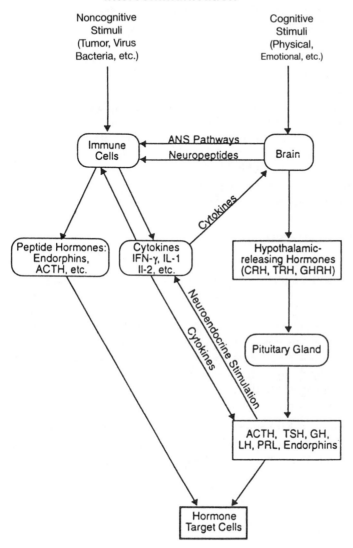

Figure 15.12 Connections between the hypothalamic–pituitary–adrenal and immune systems. Reproduced with permission Cambridge University Press.

CONCLUSION

There is clear evidence that the risk of cardiovascular disease in affluent societies rises sharply with decreasing occupational status, even among office-based workers who are not poor in the conventional sense, nor exposed to physical hazards. There is no doubt that rates of smoking and other health-related behaviours play a role in these health differences. Material and psychosocial factors associated with lower socioeconomic status have been shown to be related to levels of blood lipids, clotting factors, and carbohydrate metabolism. A unified explanation has been proposed, which links psychosocial factors with increased risk of metabolic syndrome type abnormalities. There is some evidence of direct psychoen-docrine effects which support the existence of a stress pathway. Prospective studies in the Whitehall II cohort will tell us the extent to which central obesity, and the metabolic disturbances associated with it, account for the socioeconomic gradients in cardiovascular disease.

POLICY IMPLICATIONS

The challenge for those concerned with public health is to find the means to reduce, if not to eliminate, the inequities which cause the occupational gradient in coronary risk. Ignorance of the exact mechanism by which tobacco smoking produces lung cancer did not hinder anti-smoking initia-tives. The current imperfections in our knowledge of the biological mechanisms connecting lower occupational status with higher coronary risk are likewise not a justification for a *laissez-faire* approach. Unlike smoking, the occupational hierarchy is necessarily with us to stay, but its form could be changed for the better. Though couched in anachronistic terms, John Ruskin wrote aptly on this point in 1851:

> It may be proved, with much certainty, that God intends no man to live in this world without working: but it seems to me no less evident that He intends every man to be happy in his work. It is written, 'in the sweat of thy brow', but it was never written, 'in the breaking of thine heart'.

REFERENCES

Anda, R., Williamson, D., Jones, D., Macera, C., Eaker, E.D., Glassman, A. and Marks, J. (1993) Depressed affect, hopelessness, and the risk of ischaemic heart disease in a cohort of US adults, *Epidemiology* 4: 285–294.

Baker, I.A., Sweetnam, P.M., Yarnell, J.W.G., Bainton, D. and Elwood, P.C. (1988) Haemostatic and other risk factors for ischaemic heart disease and social class: evidence from the Caerphilly and Speedwell studies, *International Journal of Epidemiology* 17: 759–765.

Barker, D.J.P. (1992) *Fetal and Infant Origins of Adult Disease*, London: British Medical Journal.

Bartley, M., Power, C., Blane, D., Davey Smith, G. and Shipley, M. (1994) Birth weight and later socioeconomic disadvantage: evidence from the 1958 British cohort study, *British Medical Journal* 309: 1475–1479.

Bjorntorp, P. (1991) Visceral fat accumulation: the missing link between psychosocial factors and cardiovascular disease?, *Journal of International Medicine* 230: 195–201.

Brunner, E.J. (1994) Social Class and Risk Factors for Coronary Heart Disease, Ph.D. thesis, University College London.

Brunner, E.J., Marmot, M.G., White, I.R., O'Brien, J.R., Etherington, M.D., Slavin, B.M., Kearney, E.M. and Davey Smith, G. (1993) Gender and employment grade differences in blood cholesterol, apolipoproteins and haemostatic factors in the Whitehall II study, *Atherosclerosis* 102: 195–207.

Checkley, S. (1992) Neuroendocrine mechanisms and the precipitation of depression by life events, *British Journal of Psychiatry* 160 (supplement 15): 7–17.

Davey Smith, G., Shipley, M.J. and Rose, G. (1990) Magnitude and causes of socioeconomic differentials in mortality: further evidence from the Whitehall study, *Journal of Epidemiology and Community Health* 44: 265–270.

Delitala, G., Palermo, M., Tomasi, P., Besser, M. and Grossman, A. (1991) Adrenergic stimulation of the human pituitary–adrenal axis is attenuated by an analog of met-enkephalin, *Neuroendocrinology* 53: 41–46.

Dohrenwend, B.P. (1990) Socioeconomic status (SES) and psychiatric disorders: are the issues still compelling?, *Social Psychiatry and Psychiatric Epidemiology* 25: 41–47.

Eschwege, E., Richard, J.L., Thibult, N., Ducimetiere, P., Warnet, J.M., Claude, J.R. and Rosselin, G.E. (1985) Coronary heart disease mortality in relation with diabetes, blood glucose and plasma insulin levels: the Paris Prospective Study, ten years later, *Hormone and Metabolic Research* supplement 15: 41–46.

Fox, A.J., Goldblatt, P.O. and Jones, D.R. (1985) Social class mortality differentials: artefact, selection or life circumstances?, *Journal of Epidemiology and Community Health* 39: 1–8.

Fuller, J.H., Shipley, M., Rose, G., Jarrett, R.J. and Keen, H. (1983) Mortality from coronary heart disease and stroke in relation to degree of glycaemia: the Whitehall study, *British Medical Journal* 287: 867–870.

Gordon, T., Kannel, W.B., Castelli, W.P. and Dawber, T.R. (1981) Lipoproteins, cardiovascular disease, and death, *Archives of Internal Medicine* 141: 1128–1131.

Gregory, J., Foster, K., Tyler, H. and Wiseman, M. (1990) *The Dietary and Nutritional Survey of British Adults*, London: HMSO.

Hein, H.O., Suadicani, P. and Gyntelberg, F. (1992) Ischaemic heart disease incidence by social class and form of smoking: the Copenhagen male study – seventeen years' follow-up, *Journal of International Medicine* 231: 477–483.

Heinrich, J., Balleisen, L., Schulte, H., Assmann, G. and van de Loo, J. (1994) Fibrinogen and factor VII in the prediction of coronary risk: results from the PROCAM study in healthy men, *Arteriosclerosis and Thrombosis* 14: 54–59.

Heiss, G., Haskell, W., Mowery, R., Criqui, M.H., Brockway, M. and Tyroler, H.A. (1980) Plasma high-density lipoprotein cholesterol and socioeconomic status, *Circulation* 62 (supplement IV): 108–115.

Hinkle, L.E., Whitney, L.H., Lehman, E.W., Dunn, J., Benjamin, B., King, R., Plakun, A. and Flehinger, B. (1968) Occupation, education and coronary heart disease, *Science* 161: 238–246.

Judge, K. (1994) Beyond health care, *British Medical Journal* 309: 1454–1455.

Kannel, W.B., Wolf, P.A., Castelli, W.P. and D'Agostino, R.B. (1987) Fibrinogen and risk of cardiovascular disease, *Journal of the American Medical Association* 258: 1183–1186.

Kaplan, G.A. and Keil, J.E. (1993) Socioeconomic factors and cardiovascular disease: a review of the literature, *Circulation* 88: 1973–1998.

Kirschbaum, C., Wust, S. and Hellhammer, D. (1992) Consistent sex differences in cortisol responses to psychological stress, *Psychosomatic Medicine* 54: 648–657.

McKeigue, P.M., Shah, B. and Marmot, M.G. (1991) Relation of central obesity and insulin resistance with high diabetes prevalence and cardiovascular risk in South Asians, *Lancet* 337: 382–386.

McLoone, P. and Boddy, F.A. (1994) Deprivation and Mortality in Scotland, 1981 and 1991, *British Medical Journal* 309: 1465–1470.

Manolio, T.A., Pearson, T.A., Wenger, N.K., Barrett-Connor, E., Payne, G.H. and Harlan, W.R. (1992) Cholesterol and heart disease in older persons and women: review of an NHLBI workshop, *Annals of Epidemiology* 2: 161–176.

Marmot, M.G. and McDowall, M.E. (1986) Mortality decline and widening social inequalities, *Lancet* ii: 274–276.

Marmot, M.G., Rose, G., Shipley, M. and Hamilton, P.J.S. (1978) Employment grade and coronary heart disease in British civil servants, *Journal of Epidemiology and Community Health* 32: 244–249.

Marmot, M.G., Davey Smith, G., Stansfeld, S., Patel, C., North, F., Head, J., White, I., Brunner, E. and Feeney, A. (1991) Health inequalities among British civil servants: the Whitehall II study, *Lancet* 337: 1387–1393.

Mascie-Taylor, C.G.N. (1990) The biology of social class, in C.G.N. Mascie-Taylor (ed.) *Biosocial Aspects of Social Class*, Oxford: Oxford University Press.

Matthews, K.A., Glass, D.C., Rosenman, R.H. and Bortner, R.W. (1977) Competitive drive, pattern A, and coronary heart disease: a further analysis of some data from the Western Collaborative Group study, *Journal of Chronic Disease* 30: 489–498.

Meade, T.W., Brozovic, M., Chakrabarti, R., Haines, A.P., Imeson, J.D., Mellows, S., Miller, G.J., North, W.R.S., Stirling, Y. and Thompson, S.G. (1986) Haemostatic function and ischaemic heart disease: principal results of the Northwick Park heart study, *Lancet* ii: 533–537.

Mendall, M.A., Goggin, P.M., Molineaux, N., Levy, J., Toosy, T., Strachan, D., Camm, A.J. and Northfield, T.C. (1994) Relation of *Helicobacter pylori* infection and coronary heart disease, *British Heart Journal* 71: 437–439.

Moyer, A.E., Rodin, J., Grilo, C.M., Cummings, N., Larson, L.M. and Rebuffe-Scrive, M. (1994) Stress-induced cortisol response and fat distribution in women, *Obesity Research* 2: 255–261.

Nanchahal, K. (1994) A Possible Mechanism underlying the Relationship between Socio-economic Status and Cardiovascular Disease, M.Sc. thesis, University College London.

Patel, P., Mendall, M.A., Khulusi, S., Northfield, T.C. and Strachan, D.P. (1994) *Helicobacter pylori* infection in childhood: risk factors and effect on growth, *British Medical Journal* 309: 1119–1123.

Phillimore, P., Beattie, A. and Townsend, P. (1994) Widening inequality of health in northern England, 1981–91, *British Medical Journal* 308: 1125–1128.

Pocock, S.J., Shaper, A.G., Cook, D.G., Phillips, A.N. and Walker, M. (1987) Social class differences in ischaemic heart disease in British men, *Lancet* ii: 197–201.

Power, C., Fogelman, K. and Fox, A.J. (1986) Health and social mobility during the early years of life, *Quarterly Journal of Social Affairs* 2: 397–413.

Pyorala, K., Savolainen, E., Kaukola, S. and Haapakoski, J. (1985) Plasma insulin as coronary heart disease risk factor: relationship to other risk factors and predictive value during nine-and-a-half-year follow-up of the Helsinki Policeman Study Population, *Acta Medica Scandinavica* 701: 38–52.

Reaven, G.M. (1988) Role of insulin resistance in human disease, *Diabetes* 37: 1595–1607.

Rose, G. and Marmot, M.G. (1981) Social class and coronary heart disease, *British Heart Journal* 45: 13–19.

Ruberman, W., Weinblatt, E., Goldberg, J.D. and Chaudhary, B.S. (1984) Psychosocial influences on mortality after myocardial infarction, *New England Journal of Medicine* 311: 552–559.

Sapolsky, R.M. and Mott, G.E. (1987) Social subordinance in wild baboons is associated with suppressed high density lipoprotein–cholesterol concentrations: the possible role of chronic social stress, *Endocrinology* 121: 1605–1610.

Siegler, I.C., Peterson, B.L., Barefoot, J.C. and Williams, R.B. (1992) Hostility during late adolescence predicts coronary risk factors at mid-life, *American Journal of Epidemiology* 136: 1–9.

Stamler, R., Shipley, M., Elliott, P., Dyer, A., Sans, S. and Stamler, J. (1992) Higher blood pressure in adults with less education: some explanations from INTERSALT, *Hypertension* 19: 237–241.

Stansfeld, S.A. and Marmot, M.G. (1992) Deriving a survey measure of social support: the reliability and validity of the Close Persons Questionnaire, *Social Science and Medicine* 35: 1027–1035.

Wilhelmsen, L., Svardsudd, K., Korsan-Bengsten, K. , Larsson, B., Welin, L. and Tibblin, G. (1984) Fibrinogen as a risk factor for stroke and myocardial infarction, *New England Journal of Medicine* 311: 501–505.

Wilkinson, R.G. (1986) Income and mortality, in R.G. Wilkinson (ed.) *Class and Health*, London: Tavistock Publications.

Wilkinson, R.G. (1992) Income distribution and life expectancy, *British Medical Journal* 304: 165–168.

Yarnell, J.W.G., Baker, I.A., Sweetnam, P.M., Bainton, D., O'Brien, J.R., Whitehead, P.J. and Elwood, P.C. (1991) Fibrinogen, viscosity and white blood cell count are major risk factors for ischemic heart disease: the Caerphilly and Speedwell Collaborative Heart Disease Studies, *Circulation* 83: 836–844.

Part V

Policy integration

Chapter 16

Health and social capital

J. Fraser Mustard

One of the striking features of the improved prosperity of countries since the industrial revolution has been the improvement of the health and well-being of populations (McKeown 1976; Fogel 1994; Frank and Mustard 1994). Dramatic as this improvement has been, the factors involved in determining the improved health status of populations have not been well understood. Some have championed improvements in medical care as the major factor in improving the health of populations while others have argued that it is better public health measures in the form of vaccination and better water systems. Important as all of these factors are, there is growing recognition that much of the improved health status following the industrial revolution was the result of prosperity and the associated social and economic changes. A society's understanding of the determinants of health has an important influence on the strategies it uses to sustain and improve the health of its population. A dominant view in developed societies today is that the main cause of premature death is cancer and heart disease and that medical science will provide cures and strategies for prevention (Mackenbach 1993). Another view that is gradually gaining prominence is that the principal influences on the health and well-being of individuals and populations are the social environment, lack of social support, poor education, poor work conditions, and stagnant economies (Marmot 1986; Evans et al. 1994).

The understanding or beliefs in a society about the determinants of health play a part in setting private and public policies in health. Theoretically the goal should be to improve the length and quality of life of everyone and to minimize avoidable differences in health status among social groups. In Canada public and private policy has moved substantially to a broad determinants of health framework, while in the United States the focus is still largely on medicine and health care. Like all countries with difficulties in financing public programmes, Canada is trying to make its health care system better managed and more efficient. Sometimes these debates get caught up in the broader determinants of health issues. When that occurs, there can often be conflict between those who see improving the environment in which people live and work as crucial to better health and those whose livelihood is dependent on health care. In the United States the debate is about the funding and control of health care costs.

SOCIOECONOMIC FACTORS AND HEALTH

McKeown (1976), and subsequently Fogel (1994), have shown that a major factor in the improvement of the health and well-being of the British population following the industrial revolution was the increased prosperity and better nutrition of the population. Fogel concluded that 50 per cent of the economic growth in the United Kingdom since the industrial revolution was directly related to better nutrition of the population. He also concluded that poor nourishment in early childhood led to poor development and increased risk of premature death in adult life, a conclusion that a number of authors are in agreement with.

In the historical analysis of Western countries, Fogel found that when the economy stagnated or declined there was a corresponding change in life expectancy. He concluded that such factors as the state of the economy, income distribution and urbanization are a significant influence on health and well-being. We know today from studies of eastern Europe (Hertzman and Ayers 1993) that countries in economic decline show adverse effects on the health and well-being of the population. The life expectancy gap between eastern and western Europe is now considered to be at least ten years.

While it is known that as the prosperity of a nation improves so does the health of its population, when a nation reaches a certain level the gains in life expectancy with increased prosperity are small (Wilkinson 1992). However, within affluent developed societies there is substantial variation in health when measured against social and economic factors. The higher people are on the socioeconomic gradient the better their health (Wilkinson 1992, 1994; Evans et al. 1994).

Kitagawa and Hauser (1973) found compelling evidence in the United States, between 1930 and 1960, of different rates of mortality by social class. Even though mortality rates in the United States have continued to decline, the social gradient in health is still present and the differences in mortality rates for individuals in the different parts of the gradient have widened. In contrast, in Scandinavian countries the gradient in health has not widened and life expectancy has increased for all social classes. Japan shows similar health outcomes to Sweden. Both countries have a high degree of income equality with social stability (Marmot and Davey Smith 1989; Pappas et al. 1993).

One of the most powerful studies to provide some clue about the factors causing these gradients in health is Michael Marmot's study (1994) of the

Whitehall civil service. The study shows that, in a working middle-class population, the higher you are in the job hierarchy the lower the risk of your dying from major causes of death such as strokes, heart attacks and smoking or non-smoking-related cancers. There is also a gradient for deaths from suicides and accidents. In all developed societies in which similar studies have been carried out there are clear non-disease-specific gradients in health as measured against social and economic markers such as job, levels of education, income, etc. These gradients do not appear to be due to lack of access to medical care, but to some underlying general susceptibility factor.

Such studies show that whatever is producing the social gradients in health affects the whole of society not just those in poverty. Although social differences in access to medical care in the United States may explain some of the health gradients in that country, it does not explain the observation in Canada and the United Kingdom, where health care is available, without financial barriers, to all members of society. Health selection has been proposed by some as the explanation of the social inequalities in health. With the exception of some mental health problems, there is no evidence to support health selection. Furthermore, longitudinal and other studies are beginning to show a relationship between early childhood and health risks in adult life and the effects of socioeconomic changes.

CHILDHOOD AND COMPETENCE AND COPING SKILLS

There is no simple explanation for how these gradients are produced, except that they must relate to the environments in which people live and work influencing biological pathways that influence disease expression (Sapolsky 1992; Reichlin 1993; Frank and Mustard 1994). Fogel showed that the mean height of a population correlated with the health of a population as measured by life expectancy. He concluded that early life experience, particularly adequacy of nutrition, influenced susceptibility to disease in adult life. In the Whitehall study (Marmot et al. 1991) there is a gradient in mean height in the civil service that could be interpreted as implying that individuals in the lower grades may not have had as advantageous an early childhood as the people in the top grades.

Although the evidence relating early childhood to health risks in adult life is far from complete, there are findings from human studies and animal experiments that illustrate the possible relationship between early childhood and health risks in adult life (Hertzman 1994). The competence and coping skills of individuals are affected by the quality of childhood, particularly early childhood. The development of the cerebral cortex is strongly influenced by the quality of the sensory stimulation nurturing received during the early period of life (including *in utero*) when the brain is most plastic (Cynader 1994). It appears that children who are well nurtured during the sensitive period of cortex development will develop cognitive and behaviourial characteristics giving them good skills for coping with adult life (Keating and Mustard 1993; Carnegie 1994). Adequate quality of nourishment is also important during this period, not only in the development of the brain, but also in the development of other organ systems.

Non-human primate studies also show the importance of nurturing in the development of competent adult animals. Several studies have shown that high-quality nurturing or stimulation of children in high-risk social and economic environments can lead to vastly improved cognitive and behaviourial performance. The findings of the small but randomized Perry pre-school intervention with children in high-risk environment have shown that the benefits of improved nurturing/education in children between the ages of three and six are manifest in their better overall performance as adults (Barrueta-Clement *et al.* 1984).

The improved understanding of the links between the brain and the endocrine and host defence systems is providing an understanding of the biological pathways that can be influenced by the social environment and thereby influence disease expression (Reichlin 1993). It is also of interest that the competence and coping skills developed before school influence school performance and drop-out rates from school (Tremblay *et al.* 1992). It also appears that the quality of early childhood is related to the incidence of crime and delinquency in male teenagers.

The improved understanding of the relationship between the quality of nurturing and nourishment in early childhood, competence and coping skills and health risks in adult life has implications not only for health policies but for the competence and coping skills of the population. Many of the provincial governments in Canada have taken steps to integrate these concepts in public policies relating to health, education and children. In the United States the health debate has not yet embraced this framework of understanding.

One of the relationships that is of increasing importance to children is the quality of the social environment in which they are brought up. In both Canada and the United States there are ample data showing a clear relationship between poor social environments and bad outcomes for children that is more than poverty. We need to understand better how economic factors influence the quality of social environments, human development and health and well-being.

ECONOMIC FORCES

How nations or regions create and distribute their resources and wealth has a major effect on the quality of their social and physical environments.

In a recent essay on economic growth, *The Economist* (1992) said, 'True enough, economists are interested in economic growth. The trouble is that even by their standards they have been terribly ignorant about it. The depth of their ignorance has long been their best kept secret.' Now that we better understand the role of technological innovation in economic growth and prosperity, particularly deep and broad changes, the issue of how societies create wealth and distribute it becomes important. This is further compounded by the globalization influence on economies and societies.

Adam Smith (1910) concluded that there were sectors of the economy that produced the wealth that made other activities in society possible. Smith described these sectors in his chapter entitled 'Of the accumulation of capital, or of productive and un-productive labour':

> The labour of some of the most respectable orders in the society is, like that of menial servants, unproductive of any value, and does not fix or realize itself in any permanent subject, or vendible commodity, which endures after that labour is past, and for which an equal quantity of labour could afterwards be procured. The sovereign, for example, with all the officers both of justice and war who serve under him, the whole army and navy, are unproductive labourers. They are the servants of the public, and are maintained by a part of the annual produce of the industry of other people. Their service, how honourable, how useful, or how necessary soever, produces nothing for which an equal quantity of service can afterwards be procured. The protection, security and defence of the commonwealth, the effect of their labour this year will not purchase its protection, security, and defence for the year to come. In the same class must be ranked, some both of the gravest and most important, and some of the most frivolous professions; churchmen, lawyers, physicians, men of letters of all kinds, players, buffoons, musicians, opera singers, opera-dancers, etc.

The new understanding of the factors determining economic growth has implications for Smith's splitting of the economy into productive and non-productive labour. Since both sectors are important to a society, the productive labour section can be considered the primary wealth-creating sector (the engine of economic growth) and the other sector, the secondary wealth-creating component (the quality of the environment in which we live and work). When the primary wealth-creating sector falters, the income that flows to the secondary sector decreases, with associated changes in our social environment that can reduce our quality of life. The old economic theory tended to treat all outputs in the economy as being equal in wealth creation. The new concept clearly brings out the importance of a better understanding of a healthy primary wealth-creating sector and the synergy between that sector and the secondary wealth-creating sector. Many activities in the secondary sector, like some aspects of education, health care, and the support of children, are key parts of the infrastructure of all innovative economies. A decline in the primary wealth-creating capacity in a region leads to a decline in its capacity to support the secondary wealth-creating sectors. This has become a serious problem in Canada.

Britain is regarded by many as a nation that has failed to make investments during this century in new technologies on the scale necessary to maintain its primary wealth-creating capacity (Dahrendorf 1982; Lazonick and Elbaum 1986; Hutton 1995). Its economy has fallen behind those of other developed countries. An interesting question is, how many of the inequalities in health in the United Kingdom, particularly in the regions of major economic decline, are products of the failure to invest in the key new technological innovations that have influenced economic growth during this century?

One of the problems associated with economic change and failure to sustain the primary wealth-creating capacity is increases in income inequality. A region or regions that fails to sustain their investment in primary wealth creation will have increased difficulty in sustaining the other sectors of their society. There is some evidence that although Britain had amassed great wealth by the turn of the century, it failed to invest effectively in the new technologies of this century, leading to progressive decline in regions that had been the sites of primary wealth production in the industrial revolution.

Britain is considered by some to have become a wealth-driven society (investing in financial markets) rather than a region investing in and creating new technologies (Porter 1990).The regions of Britain that have done poorly economically have the poorest health status, despite a national health care service. The area around London where the financial institutions are located has a better socioeconomic environment and a better overall health status for its population than the regions that were a key part of the industrial revolution. Canadian studies have shown similar relationships. Those regions with the poorest socioeconomic characteristics tend to have the poorest health (Frohlich and Mustard 1994; Provincial Health Officer 1994).

The evidence of a relationship among the economy, inequalities in income and inequalities in health has led to interest in how economic change affects individuals. One of the groups that gets hit the hardest in periods of economic change and decline is mothers and children. In Canada nearly 25 per cent of children are in single-parent families and the majority of single mothers are living in poverty with limited resources (Ross et al. 1994).

Also, many two-parent families have both parents working, with inadequate resources to care for their children. Thus a pathway by which faltering economies and increasing income inequality can affect human development and health is their effect on the quality of the nourishment and nurturing children receive during the early period of their existence. There is also increased recognition that increased income inequality in societies can become a negative factor in economic growth (*Economist* 1994). If an increased number of children are handicapped in early life, society will probably pay a high socioeconomic cost. Fogel's historical analysis of the West appears to bear this out.

There is an increasing interest in linking together our understanding of the determinants of health, human development and economic growth when considering public policy. The importance of this is brought out by Fogel's conclusion that 50 percent of the economic growth in Britain following the industrial revolution was due to better nutrition of the population.

POLICIES IN CANADA AND THE UNITED STATES

In both countries there is now substantial understanding of the importance of the quality of early childhood experiences in setting competence and coping skills for the later stages of life. In Canada the link between the early stages of life and health risk in adult life is understood in many regions of the country. Since Canada has a publicly financed health care system, it is not caught by the debate in the United States about whether there should be universal insurance coverage for all citizens. Canada, having thirty years ago accepted the social equity of a public-financed health care system, is more concerned about controlling the cost of health care in a declining economy and maintaining stable social environments that are healthy for children and building the new economy.

Since policies and procedures relating to children, communities and health are the responsibility of the provinces, many of the initiatives are being driven at the provincial level of government with support from the federal government. When the federal government is the main provider of funds it can set overall national policies. Because of its weakened financial situation, it has less capacity to set national policies and standards. Provinces that have shown a great deal of initiative in these complex areas using the new framework of understanding concerning economic growth, health and human development are New Brunswick, Quebec, Manitoba, Saskatchewan and British Columbia. Also, some of the aboriginal tribal councils that have taken control of services on their reservations are trying to work within this integrated framework. There is also considerable action and interest at the community level.

An example of how far this integration has gone can be seen from developments in Ontario. The previous Liberal government set up two advisory councils chaired by the Premier. One had to do with the economy and the other with health. After several years' work the Health Council presented a major report, *Nurturing Health* (Premier's Council 1991). This report set out the relationship among economic growth, prosperity, children and health and well-being. This set the socioeconomic environment as the major determinant of the health of the population. Meanwhile the Economic Council was also coming to grips with the issues around the determinants of economic growth, income equality and the competence and coping skills of the adult population. It too recognized the importance of early childhood. The government that followed the Liberal government (NDP) created one council that focuses on the relationship among economic growth in a sustainable environment, prosperity, early childhood/education and health and well-being. This has led to a number of reports and documents that have gradually changed understanding in the private and public sectors and led to initiatives and policies that integrate these concepts (Premier's Council 1995).

There have been a number of community initiatives that have arisen from the work of the Premier's Council. A key concept is how to keep social environments stable during a period of major socioeonomic change. Among the themes that have been picked up is Putnam's concept of a civic society or social capital.

Putnam (1993) argues that civic societies are characterized by most of the citizens being involved in local associations and following local civic affairs and engaging in politics out of programmatic conviction. He concludes from his study of Italy that

> norms of generalized reciprocity and networks of civic engagements encourage social trust and cooperation because they reduce incentives to deflect, reduce uncertainty and provide models for future cooperation . . . stocks of social capital such as trust, norms and networks tend to be self-reinforcing and cumulative. Virtuous circles result in social equilibria with high levels of cooperation, trust, reciprocity, civic engagement and collective well-being. These traits define the civic community.

In Canada there are attempts nationally, provincially and in communities, to develop social support systems that strengthen the horizontal institutions in our communities to cut across vertical structures. In some communities this involves school boards, public health and community services, recreation services and private sector groups such as the YMCA and chamber of commerce. It is too early to know how successful these developments will be, but old barriers are breaking down. All of this is taking place in a pluralistic society with many ethnic groups. Many recognize that the period of economic change will be tough and that the dominant task will be how to sustain stable social environments (social capital) with diminished resources.

In both Manitoba (Frohlich and Mustard 1994) and Ontario (Institute for Work and Health 1994) new initiatives have taken place to try and monitor health and human development and socioeconomic factors on a continuing basis. The government of Manitoba, in cooperation with the University of Manitoba and Statistics Canada, has created the Manitoba Centre for Health Policy and Evaluation. This centre uses the integrated administrative health records of 1 million citizens to track their health status as seen through the use of the health care system against their socioeconomic status from the census records. Already this system has produced major information about the health status of the population and the relative importance of health care and socioeconomic factors. It is planning to link records of early childhood to this data system. The system will also allow a continuing assessment over time of the value of different strategies and intervention to the overall health and well-being of the Manitoba population.

In Ontario initiatives have been taken to support communities trying to build health social environments for children (Ontario Ministry 1989). In particular, the focus is on interventions organized by the communities to diminish the number of children and families getting into difficulty in the early stages of life. Strategies are being put into place to measure the effects of these programmes. It is recognized that early interventions are key because of the limitations of interventions at later stages of childhood in improving outcomes.

In the United States the health debate has largely centred on reform of the health care system. The increasing inequalities in health in the United States appear to be related to the underlying socioeconomic problems in that country and the increasing inequality in income. The substantial deterioration in the quality of the social environment for children is causing major concern. Attempts to address the broader subject of the determinants of health are more fragmented than in Canada. However, many regions and states are working at community-based solutions to the issue of children at risk. One example is the work of the State of Colorado, led by its Governor, Roy Romer. A unique feature of the United States is its diversity. This may allow regions of the United States to create effective solutions to the social issues influencing health.

There is emerging a major debate around the liberal philosophy of the rights of individuals and the neglect of children (O'Neill 1994). There is understanding that building strong social capital will require some commitment of individuals to the needs of their communities and the changing social culture character of society. At present Canada has a more socially conscious society with a sense of the importance of social capital. This is one of the reasons why Canada has not yet had the degree of social breakdown of major US centres. The debate around economic growth, liberalism, social capital, communitarianism will be strong in both societies over the next decade. In these debates the relationship among economic growth, prosperity, human development and health and well-being will become an increasingly important framework for discussion, advice and policy.

The issue facing all societies in the face of global economic forces is how to maintain social environments during periods of change. Whatever the forces of globalization are, societies will be faced with the need for regions to control the quality of their social environment. Regions that fail to maintain the quality of their social environment will have major problems with the stability of society and the health and well-being of the population. It is because of this that the societies that will be successful in meeting the global change will be those that can integrate our understanding of economic growth, human development and health and well-being.

REFERENCES

Berrueta-Clement, J.R. Weikart, Schweinhart, L.J., Barnett, W.S., Epstein, A.S. and Wikart, D.P. (1984) *Changed Lives: the Effects of the Perry Preschool Program on Youths through Age 19,* Ypsilanti, Mich.: High/Scope Press.

Carnegie Corportation (1994) *Starting Points: Meeting the Needs of our Youngest Children,* the Report of the Carnegie Task Force on Meeting the Needs of Young Children, New York: Carnegie Corporation.

Cynader, Max (1994) Mechanisms of brain development and their role in health and well-being, *Daedalus* Fall 155–166.

Dahrendorf, Ralf (1982) *On Britain,* London: BBC.

Economist (1992) Economic growth: explaining the mystery, *Economist,* 4 January, 15–18.

Economist (1994) Slicing the cake, *Economist,* November, p. 13.

Evans, Robert, Barer, Morris L. and Marmor, Theodore R. (1994) *Why are some people healthy and others not? The Determinants of the Health of Populations,* New York: Aldine De Gruyter.

Fogel, Robert W. (1994) *Economic Growth, Population Theory, and Physiology: the Bearing of Long-term Processes on the Making of Economic Policy,* Cambridge, Mass.: National Bureau of Economic Research.

Frank, John and Mustard, J. Fraser (1994) The determinants of health from a population perspective, *Daedalus,* Fall.

Frohlich, Norman and Mustard, Cameron (1994) *Socio-economic Characteristics,* Winnipeg: Manitoba Centre for Health Policy and Evaluation.

Hertzman, Clyde (1994) The lifelong impact of childhood experiences: a population health perspective, *Daedalus* Fall 167–180.

Hertzman, Clyde and Ayers, W. (1993) *Environment and Health in Central and Eastern Europe,* Report for the World Bank, No. 12270-ECA, Washington, D.C.: World Bank.

Hutton, Will (1995) *The State we're in,* London: Jonathan Cape.

Institute for Work and Health (1994) *Annual Report,* Toronto: IWH.

Keating, Daniel P. and Mustard, J. Fraser (1993) *Social Economic Factors and Human Development in Family Security in Insecure Times,* National Forum on Family Security: Canadian Council on Social Development Publications.

Kitagawa, E.M. and Hauser, P.M. (1973) *Differential Mortality in the United States: a Study in Socioeconomic Epidemiology,* Cambridge, Mass.: Harvard University Press.

Lazonick, W. and Elbaum, B. (eds) (1986) *The Decline of the British Economy* Oxford: Oxford University Press.

Mackenbach, Johan P. (1993) *The Contribution of Medical Care to Mortality Decline: McKeown Revisited*, Eleventh Honda Foundation Discoveries Symposium, Proceedings, October.

McKeown, Thomas (1976) *The Modern Rise of Populations*, New York: Academic Press.

Marmot, Michael G. (1986) Social inequalities in morality: the social environment in class and health, in R.G. Wilkinson, London: Tavistock Publications.

Marmot, Michael G. (1994) Social differentials in health within and between populations, *Daedalus* Fall 197–216.

Marmot, Michael G. and Davey Smith, G. (1989) Why are the Japanese living longer? *British Medical Journal* 299: 1547–1551.

Marmot, Michael G., Davey Smith, George, *et al.* (1991) Health inequalities among British civil servants: the Whitehall II study, *Lancet* 337: 1387.

O'Neill, John (1994) *The Missing Child in Liberal Theory*, Toronto: University of Toronto Press.

Ontario Ministry of Community and Social Services (1989) *Better Beginnings, Better Futures: an Integrated Model of Primary Prevention of Emotional and Behaviour Problems*, Toronto: Queen's Printer.

Pappas, G., Queen, S., Hadden, W. and Fisher, G. (1993) The increasing disparity in mortality between socioeconomic groups in the United States, 1960 and 1986, *New England Journal of Medicine* 329: 103–110.

Porter, Michael (1990) *The Competitive Advantage of Nations*, New York: Free Press.

Premier's Council of Ontario (1995) *Ontario beyond Tomorrow*, Toronto (forthcoming).

Premier's Council on Health Strategy (1991) *Nuturing Health: a Framework on the Determinants of Health*, Toronto: Government of Ontario.

Provincial Health Officer (1994) *A Report on the Health of British Columbians*

Putnam, Robert D. (1993) *Making Democrary Work: Civic Traditions in Modern Italy*, Princeton, N.J.: Princeton University Press.

Reichlin, Seymour (1993) Neuroendocrine–immune interactions, *New England Journal of Medicine* 329: 1246.

Ross, C., Shillington, E. and Lochhead, C. (1994) *The Canadian Fact Book on Poverty 1994*, Ottawa: Canadian Council on Social Development.

Sapolsky, Robert M. (1992) *Stress, the Aging Brain, and the Mechanisms of Neuron Death*, Cambridge, Mass.: MIT Press.

Smith, Adam (1910) *The Wealth of Nations*, Everyman's Library, London: Dent, and New York: Knopf.

Tremblay, R.E., Masse, B., Perron, D. Leblanc, M. *et al.* (1992) Early disruptive behaviour, poor school achievement, delinquent behaviour, and delinquent personality: longitudinal analyses, *Journal of Consulting and Clinical Psychology* 60: 64–72.

Wilkinson, Richard G. (1992) National mortality rates: the impact of inequality? *American Journal of Public Health* 82: 1082.

Wilkinson, Richard, G. (1994) Divided we fall, *British Medical Journal* 308: 1113.

Index